Thoracic Manifestations of Rheumatic Disease

Editors

DANIELLE ANTIN-OZERKIS
KRISTIN B. HIGHLAND

CLINICS IN CHEST MEDICINE

www.chestmed.theclinics.com

September 2019 • Volume 40 • Number 3

ELSEVIER

1600 John F. Kennedy Boulevard • Suite 1800 • Philadelphia, Pennsylvania, 19103-2899

http://www.theclinics.com

CLINICS IN CHEST MEDICINE Volume 40, Number 3
September 2019 ISSN 0272-5231, ISBN-13: 978-0-323-71036-7

Editor: Colleen Dietzler
Developmental Editor: Casey Potter

Clinics in Chest Medicine (ISSN 0272-5231) is published quarterly by Elsevier Inc., 360 Park Avenue South, New York, NY 10010-1710. Months of issue are March, June, September, and December. Periodicals postage paid at New York, NY and additional mailing offices. Subscription prices are $377.00 per year (domestic individuals), $726.00 per year (domestic institutions), $100.00 per year (domestic students/residents), $423.00 per year (Canadian individuals), $902.00 per year (Canadian institutions), $484.00 per year (international individuals), $902.00 per year (international institutions), and $230.00 per year (international and Canadian students/residents). International air speed delivery is included in all Clinics subscription prices. All prices are subject to change without notice. **POSTMASTER:** Send address changes to Clinics in Chest Medicine, Elsevier Health Sciences Division, Subscription Customer Service, 3251 Riverport Lane, Maryland Heights, MO 63043. **Customer Service: Telephone: 1-800-654-2452** (U.S. and Canada); **1-314-447-8871** (outside U.S. and Canada). **Fax: 1-314-447-8029. E-mail: journalscustomerservice-usa@elsevier.com (for print support); journalsonlinesupport-usa@elsevier.com (for online support).**

Reprints. For copies of 100 or more of articles in this publication, please contact the Commercial Reprints Department, Elsevier Inc., 360 Park Avenue South, New York, NY 10010-1710. Tel.: 212-633-3874; Fax: 212-633-3820; E-mail: reprints@elsevier.com.

Clinics in Chest Medicine is covered in *MEDLINE/PubMed (Index Medicus), Current Contents/Clinical Medicine, EMBASE/ Excerpta Medica, Science Citation Index,* and *ISI/BIOMED.*

Contributors

EDITORS

DANIELLE ANTIN-OZERKIS, MD
Medical Director, Yale Interstitial Lung Disease Program, Associate Professor, Section of Pulmonary, Critical Care, and Sleep Medicine, Yale School of Medicine, New Haven, Connecticut, USA

KRISTIN B. HIGHLAND, MD, MSCR
Medical Director, Rheumatic Lung Disease Program, Departments of Pulmonary and Rheumatology, Respiratory Institute, Cleveland Clinic Foundation, Cleveland, Ohio, USA

AUTHORS

HESHAM A. ABDELRAZEK, MD
Staff Pulmonologist, Lung Transplant Program, John and Doris Norton Thoracic Institute, St. Joseph's Hospital and Medical Center, Phoenix, Arizona, USA; Assistant Professor of Medicine, Creighton University School of Medicine (Phoenix Campus), Omaha, Nebraska, USA

SANGITA AGARWAL, MD
Interstitial Lung Disease Unit, Rheumatology Department, Guy's and St Thomas' Hospital NHS Foundation Trust, London, United Kingdom

DANIELLE ANTIN-OZERKIS, MD
Medical Director, Yale Interstitial Lung Disease Program, Associate Professor, Section of Pulmonary, Critical Care, and Sleep Medicine, Yale School of Medicine, New Haven, Connecticut, USA

ANDREA V. ARROSSI, MD
Pathology and Laboratory Medicine Institute, Cleveland Clinic Foundation, Cleveland, Ohio, USA

DEMOSTHENES BOUROS, MD, PhD, FERS, FCCP, FAPSR
1st Academic Department of Respiratory Medicine, Medical School, National and Kapodistrian University of Athens, Hospital for Diseases of the Chest, "Sotiria," Athens, Greece

EVANGELOS BOUROS, MSc, PhD
1st Academic Department of Respiratory Medicine, Medical School, National and Kapodistrian University of Athens, Hospital for Diseases of the Chest, "Sotiria," Athens, Greece

ROSS M. BREMNER, MD, PhD
William Pilcher Chair, Thoracic Diseases and Transplantation, John and Doris Norton Thoracic Institute, Executive Director, Norton Thoracic Institute, St. Joseph's Hospital and Medical Center, Phoenix, Arizona, USA; Professor of Surgery, Creighton University School of Medicine (Phoenix Campus), Omaha, Nebraska, USA

SARAH G. CHU, MD
Instructor in Medicine, Division of Pulmonary and Critical Care Medicine, Brigham and Women's Hospital, Harvard Medical School, Boston, Massachusetts, USA

SONYE K. DANOFF, MD, PhD
Associate Professor, Department of Medicine, Division of Pulmonary and Critical Care Medicine, Johns Hopkins School of Medicine, Baltimore, Maryland, USA

ABHIJEET DANVE, MD, FACP, FACR
Assistant Professor of Clinical Medicine, Section of Rheumatology, Department of Medicine, Yale School of Medicine, New Haven, Connecticut, USA

PAUL F. DELLARIPA, MD
Associate Professor of Medicine, Division of
Rheumatology, Immunology and Allergy,
Brigham and Women's Hospital, Harvard
Medical School, Boston, Massachusetts, USA

VIKRAM DESHPANDE, MBBS
Department of Pathology, Massachusetts
General Hospital, Associate Professor,
Harvard Medical School, Boston,
Massachusetts, USA

TRACY J. DOYLE, MD
Assistant Professor of Medicine, Division of
Pulmonary and Critical Care Medicine,
Brigham and Women's Hospital, Harvard
Medical School, Boston, Massachusetts, USA

BRETT M. ELICKER, MD
Professor of Clinical Radiology, Department of
Radiology and Biomedical Imaging, University
of California, San Francisco, San Francisco,
California, USA

ANTHONY J. ESPOSITO, MD
Research Fellow, Division of Pulmonary and
Critical Care Medicine, Brigham and Women's
Hospital, Harvard Medical School, Boston,
Massachusetts, USA

ARYEH FISCHER, MD
Associate Professor of Medicine, Divisions of
Rheumatology, Pulmonary Sciences and
Critical Care Medicine, University of Colorado
Anschutz Medical Campus, University of
Colorado School of Medicine, Aurora,
Colorado, USA

TRAVIS S. HENRY, MD
Associate Professor of Clinical Radiology,
Department of Radiology and Biomedical
Imaging, University of California, San
Francisco, San Francisco, California, USA

KRISTIN B. HIGHLAND, MD, MSCR
Medical Director, Rheumatic Lung Disease
Program, Departments of Pulmonary and
Rheumatology, Respiratory Institute,
Cleveland Clinic Foundation, Cleveland, Ohio,
USA

MONIQUE HINCHCLIFF, MD, MS
Associate Professor, Section of
Rheumatology, Allergy and Immunology, Yale
School of Medicine, New Haven, Connecticut,
USA

CHADWICK JOHR, MD
Assistant Professor of Clinical Medicine,
Division of Rheumatology, Perelman School of
Medicine, University of Pennsylvania,
Philadelphia, Pennsylvania, USA

KIMBERLY G. KALLIANOS, MD
Assistant Professor of Clinical Radiology,
Department of Radiology and Biomedical
Imaging, University of California, San
Francisco, San Francisco, California,
USA

THEODOROS KARAMPITSAKOS, MD, MSc
1st Academic Department of Respiratory
Medicine, Medical School, National and
Kapodistrian University of Athens, Hospital for
Diseases of the Chest, "Sotiria," Athens,
Greece

MARIA KOKOSI, MD
Interstitial Lung Disease Unit, Royal
Brompton Hospital & Harefield NHS
Foundation Trust, Guy's and St Thomas'
Hospital NHS Foundation Trust, London,
United Kingdom

MARYL KREIDER, MD, MSCE
Associate Professor of Clinical Medicine,
Division of Pulmonary, Allergy and Critical
Care, Perelman School of Medicine, University
of Pennsylvania, Philadelphia, Pennsylvania,
USA

BORIS LAMS, MD
Interstitial Lung Disease Unit, Guy's and
St Thomas' Hospital NHS Foundation Trust,
London, United Kingdom

STAMATIS-NICK LIOSSIS, MD, PhD
Professor, Division of Rheumatology,
Department of Internal Medicine, Patras
University Hospital, University of Patras
Medical School, Patras, Greece

KATHRYN LONG, MD
Resident, Department of Medicine, Johns
Hopkins School of Medicine, Johns Hopkins
Hospital, Baltimore, Maryland, USA

RACHNA MADAN, MD
Instructor, Department of Radiology,
Brigham and Women's Hospital, Harvard
Medical School, Boston, Massachusetts,
USA

MARK MATZA, MD, MBA
Fellow, Rheumatology Unit, Division of
Rheumatology, Allergy, and Immunology,
Massachusetts General Hospital, Boston,
Massachusetts, USA

JAKE G. NATALINI, MD
Fellow, Division of Pulmonary, Allergy and
Critical Care, Perelman School of Medicine,
University of Pennsylvania, Philadelphia,
Pennsylvania, USA

TANMAY S. PANCHABHAI, MD
Staff Pulmonologist, Lung Transplant
Program, John and Doris Norton
Thoracic Institute, St. Joseph's Hospital
and Medical Center, Phoenix, Arizona,
USA; Associate Professor of Medicine,
Creighton University School of Medicine
(Phoenix Campus), Omaha, Nebraska,
USA

APOSTOLOS PERELAS, MD
Respiratory Institute, Cleveland Clinic
Foundation, Cleveland, Ohio, USA

CORY PERUGINO, DO
Rheumatology Unit, Division of Rheumatology,
Allergy, and Immunology, Massachusetts
General Hospital, Instructor, Harvard
Medical School, Boston, Massachusetts,
USA

AMITA SHARMA, MBBS
Department of Radiology, Massachusetts
General Hospital, Associate Professor,
Harvard Medical School, Boston,
Massachusetts, USA

ULRICH SPECKS, MD
Professor of Medicine, Thoracic Disease
Research Unit, Division of Pulmonary and
Critical Care Medicine, Mayo Clinic, Rochester,
Minnesota, USA

JOHN H. STONE, MD, MPH
Rheumatology Unit, Division of Rheumatology,
Allergy, and Immunology, Massachusetts
General Hospital, Professor, Harvard Medical
School, Boston, Massachusetts, USA

GWEN E. THOMPSON, MD, MPH
Assistant Professor of Medicine, Thoracic
Disease Research Unit, Division of Pulmonary
and Critical Care Medicine, Mayo Clinic,
Rochester, Minnesota, USA

VASSILIOS TZILAS, MD, PhD
1st Academic Department of Respiratory
Medicine, Medical School, National and
Kapodistrian University of Athens, Hospital for
Diseases of the Chest, "Sotiria," Athens,
Greece

ARGYRIS TZOUVELEKIS, MD, MSc, PhD
1st Academic Department of Respiratory
Medicine, Medical School, National and
Kapodistrian University of Athens, Hospital for
Diseases of the Chest, "Sotiria," Athens,
Greece

ZACHARY S. WALLACE, MD, MSc
Clinical Epidemiology Program, Rheumatology
Unit, Division of Rheumatology, Allergy, and
Immunology, Massachusetts General Hospital,
Assistant Professor, Harvard Medical School,
Boston, Massachusetts, USA

Contents

Systemic sclerosis (SSc) is a rare disease characterized by widespread collagen deposition resulting in fibrosis. Although skin involvement is the most common manifestation and also the one that determines the classification of disease, mortality in SSc is usually a result of respiratory compromise in the form of interstitial lung disease (ILD) or pulmonary hypertension (PH). Clinically significant ILD is seen in up to 40% of patients and PH in up to 20%. Treatment with either cyclophosphamide or mycophenolate has been shown to delay disease progression, whereas rituximab and lung transplantation are reserved for refractory cases.

Systemic lupus erythematosus (SLE) is a systemic inflammatory disease, characterized by an antibody response to nucleic antigens and involvement of any organ system. Pulmonary manifestations are frequent and include pleuritis, acute lupus pneumonitis, chronic interstitial lung disease, alveolar hemorrhage, shrinking lung syndrome, airway disease, pulmonary hypertension (PH), and thromboembolic disease. The antiphospholipid antibody syndrome (APLAS) is a systemic autoimmune disorder where different prothrombotic factors interact to induce arterial and venous thrombosis. The most common pulmonary manifestations are pulmonary thromboembolism and PH. This review will focus on the clinical presentation, diagnosis, and management of the SLE- and APLAS-associated pulmonary conditions.

Sjögren syndrome (SS) is a progressive autoimmune disease characterized by dryness, predominantly of the eyes and mouth, caused by chronic lymphocytic infiltration of the lacrimal and salivary glands. Extraglandular inflammation can lead to systemic manifestations, many of which involve the lungs. Studies in which lung involvement is defined as requiring the presence of respiratory symptoms and either radiograph or pulmonary function test abnormalities quote prevalence estimates of 9% to 22%. The most common lung diseases that occur in relation to SS are airways disease and interstitial lung disease. Evidence-based guidelines to inform treatment recommendations for lung involvement are largely lacking.

Rheumatoid arthritis (RA) is commonly associated with pulmonary disease that can affect any anatomic compartment of the thorax. The most common

and strategies of desensitization for increased antibody levels may result in approval of more patients with CTDs for lung transplant.

Imaging of the Thoracic Manifestations of Connective Tissue Disease 655

Brett M. Elicker, Kimberly G. Kallianos, and Travis S. Henry

Imaging, specifically computed tomography (CT), is a key component in the characterization, management, and follow-up of patients with connective tissue disease (CTD)-related diffuse lung disease. The main role of CT is to help direct treatment by determining the primary pattern of lung injury present. Other roles include follow-up of lung disease over time, evaluation of acute symptoms, and monitoring for treatment complications. Although diagnosis is typically made using clinical and serologic criteria, CT plays an important role when lung disease is the dominant presenting feature. This article delineates the roles of CT in patients with CTD-related lung disease.

Pulmonary Pathology in Rheumatic Disease 667

Andrea V. Arrossi

The pathology of the pulmonary manifestations of rheumatoid diseases is characterized by its histologic heterogeneity and overlap with other pulmonary diseases. All anatomic compartments are vulnerable; thus, the morphologic changes vary according to the predominant region involved. Furthermore, the histologic patterns of injury are not unique to rheumatic diseases, given their resemblance to those seen in idiopathic forms, or in lung disease associated with other conditions. The patterns of interstitial lung disease, airway disorders, pleural processes, and vascular manifestations are described. The histopathology of selected entities, including the main vasculitides affecting the lung, and Ig G4–related disease are discussed.

Autoimmune Biomarkers, Antibodies, and Immunologic Evaluation of the Patient with Fibrotic Lung Disease 679

Argyris Tzouvelekis, Theodoros Karampitsakos, Evangelos Bouros, Vassilios Tzilas, Stamatis-Nick Liossis, and Demosthenes Bouros

This review summarizes the current state of knowledge on experimental and clinical biomarkers of autoimmunity and aims to highlight important aspects of the immunologic evaluation of a patient with fibrotic lung disease.

CLINICS IN CHEST MEDICINE

SERIES OF RELATED INTEREST

Rheumatic Disease Clinics
https://www.rheumatic.theclinics.com/

THE CLINICS ARE AVAILABLE ONLINE!
Access your subscription at:
www.theclinics.com

Preface

Thoracic Manifestations of Rheumatic Disease

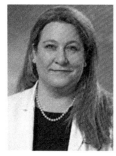 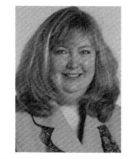

Danielle Antin-Ozerkis, MD   Kristin B. Highland, MD, MSCR

Editors

Rheum (n.): Watery or thin discharge of serum or mucus (fourteenth century)[1]

Perhaps the etymologic background of *rheumatology* foretells the intimate relationship between diseases of the chest and rheumatologic disorders, a common cause of morbidity and mortality. Close collaboration between experts in both disciplines is essential in the comprehensive assessment and management of these complex patients.

It has been nearly 10 years since *Clinics in Chest Medicine* devoted an issue to the pulmonary complications of the rheumatic disease. New antibodies have been discovered that aid in diagnosis and phenotyping of disease and give further insights into pathobiologic mechanisms. We now have criteria for interstitial pneumonia with autoimmune features, which describe individuals with both interstitial lung disease and combinations of other clinical, serologic, and/or pulmonary morphologic features, which presumably originate from an underlying systemic autoimmune condition, but who do not meet current rheumatologic criteria for a defined connective tissue disease. With translation of fundamental discoveries, we have an even greater treatment arsenal that includes new and repurposed immunosuppressive and biologic therapies, antifibrotic drugs, and agents that target vascular pathways. Data from rigorous placebo-controlled clinical trials now inform treatment decisions. In addition, a greater number of centers are willing to perform lung transplantation in highly complex patients

with outcomes mirroring those without rheumatic disease, and there is an evolving role for autologous stem-cell transplantation.

We wish to thank the impressive lineup of authors with expertise in rheumatic lung disease who have contributed to this issue of *Clinics in Chest Medicine*. We hope that it will be a helpful resource for all clinicians who care for patients with rheumatic lung disease.

Danielle Antin-Ozerkis, MD
Section of Pulmonary, Critical Care
and Sleep Medicine
Yale School of Medicine
PO Box 208057
New Haven, CT 06520-8057, USA

Kristin B. Highland, MD, MSCR
Departments of Pulmonary and Rheumatology
Cleveland Clinic Foundation
9500 Euclid Avenue, Desk A90
Cleveland, OH 44195, USA

E-mail addresses:
danielle.antin-ozerkis@yale.edu (D. Antin-Ozerkis)
highlak@ccf.org (K.B. Highland)

REFERENCE

1. Merriam-Webster.com. Available at: https://www.merriam-websster.com/dictinary/rheum. Accessed May 1, 2019.

chestmed.theclinics.com

Pulmonary Manifestations of Systemic Sclerosis and Mixed Connective Tissue Disease

Apostolos Perelas, MD[a], Andrea V. Arrossi, MD[b],
Kristin B. Highland, MD, MSCR[a],*

KEYWORDS

- Systemic sclerosis • Scleroderma • Interstitial lung disease • Pulmonary hypertension
- Mixed connective tissue disease

KEY POINTS

- Pulmonary complications of systemic sclerosis (SSc) and mixed connective tissue disease (MCTD) are a leading cause of morbidity and mortality.
- The 2 most common complications are pulmonary hypertension (PH) and interstitial lung disease (ILD), although most pulmonary manifestations have been described in SSc and MCTD.
- Early detection of ILD and PH has the potential to improve outcomes.
- The cornerstone of ILD treatment is anti-inflammatory therapies, including mycophenolate mofetil and cyclophosphamide with consideration of rituximab for those with rapidly progressive or resistant disease.
- There is evolving evidence for the role of anti-fibrotic therapy.

SYSTEMIC SCLEROSIS

Introduction

Systemic sclerosis, also known as scleroderma (SSc), is a multisystem connective tissue disease–associated with significant morbidity and mortality. It was first described in 1752 by Dr Curzio in Italy as a disease that "turned the skin into wood."[1] It is a relatively rare condition (affecting between 0.5 and 2 of 10,000 individuals), H[2] and is characterized as an orphan disease with unmet medical needs.[3] Presenting symptoms are usually nonspecific (puffy fingers, itching, myalgias, fatigue, and weakness), thus significant delays to specialist referral are the norm.[3]

The organ most commonly affected by SSc is the skin; however, this rarely results in mortality.[4,5] Gastrointestinal involvement, especially of the esophagus, is also nearly universal, with most patients reporting some degree of reflux symptoms, but this is also rarely life threatening.[4,5] In contrast, pulmonary disease has emerged as a major cause of morbidity and mortality since the effective treatment of scleroderma renal crisis with the use of angiotensin-converting enzyme (ACE) inhibitors.[6]

The diagnosis of scleroderma was revised in 2013 by the European League Against Rheumatism (EULAR) and American College of Rheumatology (**Table 1**).[7] Criteria are now more sensitive and specific, with the addition of SSc-specific

Conflict of Interest: Dr K.B. Highland receives grants and contracts, does consulting, sits on an advisory board or steering committee and/or is on the speaker's bureau of: Actelion Pharmaceuticals, Bayer HealthCare, Boehringer Ingelheim, Eiger Pharmaceuticals, Genentech, Gilead Sciences, Reata Pharmaceuticals, and United Healthcare.
[a] Respiratory Institute, Cleveland Clinic Foundation, 9500 Euclid Avenue, Desk A90, Cleveland, OH 44195, USA;
[b] Pathology and Laboratory Medicine Institute, Cleveland Clinic Foundation, Cleveland, OH, USA
* Corresponding author.
E-mail address: highlak@ccf.org

Table 1
The American College of Rheumatology/European League Against Rheumatism criteria for the classification of systemic sclerosis

Item	Sub-item	Score
Skin thickening of the fingers of both hands extending proximal to the metacarpophalangeal joints		9
Skin thickening of the fingers	Puffy fingers	2
	Sclerodactyly of the fingers	4
Fingertip lesions	Digital tip ulcers	2
	Fingertip pittings scars	3
Telangiectasia		2
Abnormal nailfold capillaries		2
Pulmonary arterial hypertension and/or interstitial lung disease	Pulmonary arterial hypertension	2
	Interstitial lung disease	2
Raynaud phenomenon		3
Scleroderma-related autoantibodies	Anticentromere	3
	Anti-topoisomerase I	3
	Anti-RNA polymerase III	3

Patients with a total score of greater than 9 are classified as having definite systemic sclerosis.
From van den Hoogen F, Khanna D, Fransen J, et al. 2013 Classification Criteria for Systemic Sclerosis: An American College of Rheumatology/European League Against Rheumatism Collaborative Initiative. *Arthritis Rheum.* 2013;65(11):2737-2747. https://doi.org/10.1002/art.38098

autoantibodies and manifestations representing important vascular changes, such as the presence of Raynaud phenomenon, telangiectasias, abnormal nailfold capillaroscopy, and/or pulmonary arterial hypertension.[7] SSc can be further divided into 3 variants: limited cutaneous scleroderma (lcSSc) is described as skin changes distal to the elbows and knees and may involve the face and neck, diffuse cutaneous scleroderma (dcSSc) has skin involvement proximal to the knees and elbows, and systemic sclerosis siné scleroderma (ssSSc) has absence of skin thickening but the occurrence of internal organ involvement and serologic abnormalities. Although skin thickening of the fingers proximal to the metacarpophalangeal joints is considered sufficient to establish a diagnosis, a significant proportion of patients do not demonstrate this finding[7]; therefore, a careful physical examination and a full laboratory investigation are important.

Interstitial lung disease (ILD) and pulmonary hypertension (PH) are the most common pulmonary manifestations found in SSc; however, any compartment of the respiratory system can be affected (**Table 2**). All pulmonary manifestations have been described in all variants of SSc, although some are more common in a particular variant of the disease.

Pathophysiology

The hallmark of scleroderma is an aberrant response to injury leading to fibrosis, which eventually leads to organ dysfunction.[8] Fibroblasts isolated from patients with SSc have a constitutively activated myofibroblast phenotype, characterized by expression of alpha-smooth muscle actin and excessive production of collagen.[9] This is the result of a complex interplay between injury to the alveolar epithelial cells, endothelial dysfunction, immune cell activation, profibrotic cytokine and autoantibody production, and deregulated matrix turnover favoring collagen accumulation.[8,9]

Endothelial dysfunction is manifested clinically as Raynaud phenomenon, digital ulcers, telangiectasias, pulmonary arterial hypertension, and scleroderma renal crisis and may result from the effect of anti–endothelial cell antibodies[9] and elevated levels of vascular endothelial growth factor (VEGF). In addition to vasoconstriction, increased endothelin levels stimulate fibroblast proliferation and differentiation into myofibroblasts[9] and result in recruitment of inflammatory cells.[10,11]

Th2 cytokines, such as interleukin (IL)-4 and IL-5 are chemotactic for fibroblasts, promote collagen deposition, and polarize macrophages toward a profibrotic M2 phenotype.[9] In addition to T-lymphocytes, B-lymphocytes are also important in SSc; they produce antibodies against endothelial cells, fibrillin-1, cardiolipin, metalloproteases, and fibroblasts[8,9,11] and are a major source of transforming growth factor (TGF)-β and IL-6, 2 important profibrotic proteins.[8,11] TGF-β is also produced by fibroblasts, and is stimulated by the

Table 2 Pulmonary manifestations of systemic sclerosis	
Interstitial lung disease	• Nonspecific interstitial pneumonia • Usual interstitial pneumonia • Organizing pneumonia • Sarcoidosis
Pulmonary hypertension	• Pulmonary arterial hypertension • Pulmonary venous occlusive disease • Post-capillary pulmonary hypertension • Pulmonary hypertension owing to disorders of the respiratory system and/or hypoxemia • Chromic thromboembolic pulmonary hypertension
Pleural disease	• Pleural thickening • Pneumothorax • Pleural effusion
Aspiration	• Recurrent pneumonia • Acute and chronic lung injury
Small airway disease	• Obstructive ventilatory defect
Lung cancer	• Non–small-cell lung cancer
Restrictive ventilatory defect	• Hide-bound chest wall • Respiratory muscle weakness
Sleep disorders	• Obstructive sleep apnea • Restless leg syndrome • Abnormal sleep architecture
Alveolar hemorrhage	• Case reports related to D-Penicillamine

increased oxidative stress seen in SSc. TGF-β is essential for fibroblast activation, and its levels correlate with the degree of collagen deposition.[9] IL-6 levels are elevated in patients with early disease, correlate with the degree of skin involvement,[8,12] are elevated in patients with ILD,[13] and seem to predict mortality. IL-6 promotes fibrosis through increased collagen production by fibroblasts and also through the generation of M2-like macrophages.[14,15]

Interstitial Lung Disease

Prevalence
Up to 90% of patients with SSc will have evidence of ILD on chest computed tomography (CT)[16–19] or autopsy.[20] However, clinically significant ILD

develops in only 30% to 40%.[21] Since the introduction of ACE inhibitors and the avoidance of high-dose corticosteroid therapy, ILD represents the most common disease-specific cause of mortality, accounting for approximately 30% of deaths.[6] Despite the progress in disease diagnosis and management, the prognosis of these patients remains poor, with a median survival of 5 to 8 years.[22] When ILD occurs, it tends to happen early after disease onset with the greatest decline in pulmonary function typically seen within the first 5 to 7 years after the first non-Raynaud symptom. Consequently, experts recommend more frequent screening for the presence of ILD during this time; and these are the patients who historically have been included in clinical trials.[23]

The feasibility of screening for ILD to facilitate early recognition and therapy has been investigated in 2 prospective studies. Suliman and colleagues[17] screened 102 patients with SSc followed at the University of Zurich with CT and pulmonary function tests. Sixty-three percent of the population demonstrated evidence of ILD; however, only 37.5% had a forced vital capacity percent predicted (FVC[%]) below 80% of predicted. In a similar study at the University of Oslo, Hoffman-Vold and colleagues[24] demonstrated evidence of ILD in 64.6% of patients with SSc, yet only 34.0% of those had abnormal spirometry. Both investigators concluded that spirometry is not sufficient for the early diagnosis of SSc-ILD, and screening with CT should be considered. The lack of sensitivity and specificity of spirometry is easily explainable considering the wide range of "normal" values, and that it may be influenced by processes not affecting the pulmonary parenchyma, such as skin thickening causing restriction of chest expansion or myopathy leading to muscle weakness.

Histopathology and imaging characteristics
The parenchymal abnormalities found on high-resolution CT (HRCT) seem to be more common and more prominent in SSc compared with other connective tissue diseases.[25] The most common finding is ground glass opacities with a basal and posterior predominance[25–27] (**Fig. 1**). Other findings include peripheral reticulations and consolidations,[25] with frank honeycombing being much less frequent (**Fig. 2**). A dilated, patulous, or fluid-filled esophagus also suggests an underlying diagnosis of scleroderma (see **Fig. 2**). These radiographic findings mirror what is found pathologically. Although many different histologic patterns have been described, nonspecific interstitial pneumonia (NSIP) seems to be the most prevalent, with fibrotic NSIP being more

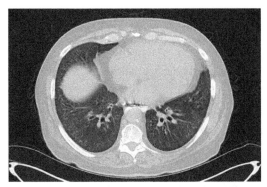

Fig. 1. Chest CT demonstrating ground glass opacities consistent with nonspecific interstitial pneumonia.

common than cellular NSIP[28] (**Fig. 3**). Usual interstitial pneumonia (UIP) has been described in a minority of cases.[29] Other histologic patterns observed include organizing pneumonia, lymphoid hyperplasia, and in rarer occasions non-necrotizing granulomas and findings suggestive of aspiration[28] (**Fig. 4**). Findings consistent with PH can be seen in patients who have both PH and ILD (**Fig. 5**).

Predictors of interstitial lung disease

The risk factors for the development of ILD are shown in **Table 3**. Demographic features associated with SSc-ILD include male sex, African American ethnicity, and the dcSSc variant.[19,30,31] ILD also should be suspected in patients with nailfold capillary abnormalities, digital ulcers, and evidence of PH on screening echocardiogram.[19,21,30,31] The presence of anti-Scl70 antibodies has been associated with increased risk

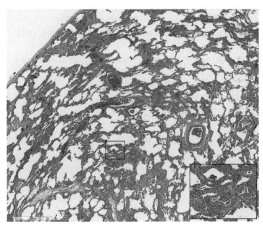

Fig. 3. Nonspecific interstitial pneumonia with diffuse homogeneous involvement of the lung parenchyma with preservation of the pulmonary architecture (hematoxylin-eosin [H&E], original magnification ×2). Inset: diffuse chronic lymphoplasmacytic infiltrates involve the alveolar interstitium (H&E, original magnification ×20).

for SSc-ILD (up to 60%–80% of patients), whereas that of anticentromere antibodies is protective.[21]

Several biomarkers are of interest in SSc-ILD. Increased fractional exhaled nitric oxide is seen in early SSc-ILD,[32] and circulating levels of lysyl oxidase, chitinase 1, serum surfactant D, tenascin-C, growth factor binding protein-15, cartilage oligomeric matrix protein, Krebs von den Lungen-6, CXCL4, and IL-6 have been associated with the presence of parenchymal abrnormalities.[32,33]

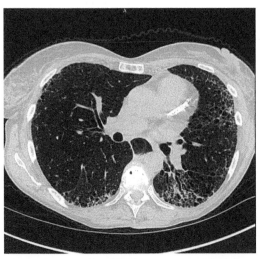

Fig. 2. Chest CT demonstrating a UIP pattern along with a dilated esophagus.

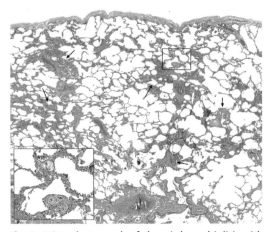

Fig. 4. Microphotograph of chronic bronchiolitis with features of aspiration in scleroderma showing centrilobular chronic inflammation (*arrows*) (H&E, original magnification ×3.0). The inset shows focal vegetable matter and hyalinized degenerated aspirated material (H&E, original magnification ×20).

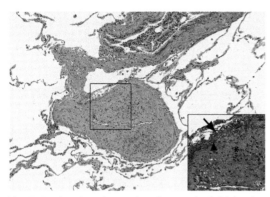

Fig. 5. PH in scleroderma showing marked thickening of the arterial wall (H&E, original magnification ×10). Inset: Pentachrome Movat stain highlights the prominent intimal fibroplasia (*asterisk*) and the tunica media delimited by the internal (*arrowhead*) and external (*arrow*) elastic laminae (Movat, original magnification ×20).

The most investigated markers of disease progression are lung physiology parameters (FVC, total lung capacity [TLC], and diffusion capacity for carbon monoxide [DLCO]). These measurements are an essential component of the evaluation and follow-up of any patient with chronic pulmonary disease and can be performed easily, quickly, and with little cost in the clinic. Both a reduced FVC(%) and low DLCO(%) at baseline predict a poor survival among patients with SSc-ILD.[34]

Although it was initially thought that the biological behavior of ILD is characterized by an initial phase of worsening followed by a period of stabilization, subsequent analysis demonstrated that this is not accurate and in fact there are distinct patient groups with different trajectories of ILD.[35] The patterns of involvement seem to be determined early in the course of the disease and are not always predicted by short-term spirometry changes.[35] However, the observation of longer term changes can be useful.[34] A decrease of more than 10% in the FVC(%) predicted or a 5% to 9% drop in the FVC(%) predicted along with a more than 15% decrease in the DLCO(%) identifies a population at high risk of death.[36]

The extent of pulmonary involvement on chest CT is also a strong predictor for mortality with a cutoff of 20% or 30% involvement being associated with a more than 300% increase in the odds of death.[37–39] There is some controversy about the prognostic significance of the predominant histologic/imaging pattern, with Takei and colleagues[40] reporting that the outcome is not dependent on the predominant entity, and Okamoto and colleagues[27] reporting worse outcomes among

patients with a UIP pattern compared with the more common NSIP.

Clinical parameters also have shown an ability to predict ILD progression. For instance, the presence of arthritis,[41] progressive skin fibrosis,[41] and/or myocardial fibrosis[42] is associated with a more progressive form SSc-ILD. Models combining clinical and laboratory data are usually more accurate than single measurements or serial measurements of a single variable. A simple model combining oxygen saturation at the end of a 6-minute walk test (SP) with the presence of arthritis (AR) (SPAR model) was able to distinguish between patients with and without ILD progression in the next 12 months with fair accuracy in a combined cohort from the Universities of Zurich, Oslo, Paris, and Berlin.[41] Another prediction model is the SADL model, based on a cohort from the University of California San Francisco and the Mayo Clinic. It combines 3 variables: ever smoking history (S), age (A), and diffusing capacity of the lung for carbon monoxide (% predicted) (DL) and demonstrated good performance in predicting the 1-year, 2-year, and 3-year all-cause mortality among patients with SSc-ILD.[43] Another staging system frequently used in SSc-ILD includes both HRCT and FVC.[38] Patients with less than 20% HRCT involvement are categorized as having "limited" SSc-ILD, whereas greater than 20% involvement is categorized as "extensive" SSc-ILD. The addition of an FVC ≥70% for patients with "intermediate" disease (10%–30% involvement on HRCT) allowed these patients to also be categorized as having "limited" SSc.

Treatment
Cyclophosphamide and mycophenolate mofetil
Two landmark studies, the Scleroderma Lung Study I (SLSI) and Scleroderma Lung Study II (SLSII), have addressed the use of immunosuppression in the treatment of SSc-ILD.

In the SLSI study, oral cyclophosphamide at a dose of up to 2 mg/kg for 1 year resulted in a small (2.5%) but statistically significant improvement in mean absolute difference in adjusted 12-month FVC(%) compared with placebo. The clinical importance of this finding was supported by improvement in dyspnea, skin thickening, functional ability, and some health-related measures of quality of life on the SF-36 (vitality and health transition).[44] The more extensive the fibrosis, the more likely the benefit from the medication.[44] Based on this information, the EULAR has recommended that "cyclophosphamide should be considered for treatment of SSc-ILD, in particular for patients with SSc with progressive ILD."[45] This is despite the accompanying editorial for

Table 3
Predictors of scleroderma-associated interstitial lung disease

Demographics	• Male sex • African American race • Early-onset disease
Signs and symptoms	• Dyspnea on exertion • Nonproductive cough • Crackles • Diffuse cutaneous systemic sclerosis ○ Progressive skin fibrosis • Arthritis • Abnormal nailfold capillaroscopy

Physiology	• Reduced forced vital capacity
	  ○ >10% reduction in forced vital capacity (FVC)
	• Reduced total lung capacity
	• Reduced diffusion capacity
	  ○ 5%–9% reduction in FVC with >15% reduction in diffusion capacity for carbon monoxide
	• Oxygen desaturation during exercise/6-minute walk test

Imaging	• >20% involvement on high-resolution computed tomography
	  ○ Ground glass opacities
	  ○ Reticulation

Comorbidities	• Digital ulcers • Pulmonary hypertension • Cardiac fibrosis
Autoantibodies	• Scl-70 (anti-topoisomerase I)
Biomarkers	• Fractional exhaled nitric oxide • Lysyl oxidase • Chitinase 1 • Serum surfactant protein D • Tenacin-C • Growth factor binding protein-15 • Cartilage oligomeric matrix protein • Krebs von den Lungen-6 • CXCL4 • Interleukin-6

SLSI that states: "Cyclophosphamide is still arguably the most toxic immunosuppressive agent currently used to treat autoimmune diseases,"[46] and data that demonstrated the benefit was lost 12 months after the discontinuation of cyclophosphamide.[47]

Recognizing the need for a safer long-term treatment option, the SLS investigators next compared 12 months of oral cyclophosphamide (up to 2 mg/kg) followed by 12 months of placebo with 24 months of mycophenolate mofetil (up to 3 g per day) in the SLSII. Improvements were seen in the FVC(%) in both groups, with no medication demonstrating superiority.[48] However, mycophenolate was better tolerated, with more patients discontinuing cyclophosphamide because of an adverse event, patient request, death, or treatment failure. Interestingly, the arm assigned to cyclophosphamide did not regress 1 year after

discontinuation of cyclophosphamide as was seen in SLSI. Although both the DLCO(%) and the DLCO/VA(%) decreased in both groups, the decrease was less in the patients who received mycophenolate, suggesting that it may be beneficial in preventing vascular remodeling that can result in PH.[48] Recently, a subsequent analysis of a subgroup of patients who participated in the SLSII trial and had serial imaging demonstrated mild, but statistically significant improvement in the fibrosis scores in both treatment arms, again with no evidence of superiority of either agent.[49] Similar to what was seen in the SLSI study, the more severe the fibrosis, the larger the effect of treatment.[49]

Rituximab Given the significant role that B cells play in the pathogenesis of SSc, their depletion with the use of the monoclonal antibody rituximab is a reasonable approach. In a randomized controlled trial in 14 patients with SSc-ILD, rituximab (4 weekly infusions followed by 4 weekly infusions at 24 weeks) was associated with significant improvement in both FVC(%) and DLCO(%) at 1 year.[50] Further evidence to support the benefits of rituximab has been demonstrated in case control studies in which anti–B-cell therapy was associated with stability or improvement in spirometric values compared with baseline, contrary to what was seen in patients not receiving rituximab.[51–53] It has been suggested that continuous therapy is warranted to maintain these benefits, and the medication seems to be well tolerated even in the long term.[52] However, a recent prospective cohort study of 254 patients treated with rituximab compared with 9575 propensity-score–matched patients showed that treated patients did not have significantly different rates of decrease in FVC or DLCO, although they were more likely to have improvement in skin fibrosis.[54] More experience is required to fully evaluate the efficacy of rituximab in SSc-ILD. Currently, there are 2 clinical trials of rituximab in patients with ILD connective tissue disease that are currently recruiting patients (clinical trials.gov: NCT02990286 and NCT01862926).

Tocilizumab The central role of IL-6 in the pathogenesis of SSc has led to the investigation of the role of the monoclonal antibody tocilizumab as a treatment option. In the phase II faSScinate clinical trial, fewer patients on tocilizumab experienced a drop in their FVC(%) values during the initial phase of the study.[55] Moreover, during the 48-week open-label period, none of the patients on tocilizumab experienced a more than 10% drop in their predicted FVC(%).[56] This was similar to findings of the phase III FocuSSced study, which also was designed to examine the effects of tocilizumab on skin fibrosis. Although the primary endpoint was again not met, the cumulative distribution of change from baseline to week 48 in FVC % favored tocilizumab over placebo (−3.9 vs −0.6, P = .0015).[56] It is important to note that patients were not screened for ILD for inclusion in either study, so the prevalence of lung disease in the study populations was unknown.[56]

Pirfenidone Pirfenidone is an antifibrotic medication that has demonstrated effectiveness in the treatment of idiopathic pulmonary fibrosis (IPF).[57] It is thought to exert its clinical efficacy through the inhibition of TGF-β activity and other inflammatory cytokines, including tumor necrosis factor-α.[58,59] In the LOTUSS trial, pirfenidone at a dose of up to 2403 mg/d was safe and well tolerated in patients with scleroderma-ILD; however, nearly 60% of patients required a dose interruption or an adjustment to a lower dose.[60] Although the duration of the study was only 16 weeks, there was no evidence of decline in lung function, demonstrated by FVC(%), DLCO(%), or dyspnea scores. Moreover, the coadministration with mycophenolate did not seem to result in more adverse effects, although a titration period longer than that used for IPF may be necessary.[60] With regard to efficacy, we await results from Scleroderma Lung Study III, which compares initial combination pirfenidone plus mycophenolate versus placebo plus mycophenolate over an 18-month period in patients with newly diagnosed SSc-ILD (clinicaltrials.gov: NCT03221257).

Nintedanib Nintedanib is a small molecule that inhibits a variety of tyrosine kinase–associated pathways, including platelet-derived growth factor receptor, fibroblast growth factor receptor, VEGF receptor, and Src.[61] It also has been approved for the treatment of IPF, having been shown to reduce the rate of FVC decline compared with placebo.[62] Preclinical studies in SSc have shown a reduction in dermal fibroblast proliferation and myofibroblast differentiation and collagen release from patients with SSc and healthy controls.[63] Nintedanib also ameliorates the extent of fibrosis in several well-established animal models of SSc.[63,64] In addition, it demonstrated a potential to prevent the development of PH by inhibiting the proliferation of pulmonary vascular smooth muscle cells, preventing the thickening of the vessel walls and the occlusion of arteries, while inhibiting the apoptosis of microvascular endothelial cells in a murine model of SSc-ILD.[64] The SENSCIS trial (REF) was a multi-national phase 3 randomized, double-blind, placebo-controlled trial that investigated the efficacy and safety of nintedanib in 580 patients with SSc-ILD. Patients were randomly assigned to receive 150mg of nintedanib twice daily or placebo. Approximately 50% of patients had diffuse cutaneous systemic sclerosis and approximately 50% were on stable background mycophenolate. There was a significant reduction in the adjusted rate of change in FVC (-52.4 ml/year in the nintedanib group versus -93.3 ml/year in the placebo group [difference, 41.0 ml/year; p = 0.04]). However, there was no significant change in the modified Rodnan skin score or the St. George Respiratory Questionnaire. Nevertheless, these data suggest a role for antiifibrotic therapy.[65]

Autologous stem cell transplantation Autologous stem cell transplantation (ASCT) has emerged as a novel treatment option for refractory SSc.[66] Although the initial studies demonstrated significant mortality associated with the procedure, its safety has improved and it is currently considered a "standard of care" treatment modality according to the American Society for Blood and Marrow Transplantation.[67] This recommendation is largely based on the outcomes of 3 randomized controlled trials, the ASSIST, SCOT, and ASTIS studies.[68–70] In the ASSIST and ASTIS trials, a significant proportion of participants had evidence of ILD based on spirometry and HRCT; however, the baseline lung involvement was significantly more severe in the former (mean FVC% of 62% vs 81%). Modest improvements were seen in TLC and FVC% on follow-up compared with the cyclophosphamide group in both studies; however, not in DLCO%.[68,69] The benefit seen was greatest in the ASSIST study, suggesting that patients with more extensive ILD may gain the most from ASTC. However, even in the ASTIS trial, the difference observed in the FVC(%) was nearly 10%, which is "clinically significant." The benefits from ASCT in lung function seem to be maintained over a 5-year follow-up period.[71]

The SCOT study randomized patients with SSc with active disease for 5 years or less and with pulmonary or renal involvement to myeloablative ASCT or cyclophosphamide. Subjects randomized to the transplantation group had better event-free survival at 54 months at a cost of increased expected toxicity.[70] Transplant-related mortality was 3% at 54 months and 6% at 72 months, which is less than what was reported in the ASTIS and ASSIST trials. This may be due to the exclusion of participants with a history of cardiac involvement or pulmonary arterial hypertension. In addition, few of the patients in the SCOT cohort had ever smoked.[69] The presence of ground glass opacities and the absence of honeycombing on the baseline chest CT seemed to predict spirometric response to stem cell transplantation,[72] and spirometric response was accompanied by reduction in the extent of parenchymal disease seen on CT.[68]

As a result of these data, EULAR recommends that "HSCT should be considered for treatment of selected patients with rapidly progressive SSc at risk of organ failure. In view of the high risk of treatment-related side effects and early treatment-related mortality, careful selection of patients with SSc for this kind of treatment and the experience of the medical team are of key importance."[45]

Pulmonary hypertension

Patients with SSc and PH have a much worse prognosis compared with patients with SSc and no PH,[73] and SSc-PH is a leading cause of morbidity and mortality, even surpassing ILD in some registries.[74] All groups of PH may occur and may even coexist in SSc, with an overall prevalence reported up to 18%.[75–78] Most patients have group 3 PH associated with underlying ILD, followed by group 1 pulmonary arterial hypertension (PAH) and then by group 2 PH owing to left heart disease, primarily diastolic dysfunction.[75,76] However, there seems to be a shift toward group 2 PH during the course of SSc, as shown in patients undergoing sequential right heart catheterizations in the PHAROS cohort.[79] Pulmonary veno-occlusive disease (PVOD) and PH as a result of chronic thromboembolic disease (group 4) also may occur.

The first association between PVOD and SSc was noted by Johnson and colleagues[80] at the University of Toronto in 2006. The group described the presence of PVOD in 4 patients with SSc and PH. This was followed by a study by Overbeek and colleagues[81] that demonstrated that a PVOD-like pattern was very common among patients with lcSSc and associated PH. Typical imaging findings of PVOD are seen in 11% to 50% of patients with SSc-PVOD and correlate well with pathology. Findings include lymphadenopathy, centrilobular ground glass opacities, pleural effusions, and septal lines.[82,83] When these features are present, they have been associated with the development of pulmonary edema after the initiation of vasodilator therapy.

Specific disease characteristics have been shown to predict the presence of SSc-PAH. Demographic and clinical features include older age, African American ethnicity, the presence of telangiectasias, abnormal nailfold capillaroscopy, long-standing disease, and late onset of disease.[16,84–87] Anticentromere antibodies, anti-pol I antibodies, antiphospholipid antibodies, and the absence of anti-Scl70 antibodies also are associated with SSc-PAH.[75,88] PAH may be seen in patients who have mild ILD,[16,77] and a DLCO less than 50% of predicted and/or an FVC%/DLCO% ratio of more than 1.6 suggest the presence of pulmonary vascular disease.[89,90] Risk factors for the presence of PAH are shown in **Table 4**.

Given the high prevalence of PH in patients with SSc, annual screening is recommended. Different algorithms have been proposed that incorporate echocardiographic findings, the presence of symptoms, spirometry, and laboratory values,[91–93] and when used have been shown to improve survival.[94] The European Cardiology Society and European Respiratory Society recommend yearly echocardiography, followed by right heart catheterization if there is an elevation in tricuspid regurgitant jet velocity or other echocardiographic

Table 4
Predictors of scleroderma-associated pulmonary arterial hypertension

Demographics	• Male sex • African American race • Older age • Long-standing disease • Late-onset disease
Signs and symptoms	• Dyspnea on exertion • Limited cutaneous systemic sclerosis • Telangiectasias • Abnormal nailfold capillaroscopy
Pulmonary function testing	• Diffusion capacity <50% predicted • FVC%/DLCO% >1.6

Echocardiographic features	• Tricuspid regurgitation jet velocity ≥2.8 m/s
	• Right ventricular enlargement
	  ○ Right ventricle/left ventricle basal diameter ratio >1.0
	• Flattening of the interventricular septum
	  ○ Left ventricular eccentricity index >1.1
	• Right ventricular outflow acceleration time <105 ms and/or midsystolic notching
	• Early diastolic pulmonary regurgitation velocity >2.2 m/s
	• Inferior cava diameter >21 mm with decreased inspiratory collapse (<50% with a sniff or <20% with quiet inspiration)
	• Right atrial area (end-systole) >18 cm^2
	• TAPSE >1.7 cm

Electrocardiogram	• Right axis deviation
Right heart catheterization	• mPAP >20 mm Hg • PVR >3 Woods units
Imaging	• Right atrial enlargement • Right ventricular enlargement • Pulmonary artery enlargement • Peripheral pruning HRCT findings of PVOD • Lymphadenopathy • Centrilobular ground glass opacities • Pleural effusions • Septal lines
Comorbidities	• Interstitial lung disease • Pulmonary hypertension • Cardiac fibrosis
Autoantibodies	• Anticentromere • RNA polymerase I antibodies • Antiphospholipid antibodies
Biomarkers	• Nt-pro BNP

Abbreviations: DLCO%, diffusion capacity for carbon monoxide %; FVC%, forced vital capacity %; HRCT, high-resolution computed tomography; mPAP, mean pulmonary artery pressure; NT-pro BNP, N-terminal pro b-type natriuretic peptide; PVOD, pulmonary veno-occlusive disease; PVR, pulmonary vascular resistance; TAPSE, tricuspid annular plane systolic excursion.

findings suggesting PH.[91,95] The DETECT algorithm has 2 steps. The first step uses risk factors for PAH to determine the need for echocardiogram, and the second step uses echocardiographic features to determine the need for right heart catheterization.[93] The Australian Screening Interest Group algorithm recommends a right heart catheterization if either N-terminal pro b-type natriuretic peptide is greater than 210 pg/mL or the DLCO is less than 70% predicted with FVC%/DLCO% ratio ≥1.8.[96] All 3 algorithms have similar sensitivity and specificity.

Despite advances in therapy, the median survival of SSc-PAH is only 3 to 4 years, which is much lower than that seen in idiopathic PAH.[77,84] In the PHAROS registry, male gender, age older than 60 years, New York Heart Association functional class IV, and DLCO less than 39% predicted at the time of diagnosis were independently associated with the risk of death.[97] Other risk factors include a reduced tricuspid annular plane systolic excursion,[98] reduced heart rate recovery on 6-minute walk,[99] the presence of ILD, higher mean pulmonary artery pressure (mPAP), digital ulcers, and renal dysfunction.[77,100] Not surprising, the nonpulmonary aspects of scleroderma blunt the ability of the 6-minute walk to measure change in lung function. Although it is somewhat sensitive to change in response to therapy, reaching target thresholds may not be as important as avoiding 6-minute walk distance deterioration.[77]

Current guidelines support the use of vasodilator therapy only for patients with PAH with the exception of riociguat, which also may be used for PH secondary to chronic thromboembolic disease. There is considerable experience in the treatment of patients with SSc-PAH with oral and parenteral agents.[78] In the first dedicated SSc-PAH trial, epoprostenol resulted in a 46-m improvement in 6-minute walk distance with a difference of 108 m compared with placebo at 12 weeks (P<.001).[101] There was also improvement in hemodynamics, functional class, and dyspnea, with a trend toward less Raynaud phenomenon and fewer digital ulcers.[101] With the newer era of clinical trials that use morbidity and mortality endpoints, patients with SSc-PAH have seen similar benefits to subjects with idiopathic PAH.[78] For instance, the GRIPHON study included 170 patients with SSc-PAH and found a 40% risk reduction in the composite morbidity/mortality endpoint in patients with SSc-PAH treated with selexipag compared with placebo.[102] Similarly, in a subgroup analysis of the AMBITION trial, combination therapy with ambrisentan and tadalafil in patients with SSc-PAH reduced the risk for clinical failure by 55%[103] compared with monotherapy with either agent. Moreover, the use of PAH-specific therapy has been associated with reduced mortality in an Australian cohort.[77] There are clinical studies addressing the usefulness of riociguat[104] and anticoagulation with apixaban[105] in patients with SSc-PAH, and we await results of the CATALYST study (clinical trials.gov: NCT02657356), a phase 3 trial exploring bardoxolone methyl, an antioxidant inflammation modulator, as a novel pathway to treat SSc-PAH.

Lung transplantation

SSc-ILD and/or SSc-PH are uncommon reasons for lung transplantation, accounting for just 1.1% of cases in the 2016 Registry of the International Society for Heart and Lung Transplantation.[106] This is related to the multiple comorbidities seen in this population that potentially increase the risk for perioperative mortality and morbidity.[107]

Esophageal dysmotility, present in up to 55% of patients with both limited and diffuse SSc, is of particular concern because it has been linked to the development of chronic rejection, the major cause of death the first year after lung transplantation.[108,109] Intestinal dysmotility can affect nutrition status and the ability to absorb medications, and the presence of muscle weakness and joint contractures may compromise the ability of patients to rehabilitate both before and after transplantation, and in some cases wean off the ventilator.[107,110] The integrity of the limbs may be jeopardized by skin fibrosis, ulcers, and poor circulation in the setting of vasopressors.[110]

Despite these barriers, the short-term and long-term outcomes are acceptable in carefully selected patients with SSc who are transplanted. The incidence of primary graft dysfunction does not seem to be increased compared with that of other groups with PH, and long-term survival is comparable to that of other patients with ILD.[111] However, the prognosis is slightly worse among female patients and patients with underlying PH.[111] To optimize pulmonary transplantation outcomes, there needs to be meticulous investigation of esophageal motility and aspiration risk and a focus on intense rehabilitation. Many centers will improve nutritional status preoperatively and postoperatively with the use of post-pyloric enteral feeding tubes to limit the risk for aspiration.[110] Steroids should be kept to a minimum because of the risk for SSc renal crisis.[110]

Other manifestations from the respiratory tract

Pleural involvement Pleural effusions are rather uncommon in SSc, being reported in only 4 of 58 patients in a combined prospective and retrospective Canadian cohort.[112] Interestingly, pleural irregularities, as detected by lung ultrasonography, are commonly described and correlate with the presence and the extent of ILD.[113] Similarly, the course of SSc is very rarely complicated by spontaneous pneumothorax.[114] When it is seen, it is thought to be caused by the rupture of subpleural cysts in patients with underlying ILD. Lung reexpansion may be slower than expected and fatalities have been reported.[115]

Aspiration The presence of an incompetent lower esophageal sphincter, along with esophageal motility problems, results in frequent aspiration episodes in patients with SSc. In a retrospective analysis of patients with SSc hospitalized at the University of Pennsylvania, aspiration events were the strongest predictors of in-hospital mortality, conferring an odds ratio for mortality of approximately 30. Of note, most of these events happened during the hospitalization and none of the patients had any concurrent risk factor for aspiration (eg, central nervous system or seizure).[116] Similar conclusions were drawn from an analysis of the 2012 to 2013 National Inpatient Sample, in which the presence of aspiration was the second strongest predictor for mortality among patients with SSc after acute renal failure.[117]

Small airway disease Although airway involvement is not one of the classic manifestations of SSc, there has been evidence of increased inflammatory cells in the sputum of patients with scleroderma, along with elevated levels of exhaled nitric oxide.[118] Moreover, Silva and colleagues[119] identified evidence of small airway dysfunction (increased closing volume to vital capacity ratio) in up to 30% of a cohort of Brazilian patients with SSc. It is unclear to what extent airway disease contributes to the respiratory morbidity and mortality seen in patients with SSc and if there is a role for therapy with inhaled corticosteroids. Interestingly, systemic immunosuppressive therapy has been associated with less inflammation in induced sputum.[118]

Malignancy Some, but not all studies have reported an increased frequency of malignancies in SSc.[120–123] The type of antibodies has been shown to predict the risk of disease, with the presence of anti-pol III conferring risk in patients with diffuse SSc, and the absence of topoisomerase, anti-pol, or anticentromere antibodies associated with increased risk in those with limited cutaneous disease.[123,124]

Non–small-cell lung cancer is the most common malignancy, being responsible for approximately 5% of deaths in the prospective multinational EUSTAR database[121] and 22% of cancer deaths in patients enrolled in the Michigan Scleroderma Registry.[120] Similar data were observed in a retrospective Italian cohort, with lung cancer complicating the course of approximately 5% of patients with SSc, most of whom will eventually succumb to the disease.[123] In general, the prevalence of lung cancer seems to be significantly increased in SSc compared with the general population.[125] Adenocarcinoma and its variants are the most common histologic subtype, followed by squamous cell cancer and then small cell lung cancer, probably reflecting the distribution of the histologic types among women who represent most patients with SSc.[120,123,126]

Smoking is the most significant risk factor for the development of lung cancer, in concordance with what is observed in the general population.[126] A forced vital capacity of less than 75% of predicted was identified as a very strong risk factor in an Italian cohort.[123] However, the presence of pulmonary fibrosis has not been linked to lung cancer in 2 large retrospective cohorts.[124,126] Large studies about the outcomes of lung cancer in patients with scleroderma are lacking, but it seems that early detection does not confer a survival benefit.[127]

Sleep-disordered breathing Lack of energy and fatigue are common among patients with SSc. Prado and colleagues[128] performed polysomnograms in 27 consecutive patients with SSc and demonstrated that SSc is associated with reduced sleep efficiency and rapid eye movement sleep. Similar results were seen in a more recent study of 18 patients with SSc and mostly mild ILD.[129] Despite that, the burden of sleep apnea is rather small, with most patients either having normal studies or just mild disease.[128,129] In contrast, the prevalence of restless leg syndrome was 3 to 4 times higher than that seen in the general population.[128]

MIXED CONNECTIVE TISSUE DISEASE

MCTD was initially described more than 45 years ago as an overlap between systemic lupus erythematosus, SSc, and polymyositis.[130] It is characterized by the presence of prominent Raynaud phenomenon along with high titers of U1-ribonucleoprotein (RNP) antibodies.[131] A definite diagnosis can be delayed, because the overlapping features of lupus, scleroderma, and myopathy may develop sequentially. Different sets of diagnostic criteria add to the confusion (**Table 5**).[131]

Pulmonary involvement is a prominent characteristic of MCTD. Depending on the methodology of screening, abnormalities have been reported in as many as 85% of patients,[132] although an estimation of 50% to 70% may be more close to clinical practice.[133–136] Nevertheless, most of them remain asymptomatic.[132]

There is some discrepancy with regard to the prominent imaging feature, with some studies reporting a high prevalence of ground glass opacities[136,137] and others indicating a much higher prevalence of fibrosis, including honeycombing[133,134] and traction bronchiectasis.[137] Whereas patients with myositis and ILD tend to have a high prevalence of consolidations.[137] Differences in disease duration, patient population, and

Table 5
Diagnostic criteria for mixed connective tissue disease

	Sharp Criteria		Kahn Criteria	Alacron-Segovia Criteria
Major Criteria	Minor Criteria		A. Serologic Criteria	A. Serologic Criteria
Myositis	Alopecia		Anti-RNP corresponding to a speckled ANA of ≥1:1200 titer	Anti-RNP with a titer of ≥1600
Pulmonary disease	Leukopenia		B. Clinical Criteria	B. Clinical Criteria
Raynaud	Anemia		Swollen fingers	Swollen hands
Esophageal dysmotility	Pleuritis		Synovitis	Synovitis
Swollen hands or sclerodactyly	Pericarditis		Myositis	Myositis
High anti-U1-RNP with negative anti-Sm	Arthritis		Raynaud phenomenon	Raynaud phenomenon
	Trigeminal neuralgia			Acrosclerosis
	Malar rash			
	Thrombocytopenia			
	Myositis			
	History of swollen hands			
Diagnosis requirements				
Definite: 4 major + serology	Probable: 3 major or 2 major +2 minor + serology		Criterion A+ Raynaud + ≥2 of remaining criteria	Criterion A+ ≥3 of clinical criteria

Abbreviations: ANA, antinuclear antibodies; RNP, ribonucleoprotein.
From Gunnarsson R, Hetlevik SO, Lilleby V, Molberg Ø. Mixed connective tissue disease. *Best Pract Res Clin Rheumatol.* 2016;30(1):95-111. https://doi.org/10.1016/j.berh.2016.03.002; with permission.

MCTD- "flavor" (SSc vs myositis) may account for these differences. Histologically, fibrosing NSIP is the predominant pattern seen in MCTD-ILD, especially among patients with myositis-MCTD, whereas those with scleroderma usually will have unclassifiable fibrosis.[137]

ILD is more common among patients with dysphagia, esophageal dysmotility, Raynaud phenomenon, anti-Ro52 antibodies, and anti-Sm antibodies.[135,138,139] Patients with arthritis and/or a positive rheumatoid factor seem to be relatively protected.[135] Among patients with established ILD, male gender, elevated U1-RNP titer, presence of anti-Ro52 antibodies and the absence of arthritis are associated with disease progression.[140] Patients with more extensive fibrosis on chest CT are also at risk of early mortality.[134,140]

Both mycophenolate mofetil and azathioprine have been used for MCTD-ILD with acceptable results, but there have been no well-designed clinical trials in MCTD-ILD.[141] Rituximab treatment has been associated with stability of pulmonary function testing in a small population with progressive disease.[142] MCTD is the most common reason for lung transplantation among patients with nonscleroderma connective tissue disease.[143] The outcomes are noninferior to those with IPF with regard to survival, acute rejection, chronic rejection, and alloimmunization.[143]

PAH is another significant and rather common pulmonary comorbidity identified in patients with MCTD. The prevalence is unknown; however, early reports estimated it to be as high as 29%,[132,144] and prevalence seems to increase with time. It is thought to be the most common cause of disease-specific morbidity and mortality in this patient population.[144,145] The treatment of MCTD-PAH follows the paradigm of connective tissue disease–associated PAH and the disease seems to respond to vasodilator therapy.[131,146] A small subset of MCTD-PAH with prominent lupus features may improve with the addition of immunosuppressive therapies, but needs to be carefully followed.[147] It is recommended that all patients with MCTD should be screened with annual echocardiography for the presence of PH, followed by right heart catheterization should suspicious findings arise.[95]

SUMMARY

Pulmonary complications of SSc and MCTD are a leading cause of morbidity and mortality. The 2 most common complications are PH and ILD, although most pulmonary manifestations have been described in SSc and MCTD. Early detection of ILD and PH has the potential to improve outcomes. The cornerstone of ILD treatment is anti-inflammatory therapies, including mycophenolate mofetil and cyclophosphamide with consideration of rituximab for those with rapidly progressive or resistant disease. However, there is accumulating data suggesting a role for antifibrotic therapy. Vasodilator therapy for PAH is able to improve exercise tolerance, functional class, hemodynamics, and survival in SSc-PAH. Lung transplantation is reserved for those with refractory disease, although patient selection, esophageal disease management, and preoperative nutritional optimization are necessary to ensure favorable outcomes.

REFERENCES

1. Suliman S, Al Harash A, Roberts WN, et al. Scleroderma-related interstitial lung disease. Respir Med Case Rep 2017;22:109–12.
2. Villaverde-Hueso A, Sánchez-Valle E, Alvarez E, et al. Estimating the burden of scleroderma disease in Spain. J Rheumatol 2007;34(11):2236–42.
3. Denton CP, Khanna D. Systemic sclerosis. Lancet 2017;390(10103):1685–99.
4. Generini S, Fiori G, Moggi Pignone A, et al. Systemic sclerosis. A clinical overview. Adv Exp Med Biol 1999;455:73–83.
5. Steen VD, Medsger TA. Changes in causes of death in systemic sclerosis, 1972-2002. Ann Rheum Dis 2007;66(7):940–4.
6. Cottin V, Brown KK. Interstitial lung disease associated with systemic sclerosis (SSc-ILD). Respir Res 2019;20(1):13.
7. van den Hoogen F, Khanna D, Fransen J, et al. 2013 classification criteria for systemic sclerosis: an American College of Rheumatology/European League Against Rheumatism collaborative initiative. Arthritis Rheum 2013;65(11):2737–47.
8. Sakkas L. Spotlight on tocilizumab and its potential in the treatment of systemic sclerosis. Drug Des Devel Ther 2016;10:2723–8.
9. Hua-Huy T, Dinh-Xuan AT. Cellular and molecular mechanisms in the pathophysiology of systemic sclerosis. Pathol Biol 2015;63(2):61–8.
10. Volkmann ER, Tashkin DP. Treatment of systemic sclerosis–related interstitial lung disease: a review of existing and emerging therapies. Ann Am Thorac Soc 2016;13(11):2045–56.
11. Eckes B, Moinzadeh P, Sengle G, et al. Molecular and cellular basis of scleroderma. J Mol Med (Berl) 2014;92(9):913–24.
12. Sato S, Hasegawa M, Takehara K. Serum levels of interleukin-6 and interleukin-10 correlate with total skin thickness score in patients with systemic sclerosis. J Dermatol Sci 2001;27(2):140–6.
13. De Lauretis A, Sestini P, Pantelidis P, et al. Serum interleukin 6 is predictive of early functional decline and mortality in interstitial lung disease associated with systemic sclerosis. J Rheumatol 2013;40(4):435–46.
14. Khan K, Xu S, Nihtyanova S, et al. Clinical and pathological significance of interleukin 6 overexpression in systemic sclerosis. Ann Rheum Dis 2012;71(7):1235–42.
15. Mauer J, Denson JL, Brüning JC. Versatile functions for IL-6 in metabolism and cancer. Trends Immunol 2015;36(2):92–101.
16. Young A, Vummidi D, Visovatti S, et al. Prevalence, treatment and outcomes of coexistent pulmonary hypertension and interstitial lung disease in systemic sclerosis. Arthritis Rheumatol 2019. https://doi.org/10.1002/art.40862.
17. Suliman YA, Dobrota R, Huscher D, et al. Brief report: pulmonary function tests: high rate of false-negative results in the early detection and screening of scleroderma-related interstitial lung disease. Arthritis Rheumatol 2015;67(12):3256–61.
18. Molberg Ø, Hoffmann-Vold A-M. Interstitial lung disease in systemic sclerosis. Curr Opin Rheumatol 2016;28(6):613–8.
19. Wangkaew S, Euathrongchit J, Wattanawittawas P, et al. Incidence and predictors of interstitial lung disease (ILD) in Thai patients with early systemic sclerosis: inception cohort study. Mod Rheumatol 2016;26(4):588–93.
20. Solomon JJ, Olson AL, Fischer A, et al. Scleroderma lung disease. Eur Respir Rev 2013;22(127):6–19.
21. Jung E, Suh C-H, Kim H-A, et al. Clinical characteristics of systemic sclerosis with interstitial lung disease. Arch Rheumatol 2018;33(3):322–7.
22. Altman RD, Medsger TA, Bloch DA, et al. Predictors of survival in systemic sclerosis (scleroderma). Arthritis Rheum 1991;34(4):403–13.
23. Schoenfeld SR, Castelino FV. Evaluation and management approaches for scleroderma lung disease. Ther Adv Respir Dis 2017;11(8):327–40.
24. Hoffmann-Vold A-M, Aaløkken TM, Lund MB, et al. Predictive value of serial high-resolution computed tomography analyses and concurrent lung function tests in systemic sclerosis. Arthritis Rheumatol 2015;67(8):2205–12.
25. Daimon T, Johkoh T, Honda O, et al. Nonspecific interstitial pneumonia associated with collagen

vascular disease: analysis of CT features to distinguish the various types. Intern Med 2009;48(10): 753–61.

26. Desai SR, Veeraraghavan S, Hansell DM, et al. CT features of lung disease in patients with systemic sclerosis: comparison with idiopathic pulmonary fibrosis and nonspecific interstitial pneumonia. Radiology 2004;232(2):560–7.

27. Okamoto M, Fujimoto K, Sadohara J, et al. A retrospective cohort study of outcome in systemic sclerosis-associated interstitial lung disease. Respir Investig 2016;54(6):445–53.

28. Fischer A, Swigris JJ, Groshong SD, et al. Clinically significant interstitial lung disease in limited scleroderma: histopathology, clinical features, and survival. Chest 2008;134(3):601–5.

29. Kim DS, Yoo B, Lee JS, et al. The major histopathologic pattern of pulmonary fibrosis in scleroderma is nonspecific interstitial pneumonia. Sarcoidosis Vasc Diffuse Lung Dis 2002;19(2):121–7.

30. Steen VD. The lung in systemic sclerosis. J Clin Rheumatol 2005;11(1):40–6.

31. Mayes MD, Lacey JV, Beebe-Dimmer J, et al. Prevalence, incidence, survival, and disease characteristics of systemic sclerosis in a large US population. Arthritis Rheum 2003;48(8):2246–55.

32. Benfante A, Messina R, Paternò A, et al. Serum surfactant protein D and exhaled nitric oxide as biomarkers of early lung damage in systemic sclerosis. Minerva Med 2018;109(2):71–8.

33. Fan M-H, Feghali-Bostwick CA, Silver RM. Update on scleroderma-associated interstitial lung disease. Curr Opin Rheumatol 2014;26(6):630–6.

34. Volkmann ER, Tashkin DP, Sim M, et al. Short-term progression of interstitial lung disease in systemic sclerosis predicts long-term survival in two independent clinical trial cohorts. Ann Rheum Dis 2019;78(1):122–30.

35. Guler SA, Winstone TA, Murphy D, et al. Does systemic sclerosis-associated interstitial lung disease burn out? Specific phenotypes of disease progression. Ann Am Thorac Soc 2018;15(12):1427–33.

36. Goh NS, Hoyles RK, Denton CP, et al. Short-term pulmonary function trends are predictive of mortality in interstitial lung disease associated with systemic sclerosis. Arthritis Rheumatol 2017;69(8): 1670–8.

37. Winstone TA, Assayag D, Wilcox PG, et al. Predictors of mortality and progression in scleroderma-associated interstitial lung disease: a systematic review. Chest 2014;146(2):422–36.

38. Goh NSL, Desai SR, Veeraraghavan S, et al. Interstitial lung disease in systemic sclerosis: a simple staging system. Am J Respir Crit Care Med 2008; 177(11):1248–54.

39. Moore OA, Goh N, Corte T, et al. Extent of disease on high-resolution computed tomography lung is a predictor of decline and mortality in systemic sclerosis-related interstitial lung disease. Rheumatology 2013;52(1):155–60.

40. Takei R, Arita M, Kumagai S, et al. Radiographic fibrosis score predicts survival in systemic sclerosis-associated interstitial lung disease. Respirology 2018;23(4):385–91.

41. Wu W, Jordan S, Becker MO, et al. Prediction of progression of interstitial lung disease in patients with systemic sclerosis: the SPAR model. Ann Rheum Dis 2018;77(9):1326–32.

42. Steen VD, Conte C, Owens GR, et al. Severe restrictive lung disease in systemic sclerosis. Arthritis Rheum 1994;37(9):1283–9.

43. Morisset J, Vittinghoff E, Elicker BM, et al. Mortality risk prediction in scleroderma-related interstitial lung disease: the SADL model. Chest 2017; 152(5):999–1007.

44. Tashkin DP, Elashoff R, Clements PJ, et al. Cyclophosphamide versus placebo in scleroderma lung disease. N Engl J Med 2006;354(25):2655–66.

45. Kowal-Bielecka O, Fransen J, Avouac J, et al. Update of EULAR recommendations for the treatment of systemic sclerosis. Ann Rheum Dis 2017;76(8): 1327–39.

46. Martinez FJ, McCune WJ. Cyclophosphamide for scleroderma lung disease. N Engl J Med 2006; 354(25):2707–9.

47. Tashkin DP, Elashoff R, Clements PJ, et al. Effects of 1-year treatment with cyclophosphamide on outcomes at 2 years in scleroderma lung disease. Am J Respir Crit Care Med 2007;176(10): 1026–34.

48. Tashkin DP, Roth MD, Clements PJ, et al. Mycophenolate mofetil versus oral cyclophosphamide in scleroderma-related interstitial lung disease (SLS II): a randomised controlled, double-blind, parallel group trial. Lancet Respir Med 2016;4(9):708–19.

49. Goldin JG, Kim GHJ, Tseng C-H, et al. Longitudinal changes in quantitative interstitial lung disease on computed tomography after immunosuppression in the scleroderma lung study II. Ann Am Thorac Soc 2018;15(11):1286–95.

50. Daoussis D, Liossis S-NC, Tsamandas AC, et al. Experience with rituximab in scleroderma: results from a 1-year, proof-of-principle study. Rheumatology 2010;49(2):271–80.

51. Jordan S, Distler JHW, Maurer B, et al. Effects and safety of rituximab in systemic sclerosis: an analysis from the European Scleroderma Trial and Research (EUSTAR) group. Ann Rheum Dis 2015; 74(6):1188–94.

52. Daoussis D, Melissaropoulos K, Sakellaropoulos G, et al. A multicenter, open-label, comparative study of B-cell depletion therapy with rituximab for systemic sclerosis-associated interstitial lung disease. Semin Arthritis Rheum 2017;46(5):625–31.

53. Sari A, Guven D, Armagan B, et al. Rituximab experience in patients with long-standing systemic sclerosis-associated interstitial lung disease: a series of 14 patients. J Clin Rheumatol 2017;23(8): 411–5.

54. Elhai M, Boubaya M, Distler O, et al. Outcomes of patients with systemic sclerosis treated with rituximab in contemporary practice: a prospective cohort study. Ann Rheum Dis 2019. https://doi.org/10.1136/annrheumdis-2018-214816.

55. Khanna D, Denton CP, Jahreis A, et al. Safety and efficacy of subcutaneous tocilizumab in adults with systemic sclerosis (faSScinate): a phase 2, randomised, controlled trial. Lancet 2016;387(10038): 2630–40.

56. Khanna D, Denton CP, Lin CJF, et al. Safety and efficacy of subcutaneous tocilizumab in systemic sclerosis: results from the open-label period of a phase II randomised controlled trial (faSScinate). Ann Rheum Dis 2018;77(2):212–20.

57. Hanta I, Cilli A, Sevinc C. The effectiveness, safety, and tolerability of pirfenidone in idiopathic pulmonary fibrosis: a retrospective study. Adv Ther 2019. https://doi.org/10.1007/s12325-019-00928-3.

58. Schaefer CJ, Ruhrmund DW, Pan L, et al. Antifibrotic activities of pirfenidone in animal models. Eur Respir Rev 2011;20(120):85–97.

59. Nakazato H, Oku H, Yamane S, et al. A novel antifibrotic agent pirfenidone suppresses tumor necrosis factor-alpha at the translational level. Eur J Pharmacol 2002;446(1–3):177–85.

60. Khanna D, Albera C, Fischer A, et al. An open-label, phase II study of the safety and tolerability of pirfenidone in patients with scleroderma-associated interstitial lung disease: the LOTUSS trial. J Rheumatol 2016;43(9):1672–9.

61. Keating GM. Nintedanib: a review of its use in patients with idiopathic pulmonary fibrosis. Drugs 2015;75(10):1131–40.

62. Bendstrup E, Wuyts W, Alfaro T, et al. Nintedanib in idiopathic pulmonary fibrosis: practical management recommendations for potential adverse events. Respiration 2019;97(2):173–84.

63. Huang J, Beyer C, Palumbo-Zerr K, et al. Nintedanib inhibits fibroblast activation and ameliorates fibrosis in preclinical models of systemic sclerosis. Ann Rheum Dis 2016;75(5): 883–90.

64. Huang J, Maier C, Zhang Y, et al. Nintedanib inhibits macrophage activation and ameliorates vascular and fibrotic manifestations in the Fra2 mouse model of systemic sclerosis. Ann Rheum Dis 2017;76(11):1941–8.

65. Distler O, Highland KB, Gahlemann M, et al. Nintedanib for systemic sclerosisassociated interstitial lung disease. New Eng J Med 2019. [Epub ahead of print].

66. Host L, Nikpour M, Calderone A, et al. Autologous stem cell transplantation in systemic sclerosis: a systematic review. Clin Exp Rheumatol 2017;35 Suppl 106(4):198–207.

67. Sullivan KM, Majhail NS, Bredeson C, et al. Systemic sclerosis as an indication for autologous hematopoietic cell transplantation: position statement from the American Society for Blood and Marrow Transplantation. Biol Blood Marrow Transplant 2018;24(10):1961–4.

68. Burt RK, Shah SJ, Dill K, et al. Autologous non-myeloablative haemopoietic stem-cell transplantation compared with pulse cyclophosphamide once per month for systemic sclerosis (ASSIST): an open-label, randomised phase 2 trial. Lancet 2011;378(9790):498–506.

69. van Laar JM, Farge D, Sont JK, et al. Autologous hematopoietic stem cell transplantation vs intravenous pulse cyclophosphamide in diffuse cutaneous systemic sclerosis. JAMA 2014;311(24): 2490.

70. Sullivan KM, Goldmuntz EA, Keyes-Elstein L, et al. Myeloablative autologous stem-cell transplantation for severe scleroderma. N Engl J Med 2018;378(1): 35–47.

71. Del Papa N, Onida F, Zaccara E, et al. Autologous hematopoietic stem cell transplantation has better outcomes than conventional therapies in patients with rapidly progressive systemic sclerosis. Bone Marrow Transplant 2017;52(1):53–8.

72. Yabuuchi H, Matsuo Y, Tsukamoto H, et al. Correlation between pretreatment or follow-up CT findings and therapeutic effect of autologous peripheral blood stem cell transplantation for interstitial pneumonia associated with systemic sclerosis. Eur J Radiol 2011;79(2):e74–9.

73. Pokeerbux MR, Giovannelli J, Dauchet L, et al. Survival and prognosis factors in systemic sclerosis: data of a French multicenter cohort, systematic review, and meta-analysis of the literature. Arthritis Res Ther 2019;21(1):86.

74. Simeón-Aznar CP, Fonollosa-Plá V, Tolosa-Vilella C, et al. Registry of the Spanish network for systemic sclerosis. Medicine (Baltimore) 2015;94(43):e1728.

75. García-Hernández FJ, Castillo-Palma MJ, Tolosa-Vilella C, et al. Pulmonary hypertension in Spanish patients with systemic sclerosis. Data from the RESCLE registry. Clin Rheumatol 2019;38(4): 1117–24.

76. Niklas K, Niklas A, Mularek-Kubzdela T, et al. Prevalence of pulmonary hypertension in patients with systemic sclerosis and mixed connective tissue disease. Medicine (Baltimore) 2018;97(28): e11437.

77. Morrisroe K, Stevens W, Huq M, et al. Survival and quality of life in incident systemic sclerosis-related

pulmonary arterial hypertension. Arthritis Res Ther 2017;19(1):122.

78. Sundaram SM, Chung L. An update on systemic sclerosis-associated pulmonary arterial hypertension: a review of the current literature. Curr Rheumatol Rep 2018;20(2):10.

79. Lammi MR, Saketkoo LA, Gordon JK, et al. Changes in hemodynamic classification over time are common in systemic sclerosis-associated pulmonary hypertension: insights from the PHAROS cohort. Pulm Circ 2018;8(2). 2045893218757404.

80. Johnson SR, Patsios D, Hwang DM, et al. Pulmonary veno-occlusive disease and scleroderma associated pulmonary hypertension. J Rheumatol 2006;33(11):2347–50.

81. Overbeek MJ, Vonk MC, Boonstra A, et al. Pulmonary arterial hypertension in limited cutaneous systemic sclerosis: a distinctive vasculopathy. Eur Respir J 2009;34(2):371–9.

82. Günther S, Jaïs X, Maitre S, et al. Computed tomography findings of pulmonary venoocclusive disease in scleroderma patients presenting with precapillary pulmonary hypertension. Arthritis Rheum 2012;64(9):2995–3005.

83. Connolly MJ, Abdullah S, Ridout DA, et al. Prognostic significance of computed tomography criteria for pulmonary veno-occlusive disease in systemic sclerosis-pulmonary arterial hypertension. Rheumatology (Oxford) 2017;56(12):2197–203.

84. Ramjug S, Hussain N, Hurdman J, et al. Idiopathic and systemic sclerosis-associated pulmonary arterial hypertension: a comparison of demographic, hemodynamic, and MRI characteristics and outcomes. Chest 2017;152(1):92–102.

85. Hurabielle C, Avouac J, Lepri G, et al. Skin telangiectasia and the identification of a subset of systemic sclerosis patients with severe vascular disease. Arthritis Care Res (Hoboken) 2016;68(7): 1021–7.

86. Chung L, Liu J, Parsons L, et al. Characterization of connective tissue disease-associated pulmonary arterial hypertension from REVEAL. Chest 2010; 138(6):1383–94.

87. Nunes JPL, Cunha AC, Meirinhos T, et al. Prevalence of auto-antibodies associated to pulmonary arterial hypertension in scleroderma – a review. Autoimmun Rev 2018;17(12):1186–201.

88. Liaskos C, Marou E, Simopoulou T, et al. Disease-related autoantibody profile in patients with systemic sclerosis. Autoimmunity 2017;50(7):414–21.

89. Steen VD, Graham G, Conte C, et al. Isolated diffusing capacity reduction in systemic sclerosis. Arthritis Rheum 1992;35(7):765–70.

90. Steen V, Medsger TA. Predictors of isolated pulmonary hypertension in patients with systemic sclerosis and limited cutaneous involvement. Arthritis Rheum 2003;48(2):516–22.

91. Galiè N, Humbert M, Vachiery J-L, et al. 2015 ESC/ERS Guidelines for the diagnosis and treatment of pulmonary hypertension. Eur Respir J 2015;46(4): 903–75.

92. Thakkar V, Stevens WM, Prior D, et al. N-terminal pro-brain natriuretic peptide in a novel screening algorithm for pulmonary arterial hypertension in systemic sclerosis: a case-control study. Arthritis Res Ther 2012;14(3):R143.

93. Coghlan JG, Denton CP, Grünig E, et al. Evidence-based detection of pulmonary arterial hypertension in systemic sclerosis: the DETECT study. Ann Rheum Dis 2014;73(7):1340–9.

94. Humbert M, Yaici A, de Groote P, et al. Screening for pulmonary arterial hypertension in patients with systemic sclerosis: clinical characteristics at diagnosis and long-term survival. Arthritis Rheum 2011;63(11):3522–30.

95. Khanna D, Gladue H, Channick R, et al. Recommendations for screening and detection of connective tissue disease-associated pulmonary arterial hypertension. Arthritis Rheum 2013; 65(12):3194–201.

96. Hao Y, Thakkar V, Stevens W, et al. A comparison of the predictive accuracy of three screening models for pulmonary arterial hypertension in systemic sclerosis. Arthritis Res Ther 2015;17(1):7.

97. Chung L, Farber HW, Benza R, et al. Unique predictors of mortality in patients with pulmonary arterial hypertension associated with systemic sclerosis in the REVEAL registry. Chest 2014; 146(6):1494–504.

98. Mathai SC, Sibley CT, Forfia PR, et al. Tricuspid annular plane systolic excursion is a robust outcome measure in systemic sclerosis-associated pulmonary arterial hypertension. J Rheumatol 2011; 38(11):2410–8.

99. Minai OA, Nguyen Q, Mummadi S, et al. Heart rate recovery is an important predictor of outcomes in patients with connective tissue disease–associated pulmonary hypertension. Pulm Circ 2015;5(3):565–76.

100. Campo A, Mathai SC, Le Pavec J, et al. Hemodynamic predictors of survival in scleroderma-related pulmonary arterial hypertension. Am J Respir Crit Care Med 2010;182(2):252–60.

101. Badesch DB, Tapson VF, McGoon MD, et al. Continuous intravenous epoprostenol for pulmonary hypertension due to the scleroderma spectrum of disease. A randomized, controlled trial. Ann Intern Med 2000;132(6):425–34.

102. Gaine S, Chin K, Coghlan G, et al. Selexipag for the treatment of connective tissue disease-associated pulmonary arterial hypertension. Eur Respir J 2017;50(2):1602493.

103. Coghlan JG, Galiè N, Barberà JA, et al. Initial combination therapy with ambrisentan and tadalafil in

connective tissue disease-associated pulmonary arterial hypertension (CTD-PAH): subgroup analysis from the AMBITION trial. Ann Rheum Dis 2017;76(7):1219–27.

104. Distler O, Pope J, Denton C, et al. RISE-SSc: riociguat in diffuse cutaneous systemic sclerosis. Respir Med 2017;122:S14–7.

105. Calderone A, Stevens W, Prior D, et al. Multicentre randomised placebo-controlled trial of oral anticoagulation with apixaban in systemic sclerosis-related pulmonary arterial hypertension: the SPHInX study protocol. BMJ Open 2016;6(12): e011028.

106. Yusen RD, Edwards LB, Dipchand AI, et al. The registry of the International Society for Heart and Lung Transplantation: thirty-third adult lung and heart–lung transplant report—2016; focus theme: primary diagnostic indications for transplant. J Hear Lung Transplant 2016;35(10):1170–84.

107. Jablonski R, Dematte J, Bhorade S. Lung transplantation in scleroderma: recent advances and lessons. Curr Opin Rheumatol 2018;30(6): 562–9.

108. Crowell MD, Umar SB, Griffing WL, et al. Esophageal motor abnormalities in patients with scleroderma: heterogeneity, risk factors, and effects on quality of life. Clin Gastroenterol Hepatol 2017; 15(2):207–13.e1.

109. Hathorn KE, Chan WW, Lo W-K. Role of gastroesophageal reflux disease in lung transplantation. World J Transplant 2017;7(2):103.

110. Shah RJ, Boin F. Lung transplantation in patients with systemic sclerosis. Curr Rheumatol Rep 2017;19(5):23.

111. Pradère P, Tudorache I, Magnusson J, et al. Lung transplantation for scleroderma lung disease: an international, multicenter, observational cohort study. J Hear Lung Transplant 2018;37(7):903–11.

112. Thompson AE, Pope JE. A study of the frequency of pericardial and pleural effusions in scleroderma. Br J Rheumatol 1998;37(12):1320–3.

113. Pinal-Fernandez I, Pallisa-Nuñez E, Selva-O'Callaghan A, et al. Pleural irregularity, a new ultrasound sign for the study of interstitial lung disease in systemic sclerosis and antisynthetase syndrome. Clin Exp Rheumatol 2015;33(4 Suppl 91):S136–41.

114. Yoon J, Finger DR, Pina JS. Spontaneous pneumothorax in scleroderma. J Clin Rheumatol 2004; 10(4):207–9.

115. Ng SC, Tan WC. Bilateral spontaneous pneumothorax in systemic sclerosis–report of two cases. J Rheumatol 1990;17(5):689–91.

116. Sehra ST, Kelly A, Baker JF, et al. Predictors of inpatient mortality in patients with systemic sclerosis: a case control study. Clin Rheumatol 2016; 35(6):1631–5.

117. Poudel DR, Jayakumar D, Danve A, et al. Determinants of mortality in systemic sclerosis: a focused review. Rheumatol Int 2018;38(10):1847–58.

118. Damjanov N, Ostojic P, Kaloudi O, et al. Induced sputum in systemic sclerosis interstitial lung disease: comparison to healthy controls and bronchoalveolar lavage. Respiration 2009;78(1): 56–62.

119. Silva BRA, Rufino R, Costa CH, et al. Ventilation distribution and small airway function in patients with systemic sclerosis. Rev Port Pneumol (2006) 2017;23(3):132–8.

120. Chatterjee S, Dombi GW, Severson RK, et al. Risk of malignancy in scleroderma: a population-based cohort study. Arthritis Rheum 2005;52(8): 2415–24.

121. Tyndall AJ, Bannert B, Vonk M, et al. Causes and risk factors for death in systemic sclerosis: a study from the EULAR Scleroderma Trials and Research (EUSTAR) database. Ann Rheum Dis 2010;69(10): 1809–15.

122. Olesen AB, Svaerke C, Farkas DK, et al. Systemic sclerosis and the risk of cancer: a nationwide population-based cohort study. Br J Dermatol 2010;163(4):800–6.

123. Colaci M, Giuggioli D, Sebastiani M, et al. Lung cancer in scleroderma: results from an Italian rheumatologic center and review of the literature. Autoimmun Rev 2013;12(3):374–9.

124. Igusa T, Hummers LK, Visvanathan K, et al. Autoantibodies and scleroderma phenotype define subgroups at high-risk and low-risk for cancer. Ann Rheum Dis 2018;77(8):1179–86.

125. Bonifazi M, Tramacere I, Pomponio G, et al. Systemic sclerosis (scleroderma) and cancer risk: systematic review and meta-analysis of observational studies. Rheumatology (Oxford) 2013;52(1): 143–54.

126. Pontifex EK, Hill CL, Roberts-Thomson P. Risk factors for lung cancer in patients with scleroderma: a nested case-control study. Ann Rheum Dis 2007; 66(4):551–3.

127. Katzen JB, Raparia K, Agrawal R, et al. Early stage lung cancer detection in systemic sclerosis does not portend survival benefit: a cross sectional study. PLoS One 2015;10(2):e0117829. Assassi S, ed.

128. Prado GF, Allen RP, Trevisani VMF, et al. Sleep disruption in systemic sclerosis (scleroderma) patients: clinical and polysomnographic findings. Sleep Med 2002;3(4):341–5.

129. Pihtili A, Bingol Z, Kiyan E, et al. Obstructive sleep apnea is common in patients with interstitial lung disease. Sleep Breath 2013;17(4): 1281–8.

130. Sharp GC, Irvin WS, Tan EM, et al. Mixed connective tissue disease–an apparently distinct

rheumatic disease syndrome associated with a specific antibody to an extractable nuclear antigen (ENA). Am J Med 1972;52(2):148–59.

131. Gunnarsson R, Hetlevik SO, Lilleby V, et al. Mixed connective tissue disease. Best Pract Res Clin Rheumatol 2016;30(1):95–111.

132. Sullivan WD, Hurst DJ, Harmon CE, et al. A prospective evaluation emphasizing pulmonary involvement in patients with mixed connective tissue disease. Medicine (Baltimore) 1984;63(2):92–107.

133. Saito Y, Terada M, Takada T, et al. Pulmonary involvement in mixed connective tissue disease: comparison with other collagen vascular diseases using high resolution CT. J Comput Assist Tomogr 2002;26(3):349–57.

134. Gunnarsson R, Aaløkken TM, Molberg Ø, et al. Prevalence and severity of interstitial lung disease in mixed connective tissue disease: a nationwide, cross-sectional study. Ann Rheum Dis 2012;71(12):1966–72.

135. Narula N, Narula T, Mira-Avendano I, et al. Interstitial lung disease in patients with mixed connective tissue disease: pilot study on predictors of lung involvement. Clin Exp Rheumatol 2018;36(4):648–51.

136. Bodolay E, Szekanecz Z, Devenyi K, et al. Evaluation of interstitial lung disease in mixed connective tissue disease (MCTD). Rheumatology 2005;44(5):656–61.

137. Yamanaka Y, Baba T, Hagiwara E, et al. Radiological images of interstitial pneumonia in mixed connective tissue disease compared with scleroderma and polymyositis/dermatomyositis. Eur J Radiol 2018;107:26–32.

138. Gunnarsson R, El-Hage F, Aaløkken TM, et al. Associations between anti-Ro52 antibodies and lung fibrosis in mixed connective tissue disease. Rheumatology 2016;55(1):103–8.

139. Fagundes MN, Caleiro MTC, Navarro-Rodriguez T, et al. Esophageal involvement and interstitial lung disease in mixed connective tissue disease. Respir Med 2009;103(6):854–60.

140. Reiseter S, Gunnarsson R, Mogens Aaløkken T, et al. Progression and mortality of interstitial lung disease in mixed connective tissue disease: a long-term observational nationwide cohort study. Rheumatology 2018;57(2):255–62.

141. Oldham JM, Lee C, Valenzi E, et al. Azathioprine response in patients with fibrotic connective tissue disease-associated interstitial lung disease. Respir Med 2016;121:117–22.

142. Lepri G, Avouac J, Airò P, et al. Effects of rituximab in connective tissue disorders related interstitial lung disease. Clin Exp Rheumatol 2016;34 Suppl 100(5):181–5.

143. Courtwright AM, El-Chemaly S, Dellaripa PF, et al. Survival and outcomes after lung transplantation for non-scleroderma connective tissue-related interstitial lung disease. J Heart Lung Transplant 2017;36(7):763–9.

144. Burdt MA, Hoffman RW, Deutscher SL, et al. Long-term outcome in mixed connective tissue disease: longitudinal clinical and serologic findings. Arthritis Rheum 1999;42(5):899–909.

145. Hajas A, Szodoray P, Nakken B, et al. Clinical course, prognosis, and causes of death in mixed connective tissue disease. J Rheumatol 2013;40(7):1134–42.

146. Yasuoka H, Shirai Y, Tamura Y, et al. Predictors of favorable responses to immunosuppressive treatment in pulmonary arterial hypertension associated with connective tissue disease. Circ J 2018;82(2):546–54.

147. Sanchez O, Sitbon O, Jaïs X, et al. Immunosuppressive therapy in connective tissue diseases-associated pulmonary arterial hypertension. Chest 2006;130(1):182–9.

Systemic Lupus Erythematosus and Antiphospholipid Antibody Syndrome

Maria Kokosi, MD[a,b],*, Boris Lams, MD[b], Sangita Agarwal, MD[b,c]

KEYWORDS

- Systemic lupus erythematosus • Antiphospholipid syndrome • Interstitial lung disease
- Pulmonary hypertension • Airways • Pleuritis • Alveolar hemorrhage • Pulmonary embolism

KEY POINTS

- Up to 50% of patients with systemic lupus erythematosus (SLE) will develop pulmonary manifestations during the course of their disease.
- Lupus pleuritis is the most common manifestation in SLE, but any part of the respiratory system can be involved.
- Treatment for pulmonary disease in SLE is based on anecdotal experience, small case series, and controlled data from other connective tissue disorders.
- Antiphospholipid antibody syndrome is mostly associated with involvement of the pulmonary vasculature in the form of acute and chronic thromboembolic disease and pulmonary hypertension.
- Despite current treatment, patients with antiphospholipid antibody syndrome still develop significant morbidity and mortality.

INTRODUCTION

Systemic lupus erythematosus (SLE) and antiphospholipid antibody syndrome (APALS) are multisystemic autoimmune disorders that can involve different parts of the pulmonary system including the pleura, airways, interstitium, and vasculature. This article reviews the recent literature on pulmonary manifestations, prevalence, risk factors, diagnosis, and management.

SYSTEMIC LUPUS ERYTHEMATOSUS

SLE is an autoimmune disease with multiorgan involvement and typical course with exacerbations and remissions. It is characterized by the production of a variety of autoantibodies and a variable clinical presentation that can include pulmonary involvement, although the more common early manifestations are arthritis, photosensitive rashes, glomerulonephritis, and cytopenias.[1] The clinical symptoms and manifestations of SLE are distinct. Early diagnosis can be difficult, and often delays occur because of the insidious onset of predominantly nonspecific constitutional symptoms such as fatigue and low-grade fever.

SLE is considered a disease of women of childbearing age, although males or females of any age can be affected. The typical age at diagnosis is between 15 and 45 years. The female-to-male ratio

[a] Interstitial Lung Disease Unit, Royal Brompton Hospital & Harefield NHS Foundation Trust, Sydney Street, London SW3 6NP, UK; [b] Interstitial Lung Disease Unit, Guy's and St Thomas' Hospital NHS Foundation Trust, Great Maze Pond, London SE1 9RT, UK; [c] Rheumatology Department, Guy's and St Thomas' Hospital NHS Foundation Trust, Great Maze Pond, London SE1 9RT, UK
* Corresponding author. Interstitial Lung Disease Unit, Royal Brompton Hospital & Harefield NHS Foundation Trust, Sydney Street, London SW3 6NP, UK
E-mail address: m.kokosi@rbht.nhs.uk

Clin Chest Med 40 (2019) 519–529
https://doi.org/10.1016/j.ccm.2019.06.001

for the development of SLE is 10:1. African Americans and Hispanic Americans have a threefold increased incidence of SLE, develop SLE at an earlier age, and have increased morbidity and mortality compared with Caucasians.[2]

Although SLE has the potential to affect any organ, the lungs are commonly involved later in the course of the disease. The most common pulmonary manifestation in SLE is pleural involvement, followed by parenchymal disease, pulmonary vascular disease, diaphragmatic dysfunction, and airway involvement. Finding the true prevalence of lung involvement with SLE is complicated by the high rates of pulmonary infections. Up to 50% of SLE patients develop pulmonary manifestations during the course of their disease.[3] Lung involvement occurring in 80% of SLE patients at autopsy, and chart review from past reports is now thought to be largely a result of infection and not directly SLE-induced. An autopsy study of 90 patients with SLE found pulmonary involvement in 97.8% of patients; the most common findings were pleuritis (77.8%), bacterial infections (57.8%), primary and secondary alveolar hemorrhage (25.6%), followed by small airway involvement (21.1%), opportunistic infections (14.4%), and pulmonary thromboembolism (7.8%).[4]

Susceptibility to SLE has a genetic component, and familial clustering of cases is seen. From 5% to 12% of first-degree relatives of SLE patients will develop the disease during their lifetime. Multiple environmental factors have been implicated as potential triggers.[5]

Data from the multicenter Latin American SLE cohort Grupo Latino Americano De Estudio del Lupus suggests that nonischemic heart disease, lupus severity of disease index more than 1, and anti-La antibody positivity at diagnosis or early in the disease course might be predictive of subsequent development of pulmonary manifestations. However, the association of anticardiolipin (aCL) antibodies, anti-RNP, anti-Ro, and anti-Sm antibodies with pulmonary manifestations described in previous studies was not confirmed.[6]

Pleural Involvement

Pleuritis with or without pleural effusions is a frequent manifestation in patients with SLE, more than in other connective tissue diseases. Up to 60% of patients with SLE will develop symptomatic pleural inflammation over the course of their disease.[7] In 5% to 10% of patients, pleuritis is an initial manifestation of their SLE. Pleural effusions in SLE tend to be bilateral but small, and may not be evident on plain chest radiograph.[8] The pleural fluid in SLE is exudative either lymphocytic or neutrophilic, with low glucose concentration (but not as low as in rheumatoid arthritis effusions), and low complement levels.[5] Serologic testing of the pleural fluid shows low complement levels and positive antinuclear antibody (ANA); however, these tests are not sufficiently sensitive to confirm the diagnosis. Lupus erythematosus cells occasionally can be found on cytologic examination of pleural fluid.[9] Differentiation of the cause of pleural effusions is important; heart failure and infection-related effusions should always be considered.[10] Biopsy is rarely performed. On rare occasions, pleural fibrosis and a trapped lung can occur as long-term complications of pleural inflammation.

The risk of pleuritis is increased by almost twofold in the presence of any of the following factors: longer disease duration, late age of diagnosis of SLE (after age of 50 years), greater cumulative damage, and seropositivity for ribonucleoprotein (RNP) and Sm antibodies.[11] A review of 2390 SLE patients in the Hopkins Lupus Cohort identified fever, Raynaud phenomenon and, anti-DNA antibodies as predictors for both pericarditis and pleurisy.[12]

Pleural disease in SLE typically responds well to nonsteroid anti-inflammatory drugs or low-dose corticosteroids. Small asymptomatic effusions usually resolve spontaneously without therapy. Occasionally, moderate- to high-dose corticosteroids are needed for resolution of the pleural inflammation, and only rarely other immunosuppressants are required for refractory or recurrent pleuritis. Pleurodesis with tetracycline or talc has been used successfully for recurrent large effusions in a limited number of cases.

Parenchymal Lung Disease

Acute lupus pneumonitis

Acute lupus pneumonitis is rare, occurring in 1% to 4% of patients, but it is 1 of the most severe complications of SLE. Patients usually present with fever, cough, pleurisy, dyspnea, hypoxia, and sometimes hemoptysis. Acute lupus pneumonitis usually occurs during SLE exacerbations with multisystem involvement such as nephritis, serositis, and arthritis. Most patients with lupus pneumonitis will be anti-dsDNA antibody positive.[13] Chest imaging shows diffuse, bilateral alveolar pulmonary infiltrates. It can be difficult to distinguish acute lupus pneumonitis from diffuse alveolar hemorrhage. Older studies suggest that the prognosis is poor for patients with acute lupus pneumonitis, with a short-term mortality of 50% and even worse outcome for postpartum lupus pneumonitis.[5] The true mortality of this condition remains unknown, and long-term morbidity includes persistent pulmonary function abnormalities and restrictive lung disease.

Bronchoalveolar lavage (BAL) is helpful to investigate for other causes of acute deterioration such as alveolar hemorrhage or infection. It is reported that eosinophilic or neutrophilic lavage fluid is predictive of a worse prognosis compared with lymphocytic fluid.[13]

There are no controlled data on treatment, which is based on anecdotal experience and case reports. Given the prognostic impact it has, the authors' practice is to use intravenous pulse corticosteroids (1 g methylprednisolone per day for 3 days) followed by oral prednisolone. In other centers, oral corticosteroids (prednisolone 1–2 mg/kg/d), are preferred as the initial treatment, and intravenous treatment is used if there is lack of response. In addition, immunosuppressants such as cyclophosphamide or rituximab should be considered. Mycophenolate mofetil and azathioprine are used as steroid-sparing agents.[7] Intravenous immunoglobulins and plasmapheresis have been used in refractory cases.[14]

Chronic interstitial lung disease

Chronic interstitial lung disease (ILD) is seen in 1% to 15% of patients with SLE,[15] primarily in patients with longstanding disease (>10 years).[16] There is an association with anti-SSA antibodies, and in 1 series anti-SSA antibodies were found in 81% of patients with lupus pneumonitis, compared with 38% for all patients with SLE. Because ILD can occur with other lupus overlap syndromes, controversy remains about the true prevalence of chronic ILD in SLE. ILD often develops insidiously, with gradually worsening nonproductive cough and dyspnea on exertion. Lung function tests show a restrictive pattern with reduced lung volumes and reduced diffusing capacity for carbon monoxide (DLCO).[5]

Nonspecific interstitial pneumonia (NSIP) (both cellular and fibrotic) (**Fig. 1**) appears to be the most common pattern in SLE–ILD, but usual interstitial pneumonia (UIP) (**Fig. 2**), organizing pneumonia (**Fig. 3**), lymphocytic interstitial pneumonia (LIP), follicular bronchiolitis, and lymphoid hyperplasia have also been reported.[15,17]

There have been no controlled treatment trials for chronic ILD in SLE. Oral corticosteroids are the first-line therapy for symptomatic patients. An open-label trial of prednisone (60 mg/d for at least 4 weeks) in 14 patients with SLE-related ILD found that respiratory symptoms in all of the patients improved. At a mean follow-up of 7.3 years, 3 of the patients had died, 2 of lung fibrosis and 1 of bacterial pneumonia, but the DLCO was improved in the majority of the survivors.[18] Beyond corticosteroids, decisions on the choice of

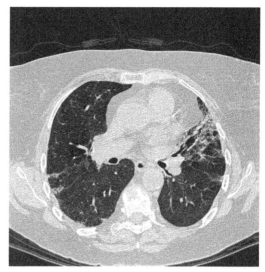

Fig. 1. High-resolution computed tomography (HRCT) in patient with SLE and fibrotic nonspecific interstitial pneumonia (NSIP) characterized by reticulation and traction bronchiectasis.

immunosuppressant treatments are guided by the scleroderma ILD experience.[19,20] The optimal choice for SLE-related ILD is uncertain, but cyclophosphamide, azathioprine, and mycophenolate have all been tried.

The prognosis is usually better than in idiopathic interstitial pneumonias (IIPs), and patients tend to have a slow course with good response to treatment.

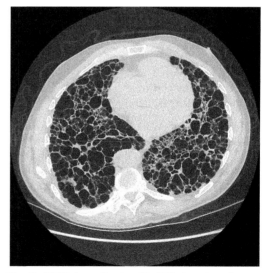

Fig. 2. HRCT in patient with SLE. Imaging demonstrates advanced fibrosis with extensive honeycombing and typical usual interstitial pneumonia (UIP) pattern.

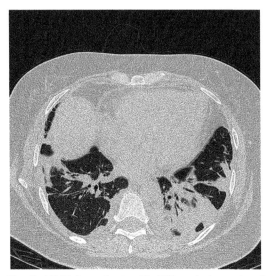

Fig. 3. HRCT in patient with SLE and dense basal consolidation bilaterally suggestive of organizing pneumonia.

Shrinking lung syndrome

The shrinking or vanishing lung syndrome (SLS) has been reported in patients with SLE who have unexplained dyspnea, elevation of the diaphragm (usually bilateral), and reduced lung volumes without evidence of ILD. Lung function tests show a restrictive defect with normal DLCO. The prevalence is reported between 0.5% and 10%.[21,22] The underlying etiology of SLS is debated but could include

- Failure of surfactant production resulting in microatelectasis
- Diaphragmatic weakness or dysfunction with decreased transdiaphragmatic pressure
- Diaphragmatic myopathy caused by corticosteroid use
- Phrenic neuropathy
- Pleural inflammation leading to impaired inspiration with decreased lung volume[6,22–25]

Factors associated with SLS include greater disease duration, positive anti-RNP antibodies, and a history of pleuritis.[11] SLS can be the presenting manifestation of SLE, or it can present later in the course of the disease.[22] Patients present with progressive dyspnea that tends to be worse in the supine position. Sixty-five percent of patients with SLS have concomitant pleuritic chest pain.[26]

Pulmonary function tests demonstrate a progressive restrictive ventilatory defect. A decrease in forced vital capacity (FVC) from sitting to the supine position can help with diagnosis.[27] High-resolution computed tomography (HRCT) usually shows elevation of the hemidiaphragms, reduced

lung volumes, and basilar atelectasis; additionally, approximately 20% of patients have pleural thickening or small pleural effusions. The main role of HRCT in SLS is to exclude parenchymal, interstitial, or vascular lung disease.[21,26] Evaluation of diaphragmatic strength reveals a decrease in maximal inspiratory pressure and maximal expiratory pressure, indicating global respiratory muscle weakness. Different diagnostic modalities have been used: electromyography with phrenic nerve conduction studies, ultrasonography and fluoroscopy, the Sniff test, and dynamic contrast-enhanced lung MRI.[26,28]

There are only case series to report the use of immunosuppression such as corticosteroids, mycophenolate mofetil, azathioprine, methotrexate, cyclophosphamide, and rituximab.[7,26,29,30] Noninvasive positive pressure ventilation at night may also be beneficial.[27] There are some patients with residual diaphragmatic weakness that may respond to surgical diaphragmatic procedures. Prognosis is good overall, with acceptable improvement in the majority of the cases.[11]

Diffuse alveolar hemorrhage

Diffuse alveolar hemorrhage (DAH) is a rare and potentially fatal complication of SLE affecting approximately 2% of patients.[7] Patients with DAH present acutely ill, often with dyspnea, cough, and hemoptysis. DAH typically presents in patients with established SLE, often in the setting of active lupus nephritis or other active organ involvement. There is usually a rapid drop of the hemoglobin of a patient with active DAH.[31] If lung function tests have been done, a significantly elevated DLCO may be suggestive of pulmonary hemorrhage. Chest imaging shows bilateral alveolar infiltrates. BAL is useful to exclude infection. The presence of persistently bloody fluid with hemosiderin-laden macrophages confirms DAH.[31] It is also important to look for other forms of pulmonary vasculitis, such as antineutrophil cytoplasmic antibody (ANCA)–associated vasculitis, and screen for coagulopathies and thrombotic thrombocytopenic purpura as part of the evaluation. Two histologic patterns have been observed: capillaritis with immune complex deposition (14% of DAH cases) and, more commonly, bland hemorrhage (72% of DAH cases).[32]

Because of the severity of the disease, aggressive treatment with high-dose corticosteroids should be initiated early (methylprednisolone 1 g for 3 consecutive days) followed by another immunosuppressive agent (usually cyclophosphamide or rituximab). High-dose corticosteroids used alone have historically been associated with a high mortality. The addition of azathioprine or mycophenolate mofetil can be considered for maintenance once remission is succeeded.[33] Recombinant factor 7 has been successfully used for pulmonary hemorrhage refractory to standard treatment.[33] Plasmapheresis has been used, although not particularly successful. Stem-cell transplantation has also been reported.[32] Mortality is reported around 30% to 40% in most recent studies.[32,34,35]

Vascular Involvement

Pulmonary hypertension

SLE is the second most common cause of CTD-related pulmonary hypertension (PH) after systemic sclerosis. Patients with SLE can have pulmonary arterial hypertension (PAH), or hypertension secondary to left heart disease, namely because of systolic and diastolic dysfunction and left-sided valvular disorders, or rarely secondary to severe ILD, or secondary to chronic thromboembolic PH (CTEPH), and finally hypertension secondary to vasculitis that has been described in SLE patients.[36]

Antiphospholipid (APL)-positive SLE patients have a higher prevalence of PAH (12.3%) versus APL-negative SLE patients (7.3%) as shown by a meta-analysis of 31 studies. The risk of PAH was the highest among lupus anticoagulant-positive and immunoglobulin G (IgG) aCL antibody-positive patients.[37] The presence of these antibodies creates a prothrombotic state that can cause a fourfold-to-fivefold increase in the risk of deep vein thrombosis and pulmonary emboli with subsequent increase in the risk for CTEPH. The prevalence of PH varies depending on the diagnostic modalities used. In the case series of SLE patients with PH where echocardiography was used for diagnosis, reported prevalence is 2.2% to 14%.[38–40] Studies that have used RHC for the diagnosis of PH report a prevalence less than 4%.[39,41]

Progressive dyspnea, chest pain, peripheral edema, and occasionally syncope are the most frequent symptoms. There is a suggestion that anti-U1-RNP antibodies might be a protective factor regarding survival in SLE–PAH patients, while the presence of anti-SSA/SSB antibodies may be a risk factor for PAH.[39] A meta-analysis of 12 studies identified anti-RNP and anti-Sm antibodies as risk factors for SLE-associated PAH.[7] Chronic hyperuricemia was found to predict the development of PH in SLE patients with normal pulmonary artery systolic pressure (PASP) at baseline.[42]

The gold standard of diagnosis remains right heart catheterization (RHC) but echocardiography has been studied extensively in the diagnosis of PH. A post hoc analysis from a cohort of patients with SLE followed over 6 years suggested that echocardiography-based definitions of PH can be useful to predict 6-year mortality in SLE patients.[43] A Japanese cohort of SLE patients was followed over 5 years and showed that 6-min walk stress echocardiography was able to detect early PH.[44]

The treatment of SLE PH is challenging. A combination of immunosuppressive therapy along with vasodilators (phosphodiesterase-5 inhibitors [PD5 inhibitors], soluble guanylate cyclase stimulators, endothelin receptor antagonists [ERAs], prostacyclin analogs and prostacyclin receptor agonists) is used. A meta-analysis of 9 clinical trials of CTD–PAH treated with vasodilators reported improvement in 6-minute walk distance.[41]

There is growing evidence to support the use of immunosuppressive therapy in SLE–PAH and a number of case series reported improvement in hemodynamics and exercise capacity. Most patients were treated with cyclophosphamide for 3 to 6 months, with or without corticosteroids, and vasodilators. Patients who responded to immunosuppressive therapy tended to have less severe disease as judged by better functional capacity, higher cardiac index, and/or lower pulmonary vascular resistance (PVR) index at presentation.[45,46] SLE–PAH patients tend to have better survival than patients with scleroderma-associated PAH.[47] Results from the French PH registry reported that patients with SLE– PAH have overall 3-year and 5-year survival rates of 89.4% and 83.9%, respectively, and anti-U1-RNP antibodies are associated with a higher survival rate.[39]

Thromboembolic disease

Patients with SLE have increased risk of venous thromboembolism, either due to inflammation or the presence of antiphospholipid antibodies.[48,49] The presence of antiphospholipid IgG and IgM antibodies increases the risk of thromboembolic events from approximately 9% to between 35% and 42% and they can be associated with a variety of clinical presentations including pulmonary embolism (PE), pulmonary infarction, PH, pulmonary arterial thrombosis, pulmonary microthrombosis, acute respiratory distress syndrome (ARDS), alveolar hemorrhage, and postpartum hemolytic-uremic syndrome.[5] Immunosuppressive therapy alone is rarely effective, and most patients are given chronic anticoagulation. Prophylactic treatment with daily aspirin is often used in SLE patients with antiphospholipid antibodies without history of thrombotic events. Patients with a known thrombotic event should be treated with anticoagulation, with heparin in the short term and coumadin in the long term.

Acute reversible hypoxemia by arterial blood gas without obvious parenchymal lung disease has been described among hospitalized patients with SLE. In a series of 22 hospitalized patients, 6 patients had episodes of hypoxemia and/or hypocapnia. Gas exchange improved within 72 hours of initiating corticosteroid therapy. Although etiology was not clear, plasma C3a levels were markedly elevated, suggesting pulmonary leukoaggregation and complement activation within pulmonary capillaries underlying the pathogenesis of this phenomenon. Most published cases report good responses to corticosteroids, either alone or in combination with aspirin.[5,35]

Airway disease

SLE can involve the upper airways but less frequently than other connective tissue disorders, ranging from laryngeal mucosal inflammation, mucosal ulcerations, and cricoarytenoiditis, to life-threatening necrotizing vasculitis with airway obstruction. Presenting symptoms can also range from cough, hoarseness, dyspnea and, much more rarely, airway obstruction. Corticosteroids are the first-line therapy, and response is good.[50,51] Bronchial wall thickening and bronchiectasis were observed in 21% of 34 patients with SLE in 1 study.[52] Similarly, in a different series, features consistent with small airway disease were found in 24% of 70 nonsmoking patients with SLE.[53]

Infectious complications

SLE patients are at increased risk for developing infections due to disease activity, end organ involvement, and treatment with immunosuppressants. Infections must always be considered in SLE patients with lung involvement. Symptoms of lupus pneumonitis can be indistinguishable from infection. Patients with SLE presenting with diffuse lung disease require bronchoscopy to evaluate for infection or alveolar hemorrhage. In 1 study, 43 pneumonia events in patients with SLE were caused by bacterial infections (75% of patients), mycobacteria (12% of patients), fungal infections (7% of patients), and viruses (5% of patients).[54] Imaging can be helpful. It is important for patients to stay up to date with influenza and pneumococcal vaccinations.

ANTIPHOSPHOLIPID ANTIBODY SYNDROME

The antiphospholipid antibody syndrome (APLAS) is an autoimmune condition in which autoantibodies directed against certain phospholipid-binding plasma proteins are associated with an increased risk of thrombosis (both venous and arterial) and pregnancy loss.[55] Other clinical manifestations can be associated with APL antibodies such as livedo reticularis, cardiac valvular disease, nephropathy, thrombocytopenia, Coombs positive hemolytic anemia, neurologic manifestations, and retinal vessel thrombosis.[56]

Primary APLAS develops in the absence of other autoimmune diseases. Secondary APLAS occurs in patients with SLE or other autoimmune diseases. APLAS usually presents in early adulthood; the median age at disease onset is 31 years. It is a rare condition, generally reported to affect approximately 1% of the general population.[57] The most common pulmonary manifestations are pulmonary thromboembolism and PH.

Acute Pulmonary Embolism

Venous thromboembolism (VTE) accounts for the vast majority of complications in this syndrome. Approximately 40% of patients with APLAS develop PE during the course of the disease, with up to 55% having documented deep venous thrombosis (DVT) of the extremities.[58] PE is often the initial clinical manifestation of APLAS.

Most of the prothrombotic risk relates to triple APL antibody positivity; lupus anticoagulant (LA), aCL antibodies IgG/IgM, and anti-beta2 glycoprotein (anti-β2GPI) IgG/IgM.[59] The risk of thrombosis is still significant when there are 2 positive tests,[60] but the significance of single APL antibody positivity is being debated.[60,61] On the other hand, among all patients who develop DVT, it is estimated that approximately 20% of them have moderate-to-high levels of APL antibodies at the time of the thrombotic event. APLAS accounts for approximately 10% to 20% of otherwise unexplained recurrent pregnancy loss.[62] A prospective study examining the incidence of complications in a multicenter cohort of 1000 patients with APLAS found that 2.1% of patients developed PE over the 5-year period of the study.[63]

The clinical presentation, course, and treatment of patients with acute PE in the setting of APS do not differ appreciably from those who suffer PE in the general population. Ventilation-perfusion (V/Q) scanning, CT pulmonary angiography (CTPA), are the most commonly used diagnostic modalities of choice, with pulmonary angiography reserved for situations in which clinical suspicion is high, but V/Q scan or CT angiography results are equivocal.[64] Lower extremity Doppler and D-dimer studies are equally useful in patients with APS as ancillary tools in the diagnosis of acute PE.[65]

The management of APS patients with VTE does not differ from the therapeutic approach used for the general population. Thrombolysis or pulmonary embolectomy should be the preferred therapeutic option for hemodynamically unstable patients, although there is limited experience with thrombolysis for PE in patients with APS.[66] The treatment consists of anticoagulation with a parenteral drug such as unfractionated heparin, low-molecular-weight heparin (LMWH), or fondaparinux. Parenteral agents are continued as a bridge to long-term anticoagulation with a vitamin K antagonist (VKA), as warfarin requires 5 to 7 days to achieve a therapeutic effect.[67] The preferred international normalized ratio (INR) is 2.0 to 3.0, but some centers prefer a target INR of 3.0 to 4.0, especially in patients with a high-risk APL antibody profile.[67] APLAS patients with a history of thrombosis should receive indefinite anticoagulation because of the high risk of recurrences. The risk of recurrent VT in APLAS patients on anticoagulation is high, being estimated as 10% to 29% per year,[68] and the risk of recurrent VT after stopping anticoagulation was estimated at 50% at 2 years and 78% at 8 years.[69] Although direct oral anticoagulants (DOACs) such as rivaroxaban, apixaban, dabigatran and edoxaban, are widely used for the secondary prevention of VTE in the general population,[70,71] their role in APLAS has not been fully investigated.[67,72–74] Available data suggest that the use of DOACs should be reserved for patients with adverse reactions or other contraindications to heparins.[67]

In case of recurrence despite adequate anticoagulation, the alternative strategies are increasing the INR from 3.0 to 4.0, switching to long-term LMWH, or adding intravenous immunoglobulins (IVIGs).[67] Besides anticoagulation, hydroxychloroquine (HCQ),[75] statins, and vitamin D supplementation have shown a potential antithrombotic role[67] and have been used in individual cases.

Pulmonary Hypertension

The prevalence of PH in APLAS is reported between 1.8% and 3.5%.[76,77] In the largest published series of 1000 APLAS patients, the rate of PH was 2.2%.[55] It is believed that PH prevalence is higher in primary than secondary APLAS, 3.5% versus 1.8%.[78]

Patients with APLAS can develop PH following a PE, or they might develop PAH associated with systemic sclerosis (SSc), SLE, or other connective tissue disease (CTD); alternatively, they might develop pulmonary venous hypertension associated with valve disease such as Libman–Sacks endocarditis.[77] Although PH in the context of APLAS might be due to several causes, underlying thrombotic mechanisms are the most common etiologies.[77]

0.5% to 2% of patients who suffer acute pulmonary emboli will develop permanent pulmonary vascular changes and chronic thromboembolic PH (CTEPH).[79] The precise mechanisms for the development of CTEPH are unclear but are thought to be caused by incomplete resolution of acute clot and endothelial damage precipitated by acute PE that sets off a cascade of vascular remodeling events including the development of in situ microthrombosis. The rate of APL antibody positivity in CTEPH ranges from 10% to 63.6%. A recent meta-analysis estimated a rate of APL antibody positivity in CTEPH patients of 12.06%.[80] Anti–β2GPI antibodies were positive in 36.4% of patients with CTEPH.[81] However, patients with CTEPH do not have a higher prevalence of extrapulmonary thrombophilic disorders.

The manifestations of CTEPH are the same as those of PH attributable to any etiology. Progressive exertional dyspnea is common, and as right heart failure progresses, lower extremity edema, ascites, dizziness with exertion, and syncope may develop. Chest pain and palpitations may be present also, but are less common. The absence of a documented history of acute PE does not rule out the presence of CTEPH. Elevation of the tricuspid regurgitant jet and signs of right ventricular and/or right atrial volume or pressure overload on echocardiography are often the first clues to the presence of PH. PH must be confirmed via right heart catheterization. This is critical in differentiating between PAH and PVH, as PVR can be determined. PAH is present if the mean pulmonary artery pressure (mPAP) on right heart catheterization is 25 mm Hg or higher, the pulmonary capillary wedge pressure (PCWP) is 15 mm Hg or lower, and the PVR is 3.0 or more Wood units. Provocative testing such as inhalation of nitric oxide, exercise challenges, or systemic vasodilators can also help to assess for vasoreactivity and to differentiate PAH from PVH.

All patients with PH should undergo V/Q scanning to screen for chronic thromboemboli, and if significant ventilation perfusion mismatching is detected, formal pulmonary angiography should be performed. Pulmonary angiography is important in that it allows for the determination of the extent of the disease (major vessel, segmental, or subsegmental pulmonary artery branches) and provides information as to the feasibility of pulmonary thromboendarterectomy (PTE).

PTE is the treatment of choice for CTEPH, with low mortality in experienced centers. Significant improvements in pulmonary hemodynamics are usually observed, as PVR is reduced by the removal of chronic clot. Approximately, 20% to 40% of CTEPH patients are not operable because of the distal nature of the lesions or comorbidities. Persistence or reoccurrence after PTE is described in up to 35% of patients.[82] Medical management for CTEPH includes diuretics, and oxygen therapy in cases of heart failure or hypoxemia.[83] APLAS patients with PAH or CTEPH, including those undergoing PTE, should be commenced on lifelong anticoagulation.

Despite the availability of several vasodilators for the treatment of PAH, none has been shown to be invariably effective in the treatment of CTEPH. Patients have been treated with riociguat, with a significant improvement.[84] Bosentan has been evaluated in 157 patients with inoperable CTEPH or persistent/recurrent PH after PTE over 16 weeks; the primary endpoint of a decrease in PVR and an increase in the 6-minute walk distance was not met.[85,86] In cases of severe CTEPH in APLAS patients, continuous intravenous prostacyclin infusion with a pump has been used.[87,88] Cyclophosphamide has been tried as a treatment for APL antibody-associated PH, with success in individual cases.[89] PAH in the context of APLAS should be treated as in other connective tissue diseases (already discussed in the SLE section). In pulmonary venous hypertension caused by valve disease, valve replacement can be considered in the case of severe heart failure.

Catastrophic Antiphospholipid Syndrome

Catastrophic antiphospholipid syndrome (CAPS) is rare but fulminant presentation of APLAS. It is characterized by rapidly progressive multiorgan failure, multiple small-vessel occlusions on tissue biopsy, and circulating APL antibodies. This syndrome only occurs in about 1% of patients with APLAS, but is characterized by a 50% mortality[90]; 70% of cases occur in women. The main pulmonary complication is ARDS, and PE and alveolar hemorrhage are less common. Cytokine activation creates a proinflammatory state that clinically is much like systemic inflammatory response syndrome. Laboratory features are suggestive of microangiopathy. Thrombocytopenia and schistocytes on peripheral blood smear are frequent findings, although schistocytes are less than in thrombotic thrombocytopenic purpura.[91,92] CAPS can be associated with either IgG or IgM aCL antibodies. Once correctly identified, treatment of CAPS includes anticoagulation with heparin, corticosteroid therapy and other immunosuppression such as cyclophosphamide[93] and rituximab,[94] plasma exchange, and intravenous immunoglobulins.[91]

SUMMARY

Pulmonary involvement may complicate SLE and APLAS and is an important cause of morbidity and mortality. Early detection of pulmonary disease is important, because therapy ranges from aggressive immunosuppression for lupus pneumonitis, to anticoagulation for antiphospholipid antibody syndrome, to lowering immunosuppression and antimicrobial therapy in settings where infection is the cause. Treatment strategies for pulmonary disease in SLE are based on limited data (primarily small, uncontrolled series and case reports) and the experience from other connective tissue disorders.

REFERENCES

1. Stojan G, Petri M. Epidemiology of systemic lupus erythematosus: an update. Curr Opin Rheumatol 2018;30(2):144–50.
2. Tsokos GC. Systemic lupus erythematosus. N Engl J Med 2011;365(22):2110–21.
3. Pines A, Kaplinsky N, Olchovsky D, et al. Pleuro-pulmonary manifestations of systemic lupus erythematosus: clinical features of its subgroups. Prognostic and therapeutic implications. Chest 1985;88(1):129–35.
4. Quadrelli SA, Alvarez C, Arce SC, et al. Pulmonary involvement of systemic lupus erythematosus: analysis of 90 necropsies. Lupus 2009;18(12):1053–60.
5. Kamen DL, Strange C. Pulmonary manifestations of systemic lupus erythematosus. Clin Chest Med 2010;31(3):479–88.
6. Haye Salinas MJ, Caeiro F, Saurit V, et al. Pleuropulmonary involvement in patients with systemic lupus erythematosus from a Latin American inception cohort (GLADEL). Lupus 2017;26(13):1368–77.
7. Lopez Velazquez M, Highland KB. Pulmonary manifestations of systemic lupus erythematosus and Sjogren's syndrome. Curr Opin Rheumatol 2018; 30(5):449–64.
8. Bouros D, Pneumatikos I, Tzouvelekis A. Pleural involvement in systemic autoimmune disorders. Respiration 2008;75(4):361–71.
9. Small P, Frank H, Kreisman H, et al. An immunological evaluation of pleural effusions in systemic lupus erythematosus. Ann Allergy 1982;49(2):101–3.
10. Palavutitotai N, Buppajarntham T, Katchamart W. Etiologies and outcomes of pleural effusions in patients with systemic lupus erythematosus. J Clin Rheumatol 2014;20(8):418–21.
11. Mittoo S, Fell CD. Pulmonary manifestations of systemic lupus erythematosus. Semin Respir Crit Care Med 2014;35(2):249–54.
12. Ryu S, Fu W, Petri MA. Associates and predictors of pleurisy or pericarditis in SLE. Lupus Sci Med 2017; 4(1):e000221.

13. Witt C, Dorner T, Hiepe F, et al. Diagnosis of alveolitis in interstitial lung manifestation in connective tissue diseases: importance of late inspiratory crackles, 67 gallium scan and bronchoalveolar lavage. Lupus 1996;5(6):606–12.

14. Mulhearn B, Bruce IN. Indications for IVIG in rheumatic diseases. Rheumatology (Oxford) 2015; 54(3):383–91.

15. Mathai SC, Danoff SK. Management of interstitial lung disease associated with connective tissue disease. BMJ 2016;352:h6819.

16. Memet B, Ginzler EM. Pulmonary manifestations of systemic lupus erythematosus. Semin Respir Crit Care Med 2007;28(4):441–50.

17. Vivero M, Padera RF. Histopathology of lung disease in the connective tissue diseases. Rheum Dis Clin North Am 2015;41(2):197–211.

18. Weinrib L, Sharma OP, Quismorio FP Jr. A long-term study of interstitial lung disease in systemic lupus erythematosus. Semin Arthritis Rheum 1990;20(1): 48–56.

19. Tashkin DP, Roth MD, Clements PJ, et al. Mycophenolate mofetil versus oral cyclophosphamide in scleroderma-related interstitial lung disease (SLS II): a randomised controlled, double-blind, parallel group trial. Lancet Respir Med 2016;4(9):708–19.

20. Tashkin DP, Elashoff R, Clements PJ, et al. Cyclophosphamide versus placebo in scleroderma lung disease. N Engl J Med 2006;354(25):2655–66.

21. Deeb M, Tselios K, Gladman DD, et al. Shrinking lung syndrome in systemic lupus erythematosus: a single-centre experience. Lupus 2018;27(3):365–71.

22. Borrell H, Narvaez J, Alegre JJ, et al. Shrinking lung syndrome in systemic lupus erythematosus: a case series and review of the literature. Medicine (Baltimore) 2016;95(33):e4626.

23. Hardy K, Herry I, Attali V, et al. Bilateral phrenic paralysis in a patient with systemic lupus erythematosus. Chest 2001;119(4):1274–7.

24. Martens J, Demedts M, Vanmeenen MT, et al. Respiratory muscle dysfunction in systemic lupus erythematosus. Chest 1983;84(2):170–5.

25. Laroche CM, Mulvey DA, Hawkins PN, et al. Diaphragm strength in the shrinking lung syndrome of systemic lupus erythematosus. Q J Med 1989; 71(265):429–39.

26. Duron L, Cohen-Aubart F, Diot E, et al. Shrinking lung syndrome associated with systemic lupus erythematosus: a multicenter collaborative study of 15 new cases and a review of the 155 cases in the literature focusing on treatment response and long-term outcomes. Autoimmun Rev 2016; 15(10):994–1000.

27. Panchabhai TS, Bandyopadhyay D, Highland KB, et al. A 26-year-old woman with systemic lupus erythematosus presenting with orthopnea and restrictive lung impairment. Chest 2016;149(1):e29–33.

28. Nemec M, Pradella M, Jahn K, et al. Magnetic resonance imaging-confirmed pleuritis in systemic lupus erythematosus-associated shrinking lung syndrome. Arthritis Rheumatol 2015;67(7):1880.

29. Goswami RP, Mondal S, Lahiri D, et al. Shrinking lung syndrome in systemic lupus erythematosus successfully treated with rituximab. QJM 2016; 109(9):617–8.

30. Langenskiold E, Bonetti A, Fitting JW, et al. Shrinking lung syndrome successfully treated with rituximab and cyclophosphamide. Respiration 2012;84(2): 144–9.

31. Martinez-Martinez MU, Abud-Mendoza C. Diffuse alveolar hemorrhage in patients with systemic lupus erythematosus. Clinical manifestations, treatment, and prognosis. Reumatol Clin 2014;10(4):248–53.

32. Ednalino C, Yip J, Carsons SE. Systematic review of diffuse alveolar hemorrhage in systemic lupus erythematosus: focus on outcome and therapy. J Clin Rheumatol 2015;21(6):305–10.

33. Alabed IB. Treatment of diffuse alveolar hemorrhage in systemic lupus erythematosus patient with local pulmonary administration of factor VIIa (rFVIIa): a case report. Medicine (Baltimore) 2014;93(14):e72.

34. Andrade C, Mendonca T, Farinha F, et al. Alveolar hemorrhage in systemic lupus erythematosus: a cohort review. Lupus 2016;25(1):75–80.

35. Abramson SB, Dobro J, Eberle MA, et al. Acute reversible hypoxemia in systemic lupus erythematosus. Ann Intern Med 1991;114(11):941–7.

36. Simonneau G, Gatzoulis MA, Adatia I, et al. Updated clinical classification of pulmonary hypertension. J Am Coll Cardiol 2013;62(25 Suppl):D34–41.

37. Zuily S, Domingues V, Suty-Selton C, et al. Antiphospholipid antibodies can identify lupus patients at risk of pulmonary hypertension: a systematic review and meta-analysis. Autoimmun Rev 2017;16(6):576–86.

38. Elalouf O, Fireman E, Levartovsky D, et al. Decreased diffusion capacity on lung function testing in asymptomatic patients with systemic lupus erythematosus does not predict future lung disease. Lupus 2015;24(9):973–9.

39. Hachulla E, Jais X, Cinquetti G, et al. Pulmonary arterial hypertension associated with systemic lupus erythematosus: results from the French pulmonary hypertension registry. Chest 2018;153(1):143–51.

40. Thakkar V, Lau EM. Connective tissue disease-related pulmonary arterial hypertension. Best Pract Res Clin Rheumatol 2016;30(1):22–38.

41. Schreiber BE, Connolly MJ, Coghlan JG. Pulmonary hypertension in systemic lupus erythematosus. Best Pract Res Clin Rheumatol 2013;27(3):425–34.

42. Castillo-Martinez D, Marroquin-Fabian E, Lozada-Navarro AC, et al. Levels of uric acid may predict the future development of pulmonary hypertension in systemic lupus erythematosus: a seven-year follow-up study. Lupus 2016;25(1):61–6.

43. Hubbe-Tena C, Gallegos-Nava S, Marquez-Velasco R, et al. Pulmonary hypertension in systemic lupus erythematosus: echocardiography-based definitions predict 6-year survival. Rheumatology (Oxford) 2014;53(7):1256–63.

44. Kusunose K, Yamada H, Hotchi J, et al. Prediction of future overt pulmonary hypertension by 6-min walk stress echocardiography in patients with connective tissue disease. J Am Coll Cardiol 2015;66(4):376–84.

45. Kommireddy S, Bhyravavajhala S, Kurimeti K, et al. Pulmonary arterial hypertension in systemic lupus erythematosus may benefit by addition of immunosuppression to vasodilator therapy: an observational study. Rheumatology (Oxford) 2015;54(9):1673–9.

46. Qian J, Wang Y, Huang C, et al. Survival and prognostic factors of systemic lupus erythematosus-associated pulmonary arterial hypertension: a PRISMA-compliant systematic review and meta-analysis. Autoimmun Rev 2016;15(3):250–7.

47. Bazan IS, Mensah KA, Rudkovskaia AA, et al. Pulmonary arterial hypertension in the setting of scleroderma is different than in the setting of lupus: a review. Respir Med 2018;134:42–6.

48. Yusuf HR, Hooper WC, Grosse SD, et al. Risk of venous thromboembolism occurrence among adults with selected autoimmune diseases: a study among a U.S. cohort of commercial insurance enrollees. Thromb Res 2015;135(1):50–7.

49. Ahlehoff O, Wu JJ, Raunso J, et al. Cutaneous lupus erythematosus and the risk of deep venous thrombosis and pulmonary embolism: a Danish nationwide cohort study. Lupus 2017;26(13):1435–9.

50. Teitel AD, MacKenzie CR, Stern R, et al. Laryngeal involvement in systemic lupus erythematosus. Semin Arthritis Rheum 1992;22(3):203–14.

51. Langford CA, Van Waes C. Upper airway obstruction in the rheumatic diseases. Rheum Dis Clin North Am 1997;23(2):345–63.

52. Fenlon HM, Doran M, Sant SM, et al. High-resolution chest CT in systemic lupus erythematosus. AJR Am J Roentgenol 1996;166(2):301–7.

53. Keane MP, Lynch JP 3rd. Pleuropulmonary manifestations of systemic lupus erythematosus. Thorax 2000;55(2):159–66.

54. Kinder BW, Freemer MM, King TE Jr, et al. Clinical and genetic risk factors for pneumonia in systemic lupus erythematosus. Arthritis Rheum 2007;56(8):2679–86.

55. Miyakis S, Lockshin MD, Atsumi T, et al. International consensus statement on an update of the classification criteria for definite antiphospholipid syndrome (APS). J Thromb Haemost 2006;4(2):295–306.

56. Meroni PL, Chighizola CB, Rovelli F, et al. Antiphospholipid syndrome in 2014: more clinical manifestations, novel pathogenic players and emerging biomarkers. Arthritis Res Ther 2014;16(2):209.

57. Cervera R, Piette JC, Font J, et al. Antiphospholipid syndrome: clinical and immunologic manifestations and patterns of disease expression in a cohort of 1,000 patients. Arthritis Rheum 2002;46(4):1019–27.

58. Ford HJ, Roubey RA. Pulmonary manifestations of the antiphospholipid antibody syndrome. Clin Chest Med 2010;31(3):537–45.

59. Ginsburg KS, Liang MH, Newcomer L, et al. Anticardiolipin antibodies and the risk for ischemic stroke and venous thrombosis. Ann Intern Med 1992;117(12):997–1002.

60. Galli M, Borrelli G, Jacobsen EM, et al. Clinical significance of different antiphospholipid antibodies in the WAPS (warfarin in the antiphospholipid syndrome) study. Blood 2007;110(4):1178–83.

61. Pengo V, Biasiolo A, Pegoraro C, et al. Antibody profiles for the diagnosis of antiphospholipid syndrome. Thromb Haemost 2005;93(6):1147–52.

62. Branch DW, Khamashta MA. Antiphospholipid syndrome: obstetric diagnosis, management, and controversies. Obstet Gynecol 2003;101(6):1333–44.

63. Cervera R, Khamashta MA, Shoenfeld Y, et al. Morbidity and mortality in the antiphospholipid syndrome during a 5-year period: a multicentre prospective study of 1000 patients. Ann Rheum Dis 2009;68(9):1428–32.

64. Lim W, Le Gal G, Bates SM, et al. American Society of Hematology 2018 guidelines for management of venous thromboembolism: diagnosis of venous thromboembolism. Blood Adv 2018;2(22):3226–56.

65. Tritschler T, Kraaijpoel N, Le Gal G, et al. Venous thromboembolism: advances in diagnosis and treatment. JAMA 2018;320(15):1583–94.

66. Prashanth P, Mukhaini MK. Primary antiphospholipid syndrome with recurrent coronary thrombosis, acute pulmonary thromboembolism and intracerebral hematoma. J Invasive Cardiol 2009;21(12):E254–8.

67. Chighizola CB, Andreoli L, Gerosa M, et al. The treatment of anti-phospholipid syndrome: a comprehensive clinical approach. J Autoimmun 2018;90:1–27.

68. Galli M, Luciani D, Bertolini G, et al. Lupus anticoagulants are stronger risk factors for thrombosis than anticardiolipin antibodies in the antiphospholipid syndrome: a systematic review of the literature. Blood 2003;101(5):1827–32.

69. Derksen RH, de Groot PG, Kater L, et al. Patients with antiphospholipid antibodies and venous thrombosis should receive long term anticoagulant treatment. Ann Rheum Dis 1993;52(9):689–92.

70. Investigators E, Bauersachs R, Berkowitz SD, et al. Oral rivaroxaban for symptomatic venous thromboembolism. N Engl J Med 2010;363(26):2499–510.

71. Agnelli G, Buller HR, Cohen A, et al. Oral apixaban for the treatment of acute venous thromboembolism. N Engl J Med 2013;369(9):799–808.

72. Cohen H, Hunt BJ, Efthymiou M, et al. Rivaroxaban versus warfarin to treat patients with thrombotic antiphospholipid syndrome, with or without systemic lupus erythematosus (RAPS): a randomised, controlled, open-label, phase 2/3, non-inferiority trial. Lancet Haematol 2016;3(9):e426–36.

73. Pengo V, Denas G, Zoppellaro G, et al. Rivaroxaban vs warfarin in high-risk patients with antiphospholipid syndrome. Blood 2018;132(13):1365–71.

74. Woller SC, Stevens SM, Kaplan DA, et al. Apixaban for the secondary prevention of thrombosis among patients with antiphospholipid syndrome: study rationale and design (ASTRO-APS). Clin Appl Thromb Hemost 2016;22(3):239–47.

75. Schmidt-Tanguy A, Voswinkel J, Henrion D, et al. Antithrombotic effects of hydroxychloroquine in primary antiphospholipid syndrome patients. J Thromb Haemost 2013;11(10):1927–9.

76. Espinosa G, Cervera R, Font J, et al. The lung in the antiphospholipid syndrome. Ann Rheum Dis 2002; 61(3):195–8.

77. Kanakis MA, Kapsimali V, Vaiopoulos AG, et al. The lung in the spectrum of antiphospholipid syndrome. Clin Exp Rheumatol 2013;31(3):452–7.

78. Vianna JL, Khamashta MA, Ordi-Ros J, et al. Comparison of the primary and secondary antiphospholipid syndrome: a European Multicenter Study of 114 patients. Am J Med 1994;96(1):3–9.

79. Maioli G, Calabrese G, Capsoni F, et al. Lung disease in antiphospholipid syndrome. Semin Respir Crit Care Med 2019;40(2):278–94.

80. Cheng CY, Zhang YX, Denas G, et al. Prevalence of antiphospholipid (aPL) antibodies among patients with chronic thromboembolic pulmonary hypertension: a systematic review and meta-analysis. Intern Emerg Med 2019;14(4):521–7.

81. Martinuzzo ME, Pombo G, Forastiero RR, et al. Lupus anticoagulant, high levels of anticardiolipin, and anti-beta2-glycoprotein I antibodies are associated with chronic thromboembolic pulmonary hypertension. J Rheumatol 1998;25(7):1313–9.

82. Smith ZR, Makowski CT, Awdish RL. Treatment of patients with chronic thrombo embolic pulmonary hypertension: focus on riociguat. Ther Clin Risk Manag 2016;12:957–64.

83. Galie N, Humbert M, Vachiery JL, et al. 2015 ESC/ERS guidelines for the diagnosis and treatment of pulmonary hypertension. Rev Esp Cardiol (Engl Ed) 2016;69(2):177.

84. Ghofrani HA, D'Armini AM, Grimminger F, et al. Riociguat for the treatment of chronic thromboembolic pulmonary hypertension. N Engl J Med 2013; 369(4):319–29.

85. Naclerio C, D'Angelo S, Baldi S, et al. Efficacy of bosentan in the treatment of a patient with mixed connective tissue disease complicated by pulmonary arterial hypertension. Clin Rheumatol 2010;29(6): 687–90.

86. Jais X, D'Armini AM, Jansa P, et al. Bosentan for treatment of inoperable chronic thromboembolic pulmonary hypertension: BENEFiT (Bosentan Effects in iNopErable Forms of chronIc Thromboembolic pulmonary hypertension), a randomized, placebo-controlled trial. J Am Coll Cardiol 2008; 52(25):2127–34.

87. de la Mata J, Gomez-Sanchez MA, Aranzana M, et al. Long-term iloprost infusion therapy for severe pulmonary hypertension in patients with connective tissue diseases. Arthritis Rheum 1994;37(10): 1528–33.

88. Humbert M, Sanchez O, Fartoukh M, et al. Treatment of severe pulmonary hypertension secondary to connective tissue diseases with continuous IV epoprostenol (prostacyclin). Chest 1998;114(1 Suppl): 80S–2S.

89. Tam LS, Li EK. Successful treatment with immunosuppression, anticoagulation and vasodilator therapy of pulmonary hypertension in SLE associated with secondary antiphospholipid syndrome. Lupus 1998;7(7):495–7.

90. Asherson RA, Cervera R, Piette JC, et al. Catastrophic antiphospholipid syndrome: clues to the pathogenesis from a series of 80 patients. Medicine (Baltimore) 2001;80(6):355–77.

91. Bucciarelli S, Espinosa G, Cervera R, et al. Mortality in the catastrophic antiphospholipid syndrome: causes of death and prognostic factors in a series of 250 patients. Arthritis Rheum 2006;54(8):2568–76.

92. Espinosa G, Bucciarelli S, Cervera R, et al. Thrombotic microangiopathic haemolytic anaemia and antiphospholipid antibodies. Ann Rheum Dis 2004; 63(6):730–6.

93. Bayraktar UD, Erkan D, Bucciarelli S, et al, Catastrophic Antiphospholipid Syndrome Project Group. The clinical spectrum of catastrophic antiphospholipid syndrome in the absence and presence of lupus. J Rheumatol 2007;34(2):346–52.

94. Berman H, Rodriguez-Pinto I, Cervera R, et al. Rituximab use in the catastrophic antiphospholipid syndrome: descriptive analysis of the CAPS registry patients receiving rituximab. Autoimmun Rev 2013; 12(11):1085–90.

Pulmonary Involvement in Sjögren Syndrome

Jake G. Natalini, MD[a], Chadwick Johr, MD[b], Maryl Kreider, MD, MSCE[a],*

KEYWORDS

- Sjögren syndrome • Autoimmune • Lung • Airways

KEY POINTS

- SS can frequently affect the respiratory systems.
- A variety of manifestations have been described ranging from airways disease to interstitial lung disease to lymphoma and pseudolymphoma. Symptoms are common and non-specific.
- Sjogren's patients therefore should be regularly screened for respiratory involvement.

INTRODUCTION

Sjögren syndrome (SS) is an autoimmune disease characterized by dryness, mainly of the eyes and mouth, caused by chronic lymphocytic infiltration of the lacrimal and salivary glands. Aside from these sicca symptoms, other typical features include chronic fatigue, arthralgias, and cognitive dysfunction, frequently described as brain fog. Extraglandular manifestations may include the skin, joints, muscles, blood, kidneys, peripheral nerves, brain, and the gastrointestinal and respiratory tracts. SS has been described as the second most common autoimmune connective tissue disease after rheumatoid arthritis, with an estimated prevalence between 0.2% and 1.4% of the general population.[1] As with systemic lupus erythematosus (SLE), SS more commonly affects women, with approximately a 9:1 female/male ratio. However, unlike SLE,SS tends to be diagnosed later in life, typically between the ages of 30 and 60 years. Although most patients with SS live a normal lifespan, quality of life is significantly limited by burdensome chronic symptoms that are often refractory to treatment.[2,3] The most serious complication of SS is non-Hodgkin lymphoma, which can occur in 5% to 10% of patients and is the main contributor to increased mortality.[4–6]

Diagnosing SS is complicated by the symptoms being nonspecific, and obtaining objective evidence of the disease often requires input from multiple specialists. Although the gold standard for diagnosis, as with most rheumatologic conditions, is expert opinion, classification criteria are available for guidance.[7–9] Essentially, there are 3 main pieces to the diagnostic puzzle, and obtaining any 2 of them in someone with suspected SS can make the diagnosis: an objective measure of lacrimal or salivary gland dysfunction, significant autoimmune serologic testing, and a positive minor salivary gland biopsy (commonly referred to as a lip biopsy because the sample is taken from the inside of the lower lip).

Objective measures of lacrimal or salivary gland dysfunction may include any of the following: decreased tear production, as shown by an unanesthetized Schirmer test; decreased saliva production, as shown by a reduced unstimulated whole-mouth salivary flow rate; damage to the surface of the eye, as shown by an ocular staining score; or abnormal salivary gland uptake or discharge, as shown using salivary scintigraphy. Significant autoimmune serologic testing may include either of the following: a positive anti-Ro SSA antibody; or a positive antinuclear antibody

Disclosure: Dr. Natalini is supported on NIH grant T32HL007891.

[a] Division of Pulmonary, Allergy and Critical Care, Perelman School of Medicine, University of Pennsylvania, 3400 Spruce Street, 836 W. Gates Building, Philadelphia, PA 19104, USA; [b] Division of Rheumatology, Perelman School of Medicine, University of Pennsylvania, 3737 Market Street, 8th floor, Philadelphia, PA 19104, USA
* Corresponding author.
E-mail address: maryl.kreider@uphs.upenn.edu

Clin Chest Med 40 (2019) 531–544
https://doi.org/10.1016/j.ccm.2019.05.002

(ANA) at a titer of 1:320 or greater along with a positive rheumatoid factor (RF).

The minor salivary gland biopsy is invasive and is therefore typically reserved for instances in which a patient with suspected SS does not have both an objective measure of lacrimal or salivary gland dysfunction and a significant autoimmune serologic test result. It is a minor outpatient procedure akin to getting a dental filling, typically involving local anesthesia, a small incision, and a few sutures. The most troublesome complication of this procedure is persistent lower lip numbness. Although this is estimated to occur in up to 6% of biopsy cases, when a minimally invasive technique is used, the risk is mitigated to less than 1%.[10] A positive minor salivary gland biopsy result is one in which there is at least 1 cluster of 50 mononuclear lymphoid cells per 4 mm^2 of glandular tissue (which correlates to a focus score of 1 or greater).

PREVALENCE AND IMPACT OF LUNG DISEASE IN SJÖGREN SYNDROME

Extraglandular involvement of SS is common and can manifest in several ways. In particular, several pulmonary abnormalities have been described (**Box 1**). Multiple studies have tried to characterize the exact prevalence of lung involvement in SS, with estimates ranging widely from 9% to 75%.[11–18] In general, studies in which lung involvement is defined as requiring the presence of respiratory symptoms and either radiograph or pulmonary function test (PFT) abnormalities quote estimates of 9% to 22%.[11,14–17]

Lung involvement carries serious implications for patients with SS, with previous studies showing a significant impact on health-related quality of life (HRQL) and mortality.[17,19] In one study of 110 patients with primary SS (pSS), HRQL was measurably worse across several physical and emotional domains of the Short Form Health Survey (SF-36) in patients with lung involvement compared with those without lung involvement.[19] Similarly, another study of patients with pSS enrolled in the Norwegian Systemic Connective Tissue Disease and Vasculitis Registry noted significant differences in the physical functioning domain of the SF-36 between patients with pSS with and without lung disease. The presence of pulmonary involvement also carried a 4-fold increased risk of mortality within 10 years of disease onset (17% vs 4.5%).[17]

Identifying those patients with pSS who are at risk of having lung involvement remains a challenge. Strimlan and colleagues[11] initially described an increased frequency of hypergammaglobulinemia (73%) and an increased ANA or RF titer (74%)

Box 1
Described pulmonary manifestations of Sjögren syndrome

Respiratory symptoms
- Cough
- Dyspnea
- Nasal dryness
- Epistaxis
- Smell and taste disorders
- Dysphagia

Airways disease
- Rhinitis sicca
- Xerostomia
- Xerotrachea
- Xerobronchitis
- Bronchiectasis
- Follicular bronchiolitis
- Chronic bronchiolitis
- Bronchiolitis obliterans

Interstitial lung disease
- Nonspecific interstitial pneumonia
- Usual interstitial pneumonia
- Lymphocytic interstitial pneumonia
- Organizing pneumonia
- Cystic lung disease

Lymphoma

Pseudolymphoma

Pulmonary amyloidosis

Venous thromboembolism

Pulmonary hypertension

Pleuritis

Shrinking lung syndrome

Sarcoidosis

Lung cancer

in patients with documented pulmonary involvement of their SS. Subsequent studies have yielded conflicting results on the significance of a positive ANA test. For example, only 2 other studies have shown an association between the presence of lung involvement and an increased ANA titer,[14,20] whereas another recent study showed a trend for a higher occurrence of pleuropulmonary disease in ANA-negative cases.[21] Yazisiz and colleagues[16] also showed an association with hypergammaglobulinemia and an increased RF titer, as well as the presence of lymphopenia and anti-Ro SSA and anti-La SSB autoantibodies. Although highly specific, these findings lacked adequate sensitivity to detect pSS-associated lung disease. Other studies exploring the predictive utility of anti-SSA and anti-SSB antibodies have yielded conflicting results. For example, Davidson and colleagues[22] found that patients with anti-SSA antibodies were more likely to have lung involvement, whereas Ramos-Casals and colleagues[15] did not find any relationship with serologic status. Other studies focused on patient characteristics have suggested that male sex, older age, smoking, and longer disease duration are associated with a higher risk of lung involvement.[15–17,20,23,24]

CLINICAL MANIFESTATIONS

Cough and dyspnea are commonly reported symptoms among patients with SS and sometimes occur even in the absence of distinct pathologic processes. The prevalence of cough has been estimated at between 41% and 50%[13,25–27] and has a significant impact on quality of life.[26] In a series of 36 consecutively screened patients with pSS, 28% complained of dyspnea.[13] Reports of dyspnea were even more common in a recent cohort of consecutively enrolled patients with pSS, with an estimated prevalence of 42%.[27] In a larger series of 100 patients with pSS, 43% reported respiratory symptoms when evaluated within 6 months of diagnosis. Four years after diagnosis, symptoms were reported in 57% of patients, suggesting that pulmonary involvement may become increasingly common throughout the duration of illness.[28] In addition, dryness in the nasal and oropharyngeal mucosa can lead to smell and taste disorders, epistaxis, sinusitis, swallowing difficulties, and symptoms of globus, hoarseness, and excessive throat clearing.[29,30]

RADIOGRAPH AND PULMONARY FUNCTION TEST ABNORMALITIES

Radiograph and PFT abnormalities are commonly described in patients with SS, although PFT and imaging findings do not uniformly correlate with one another. The most commonly described PFT impairment is a reduced diffusing capacity of the lungs for carbon monoxide (DLCO).[13,17,18,22,31,32] Although some studies more commonly report a restrictive pattern,[32,33] others suggest that obstruction may be more common.[12,13,18,25] In particular, diseases of the small airways are fairly common, as supported by 3 studies that noted significant reductions (23%–44% predicted) in the maximal expiratory flow at 25% of vital

capacity (MEF25).[12,13,33] PFT abnormalities among patients with SS are typically mild.

Changes by plain chest radiograph (CXR) are frequently described but lack specificity.[11,13] High-resolution computed tomography (HRCT) may provide improved sensitivity for the detection of lung involvement. Several radiographic abnormalities have been described in patients with SS, such as airway-related changes, interstitial changes with reticulation, cystic changes, ground-glass opacities, consolidation, pulmonary nodules, or any combination thereof. Several studies have attempted to characterize the prevalence of these radiographic abnormalities, but findings have been inconsistent, probably because of underlying differences in pulmonary manifestations across various study populations. **Table 1** summarizes various studies reporting on HRCT findings.

Despite improved sensitivity in the detection of lung involvement with HRCT, radiographic abnormalities are often not predictive of physiologic impairments noted on PFT measurements. For example, a recent study of 44 patients with pSS by Chen and colleagues[32] showed a negative correlation between the extent of HRCT findings (measured using a dedicated scoring system) and DLCO but not with other PFT measurements such as forced vital capacity (FVC) or forced expiratory volume in 1 second (FEV$_1$). However, the investigators note that reductions in FVC and FEV$_1$ were associated with an increased risk for mortality. Similarly, having a higher HRCT score was an independent risk factor for mortality, even after adjustment for PFT results.[32] Another study of 66 patients with SS who underwent routine CXR screening noted a diffuse reticulonodular pattern, predominantly in the lower lobes, in 43% of patients with pSS and 62% of patients with secondary SS (sSS); however, these changes often did not correlation with PFT abnormities or the presence of respiratory symptoms.[33]

UTILITY OF BRONCHOALVEOLAR LAVAGE

The utility of bronchoalveolar lavage (BAL) in the evaluation of SS-related lung disease remains unknown, although studies have uniformly shown an increased presence of lymphocytosis on BAL specimens.[18,34,35] In a study of patients with pSS performed by Dalavanga and colleagues,[35] lymphocytosis on BAL was associated with the presence of dyspnea and cough, restriction on PFTs, and radiographic findings suggestive of pSS-associated interstitial lung disease (ILD). A later study of that same patient cohort reported that the presence of lymphocytosis of BAL

Table 1
High-resolution computed tomography studies in Sjögren syndrome

Study	Normal (%)	Airway Findings	Interstitial Findings	Other
Gardiner et al,[18] 1993 (n = 16)	47	7% bronchiectasis	20% fibrosis 13% reticulation	20% pleural changes 14% cysts
Franquet et al,[53] 1997 (n = 50)	66	22% bronchiolar abnormalities	22% reticulation 14% ground glass 8% honeycombing	2% airspace consolidation 64% of those with bronchiolar changes also had parenchymal changes
Papiris et al,[25] 1999 (n = 61)	69	22% airway thickening	6% interstitial changes	9% cysts
Franquet et al,[79] 1999 (n = 34)	NR	32% bronchiolar abnormalities	—	—
Uffmann et al,[12] 2001(n = 37)	35	—	24% interlobular septal thickening 10% ground-glass opacities	24% micronodules 14% cysts
Taouli et al,[54] 2002 (n = 35)	6	54% airways disease	20% pulmonary fibrosis 14% LIP	—
Matsuyama et al,[55] 2003 (n = 107)	42	33% in pSS; 16% in sSS	50% in pSS; 74% in sSS	13% lymphoproliferative pattern (only in pSS) 5% BOOP pattern (only in sSS)
Lohrman et al,[48] 2004 (n = 24)	22	46% bronchiectasis	38% ground-glass opacities 29% interlobular septal thickening 25% honeycombing	46% cysts 46% small nodules
Watanabe et al,[49] 2010 (n = 80)	10	23% bronchiectasis	70% interlobular septal thickening 14% honeycombing	38% cysts
Yazisiz et al,[16] 2010 (n = 213)	NR	50% bronchiectasis	64% ground-glass opacities 50% reticulation 43% honeycombing	50% lymphadenopathy 7% cysts
Mandl et al,[50] 2012 (n = 41)	—	44% bronchiectasis	54% interstitial changes 7% ground-glass opacities	7% emphysema
Palm et al,[17] 2013 (n = 117)	50	22% air trapping	44% reticulation	42% cysts
Dong et al,[57] 2018 (n = 206)	NR	12% bronchiectasis	36% reticulation 34% ground-glass opacities 8% honeycombing	13% airspace 10% cysts 12% nodules 12%

Abbreviations: BOOP, bronchiolitis obliterans organizing pneumonia; LIP, lymphocytic interstitial pneumonia; NR, not reported; pSS, primary SS; sSS, secondary SS.

predicted an increased need for immunologic therapy, as well as a higher risk for mortality.[36] However, increased mortality was not driven by respiratory failure, so it is difficult to attribute a causal explanation to this observed phenomenon. In contrast, Salaffi and colleagues[37] showed that lymphocytosis on BAL tended to predict a better prognosis, even if other findings of lung disease were noted, whereas patients with neutrophilic BAL had less favorable outcomes.

AIRWAYS DISEASE IN SJÖGREN SYNDROME

Upper airway inflammation and dryness are hallmark features of SS and partly explain why certain symptoms, such as cough and nasal irritation, are particularly common. In general, pathologic changes within the airways mimic the hallmark pathologic changes described within the exocrine glands, in which there is an increase in lymphocytic infiltration that eventually leads to glandular dysfunction and desiccation of the airway mucosa. Even in patients without evidence of airway involvement, inflammation within the trachea and bronchi is often detected. For example, Papiris and colleagues[38] examined lobar bronchial biopsies in 10 patients with SS and compared them with biopsies from 10 healthy volunteers. Among patients with SS, the investigators uniformly found an increase in the presence of CD4-positive lymphocytes within the bronchial mucosa. Similar findings were noted by Gardiner and colleagues,[18] who described lymphocytic bronchial changes by transbronchial biopsy in 5 of 16 patients with SS with symptomatic dyspnea. In the setting of long-standing inflammation, patients can develop both dryness of the trachea (xerotrachea) and of the large airways (xerobronchitis), which, in turn, can impair mucociliary clearance mechanisms and lead to the development of chronic cough.[13,25–27,39]

Bronchiolitis is another frequently described pulmonary manifestation involving the airways. In one series of 14 patients with pSS who underwent surgical lung biopsy, 29% of patients were reported to have histopathologic changes consistent with follicular bronchiolitis. Another 21% of patients had findings consistent with chronic bronchiolitis, and an additional 7% of patients had findings consistent with bronchiolitis obliterans.[40] Many of these patients' biopsies showed concomitant interstitial changes. In contrast, Nakanishi and colleagues[41] found chronic bronchiolitis to be more common than follicular bronchiolitis. Another study of pathology specimens taken from 33 patients (31 surgical lung biopsies and 2 autopsies) showed the presence of bronchiolitis in 12% of patients.[34] In some instances, the development of bronchiolitis can predate the onset of sicca symptoms. For example, in a retrospective review of 11 patients with pSS and bronchiolitis obliterans, bronchiolitis obliterans was the presenting manifestation of pSS in 36% of cases. Patients in this study generally did not respond well to immunosuppressive therapy.[42]

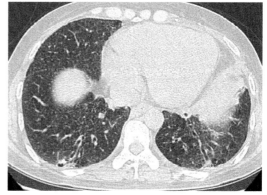

Fig. 1. A 32-year-old woman, nonsmoker, with SS who presented with dry cough and dyspnea for 5 years. HRCT shows a combination of centrilobular nodules with occasional tree-in-bud morphology, patchy consolidation and ground-glass opacities, subpleural cysts, and bronchiectasis in both lower lobes. Surgical lung biopsy confirmed a diagnosis of follicular bronchiolitis.[114] (From Lu J, Ma M, Zhao Q, et al. The Clinical Characteristics and Outcomes of Follicular Bronchiolitis in Chinese Adult Patients. Scientific reports 2018;8:7300.)

Follicular bronchiolitis has been specifically linked to certain connective tissue diseases, such as SS and rheumatoid arthritis (**Fig. 1**). It is characterized by the presence of hyperplastic lymphoid follicles with reactive germinal centers distributed along bronchovascular bundles.[43,44] It traditionally presents with cough and dyspnea. PFT findings may be normal or show either a restrictive or obstructive pattern. Radiographically, it appears as a reticular or reticulonodular pattern on HRCT.[45] In a review of 12 cases seen over a 9-year period at the Mayo Clinic, only 1 patient was thought to have follicular bronchiolitis in association with SS.[23] Most patients experienced a fairly stable course, with most showing a partial response to immunosuppressive therapy, as shown by improvement in symptoms, PFTs, and/or radiographic findings.[23]

Although bronchiolitis in association with SS has mostly been reported as being fairly mild, a 2011 case series describes 5 patients with severe chronic bronchiolitis that was thought to be a presenting manifestation of pSS. Four of the 5 patients improved on a combination of inhaled corticosteroids, inhaled long-acting beta-agonists, and a low dose of erythromycin.[46] In general, there are minimal data to guide treatment of bronchiolitis in SS. In the Mayo series on follicular bronchiolitis, the patient with pSS-associated follicular bronchiolitis responded favorably to corticosteroids.[23] In the retrospective review of 11 patients with bronchiolitis obliterans, 2 patients showed either stability or improvement on a combination of hydroxychloroquine and mycophenolate mofetil (MMF), and another patient treated with methylprednisolone alone showed symptomatic improvement.[42] Rituximab has been used successfully at least once in bronchiolitis associated with SS.[47]

In addition, radiographically evident bronchiectasis has been described in 23% to 54% of patients with SS.[16,48–50] In a 2010 study of 507 patients with pSS, 8% were thought to have pSS-associated bronchiectasis. These patients tended to be older at pSS diagnosis and had a higher frequency of hiatal hernia.[51] Most patients with bronchiectasis had cylindrical, lower lobe–predominant disease. In addition, patients with bronchiectasis had a higher frequency of respiratory infections (56% vs 3%) and pneumonia (29% vs 3%).[51]

INTERSTITIAL LUNG DISEASE IN SJÖGREN SYNDROME

ILD is a frequently described pulmonary manifestation of SS, with prevalence estimates ranging widely between 6% and 79%.[12,16–18,20,48–50,52–57] Older age, smoking, an increased ANA or RF titer, and increases in C-reactive protein level have all been described as potential risk factors for the development of ILD.[20,24] In another review of 315 patients with pSS, the presence of anti-SSA antibodies and low levels of circulating C3 were associated with ILD,[58] although no other studies have produced similar findings. A recent retrospective review of 102 patients with pSS-ILD found that those with non–sicca-onset pSS-ILD less commonly had hypergammaglobulinemia, an increased RF titer, or positive anti-SSA and anti-SSB antibodies compared with patients with sicca-onset pSS-ILD.[59] Pulmonary complications tended to be more progressive and severe in the non–sicca-onset patients.

Although lymphocytic interstitial pneumonia (LIP) has been classically linked to SS,[60] more recent studies have suggested that alternative histopathologic patterns of ILD, such as nonspecific interstitial pneumonia (NSIP) and usual interstitial pneumonia (UIP), may be more common (**Table 2**). For example, a recent retrospective analysis of 527 Chinese patients with pSS described the presence of pSS-ILD in 39% of cases. Of those, 42% had NSIP, 11% had UIP, 4% had LIP, and 4% had organizing pneumonia (OP). An additional 25% had multiple HRCT patterns in which NSIP was the predominant pattern. The remaining 14% had multiple HRCT patterns in which UIP, OP, or LIP was the

predominant pattern.[57] In almost all cases, there was bilateral involvement (99%). In addition, lower lobe involvement was reported in 89% of cases.[57] In another retrospective review of 165 Chinese patients with pSS-ILD in which 69 patients underwent HRCT, NSIP was again the predominant pattern seen on HRCT (39%), followed by an indeterminate pattern (19%), an LIP pattern (17%), a UIP pattern (16%), an admixed NSIP and LIP pattern (6%), an OP pattern (1%), and a respiratory bronchiolitis-ILD pattern (1%).[24] In a prospective cohort of 201 newly diagnosed patients with pSS, the prevalence of pSS-ILD was 78.6%. NSIP was the most common pattern seen on HRCT, present in 46% of cases.[20]

In a Japanese series of patients with SS who underwent surgical lung biopsy, 61% had NSIP, 12% had bronchiolitis, 12% had lymphoma, 6% had amyloidosis, and 3% had honeycomb changes.[34] Not a single patient had LIP. Similarly, Shi and colleagues[40] also found that NSIP was the most common histopathologic pattern on biopsy, followed by OP. A third series of 18 patients with pSS followed at the Mayo Clinic who underwent surgical lung biopsy again found NSIP to be the most common histopathologic pattern (28%), followed by OP (22%), UIP (17%), LIP (17%), lymphoma (11%), and amyloidosis (6%).[61]

Although LIP is likely not the most common histopathologic pattern seen in pSS-ILD, it is a fairly unusual pattern and carries a strong association with pSS (**Fig. 2**). One of the earliest descriptions of LIP was provided by Liebow and Carrington[60] in 1973, in which they report on 18 cases of LIP, 28% of which were associated with SS. In a more recent series of 15 patients with LIP, 53% had SS.[62] Classically described HRCT findings include the presence of ground-glass opacities and poorly defined centrilobular nodules that are thought to evolve into cystic changes over time.[63,64] Although cystic changes may be suggestive of LIP, there are cases of lymphoma and amyloidosis presenting with a radiographic pattern similar to LIP,[34,61,65] and caution should be used in making the diagnosis of LIP based solely on imaging findings.

Data on the natural history and treatment of pSS-ILD are limited. Five-year survival rates have been estimated at as high as 83% to 89%[24,34]; however, other studies have described much worse outcomes. For example, the investigators of the Mayo series reported that 39% of their cohort had died during a median follow-up of about 3 years, with 3 deaths attributed to acute exacerbations of ILD (AEILD).[61] Suda and

Table 2
Frequency of interstitial lung disease patterns in Sjögren syndrome

Study	Method	Predominant Pattern				
		Nonspecific Interstitial Pneumonia	UIP	LIP	Organizing Pneumonia	Other
Ito et al,[34] 2005 (n = 31)	HRCT	55%	13%	3%	—	13% bronchiolitis 10% cysts 6% other
	Pathology	61%	—	—	—	13% bronchiolitis 10% lymphoma 6% amyloidosis 6% atelectatic fibrosis 3% honeycomb changes only
Parambil et al,[61] 2006 (n = 18)	Pathology	28%	17%	17%	22%	11% lymphoma 6% amyloidosis
Shi et al,[40] 2009 (n = 7)	Pathology	57% (25% admixed with LIP, OP, or bronchiolitis)	—	—	—	43% bronchiolitis (14% admixed with NSIP)
Dong et al,[57] 2018 (n = 206)	HRCT	67% (25% admixed with UIP, LIP, or OP)	17% (6% admixed with NSIP, LIP, or OP)	6% (2% admixed with NSIP, UIP, or OP)	10% (6% admixed with NSIP or UIP)	—
Gao et al,[24] 2018 (n = 69)	HRCT	45% (6% admixed with LIP)	16%	17%	1%	19% indeterminate 1% RB-ILD
Wang et al,[20] 2018(n = 201)	HRCT	46%	10%	8%	4%	25% unclassifiable

Abbreviations: OP, organizing pneumonia; RB-ILD, respiratory bronchiolitis ILD.

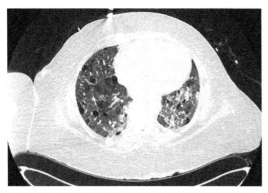

Fig. 2. 70-year-old woman who presented with dry eyes and dyspnea on exertion. Laboratory testing confirmed the presence of anti-SSA antibodies. HRCT demonstrates bilateral thin-walled cystic changes, as well as poorly defined multifocal nodules.[115]

colleagues[66] reported a lower incidence of AEILD (6%) but showed a similar risk for mortality from AEILD in connective tissue disease–associated ILD compared with AEILD in idiopathic pulmonary fibrosis.

Studies to guide treatment decisions in pSS-ILD are limited. In the Mayo series, 15 of the 18 patients were treated with corticosteroids and often another agent, such as hydroxychloroquine, azathioprine, or cyclophosphamide.[61] During longitudinal follow-up, 50% of patients had a significant improvement in FVC and/or DLCO, whereas 28% had significant decline. Deheinzelin and colleagues[52] described their experiences using azathioprine to treat SS-ILD in 11 patients and found a favorable response overall, with 7 patients showing improvement in FVC by more than 10%. In 2013, Fischer and colleagues[67] reported on their experiences using MMF to treatment connective tissue disease–associated ILD. Among the 125 patients treated with MMF, only 5 patients were thought to have pSS-ILD. Nonetheless, MMF was associated with significant interval improvements in FVC, measured at 52, 104, and 156 weeks after initiation of therapy. In their subgroup analyses, patients with a UIP pattern were found to have stability in FVC and DLCO but did not show considerable improvement, whereas patients with an NSIP had a more favorable response. In a more recent retrospective study of 21 patients with pSS-ILD, all 21 patients received steroids, 1 patient received cyclophosphamide, 4 patients received azathioprine, and 1 patient received rituximab. Response to treatment was variable, in which 16% improved, 47% showed stabilization of disease, and 37% deteriorated. Older age and esophageal disease were associated with poorer outcomes.[56] A 2013 review of the Autoimmune and Rituximab Registry in France reported on 9 patients with SS with lung involvement who received rituximab therapy.[47] Of those, 8 out of 9 had ILD and 6 of those 8 improved with the first cycle of therapy. Adverse events occurred infrequently. Isaksen and colleagues[68] summarize available literature describing experiences using rituximab for the treatment of SS, with good efficacy and safety reported among patients with extraglandular involvement.

In addition, cystic lung disease (CLD), even in the absence of interstitial changes, has been described in 2 separate retrospective studies. In the first study of 84 patients with SS (both primary and secondary), 15.4% of patients were found to have CLD on either computed tomography (CT) or CXR. Among patients who underwent CT, 31% of patients were found to have CLD, suggesting that cystic changes frequently go undetected on CXR. Six patients had cysts without other radiographic findings present.[69] The other study reported the presence of cysts in 23% of patients who underwent CT. Cystic changes were predominantly bilateral (52%) and mostly located in the middle long zones (76%). A small subset of patients were again noted to have cysts in the absence of other radiographic findings.[70] Both studies describe little to no progression of CLD during several years of longitudinal follow-up.[69,70]

LYMPHOMA AND PSEUDOLYMPHOMA

Patients with SS are at higher risk for the development of non-Hodgkin lymphoma (NHL). Over time, lymphocytic infiltration of polyclonal B and T cells can evolve into a monoclonal B-cell proliferation characteristic of lymphoma. The most commonly reported histologic subtypes of NHL include diffuse large B-cell lymphoma and mucosa-associated lymphoid tissue lymphoma,[71–74] although follicular and lymphoplasmacytoid lymphoma have also been previously described.[75] In a large cohort study of 676 patients with pSS, the standardized incidence ratio of NHL was 8.7.[76] In another study of patients with pSS according to the American-European Consensus Criteria, the standardized incidence ratio of NHL was nearly 16. In this study, CD4+ T-cell lymphocytopenia was a strong risk factor for the development of lymphoma.[71] Other risk factors include markers for severe SS such as parotid enlargement, hypocomplementemia, cryoglobulinemia, and palpable purpura.[71,74,77,78]

The prevalence of primary pulmonary lymphoma is estimated at between 1% and 2% in patients with pSS,[79] with lymphoma more frequently described in the lymph nodes and salivary and lacrimal glands.[80] Symptoms of pulmonary NHL generally include cough, dyspnea, and traditional B symptoms, such as fever, night sweats, and weight loss. Radiographic findings are varied, with solitary or multifocal nodules, bilateral alveolar infiltrates, and interstitial opacities all having been described. Mediastinal lymphadenopathy and pleural effusions may accompany parenchymal abnormalities.[75]

Pseudolymphoma, or pulmonary nodular lymphoid hyperplasia, is a benign lesion characterized by infiltration of mature polyclonal lymphocytes and plasma cells[81] and is most commonly seen in patients with isolated sicca symptoms.[75] It is typically asymptomatic, although it can present with cough and dyspnea. It generally appears as a solitary nodule or mass on CT; however, it can also present as parenchymal consolidation with air bronchograms or even as multiple nodules. If mediastinal lymphadenopathy or the presence of pleural effusions is noted, a diagnosis of lymphoma should be considered.[75] There is debate as to whether pseudolymphoma and extranodal marginal zone B-cell lymphoma are distinct clinical entities. Immunohistochemical and molecular studies are needed to distinguish pseudolymphoma from other lymphoproliferative disorders.[82] Pseudolymphoma generally regresses after treatment with corticosteroids or immunosuppressive therapy, but rarely it progresses to frank lymphoma.[83]

OTHER PULMONARY MANIFESTATIONS OF SJÖGREN SYNDROME

Pulmonary amyloidosis is a rare complication of pSS and occurs almost exclusively in women. Clinical symptoms generally include cough and dyspnea, along with fatigue, weakness, hemoptysis, and pleurisy.[84] Other associated abnormalities include idiopathic thrombocytopenic purpura,[85] cryoglobulinemia,[86,87] Raynaud phenomenon,[88] antiphospholipid antibody syndrome,[84] and lymphoma.[85,89,90] Large, calcified, randomly distributed, irregular, smooth-bordered nodules may be the sole radiological abnormality or may occur in association with multiple cysts, septal thickening, and smaller nodules as seen in LIP.[84,90] Surgical lung biopsy is generally required to establish the diagnosis and rule out lymphoma. The prognosis of pSS-related pulmonary amyloidosis is unknown, and there are no data to support any definitive therapeutic options.

Patients with pSS are thought to be at increased risk for venous thromboembolism (VTE), which may be related to the presence of antiphospholipid antibodies in up to 30% of patients.[91] In a recent population-based study of 1175 incident pSS cases, multivariable hazard ratios for pulmonary embolism, deep vein thrombosis, and VTE among SS cases were 4.1, 2.8, and 2.9, respectively, compared with non-SS controls.[92] Risk was highest during the first year after pSS diagnosis.

Pulmonary hypertension (PH) in association with SS can occur as a result of an arteriopathy, pulmonary veno-occlusive disease,[93] valvular heart disease,[94] or ILD.[95] Hypergammaglobulinemia and increases in ANA and RF titers, as well as the presence of anti-SSA, anti-SSB, and anti-RNP autoantibodies, have all been associated with the development and progression of PH.[95] Patients with pSS-associated pulmonary arterial hypertension (PAH) are more likely to have Raynaud phenomenon, cutaneous vasculitis, and ILD.[95] Together, these data suggest that systemic vasculopathy, B-cell activation, and autoimmunity contribute to the pathogenesis of pSS-associated PAH. Typically, pSS precedes the diagnosis of pulmonary hypertension,[95] although PH can be a presenting manifestation of pSS in up to 41% of patients.[96] Although the exact prevalence of PH is unknown, one study reported echocardiographic evidence of PH in 22% of patients with pSS.[94] Published case reports often describe women in their third and fourth decades of life and most often of Japanese descent.[95,97,98] The degree of sicca symptoms is not predictive of PH severity.[95,99] Survival estimates are as low as 73% at 1 year and 66% at 3 years, probably in part because of delays in diagnosis.

Lymphocytic pleuritis with or without pleural effusion and/or pleural thickening has rarely been described in pSS.[18,100] The pleural fluid is a lymphocytic-predominant exudate with a normal glucose level and pH. Laboratory analyses may show increased plasma and pleural levels of RF, anti-SSA, and anti-SSB autoantibodies, along with hypocomplementemia.[101] The presence of a coexisting autoimmune disease, such as rheumatoid arthritis or SLE, must be excluded.

Certain neuromuscular diseases have also been described. For example, shrinking lung syndrome, although more traditionally associated with SLE, has been reported in association with SS.[102,103] It is characterized by small lung volumes, elevation of the diaphragm, and restrictive physiology without evidence of parenchymal disease. Respiratory muscle weakness with or without failure can be a consequence of hypokalemic periodic paralysis associated with a distal renal tubular acidosis[104–106] or rarely as a consequence of proximal skeletal myopathy.[107–109]

Sarcoidosis and SS share a number pathogenic, immunogenic, and clinical features, making it difficult to distinguish between the two clinical entities. To date, more than 70 cases of overlap have been reported. The prevalence of sarcoidosis in patients with pSS has been estimated at between 1% and 2%, which is significantly higher than the general population.[110,111] In a case series of 59 patients with suspected coexistent sarcoidosis and pSS, the main clinical features at initial presentation included sicca syndrome, parotidomegaly, respiratory symptoms, cutaneous involvement, articular involvement, and fatigue. In patients in whom pSS was first diagnosed, the development of hilar adenopathy, uveitis, and hypercalcemia most often led to a concomitant diagnosis of sarcoidosis. The presence of autoantibodies was also closely tied to the coexistence of sarcoidosis and pSS.[112]

In addition, a retrospective review of patients with pSS suggested that the incidence of lung cancer may be higher with respect to the general population. Of the types of cancers reported in this study, adenocarcinoma accounted for 90% of cases.[113] No other studies to date have shown an association between pSS and lung cancer.

SUMMARY

Extraglandular manifestations of SS frequently implicate the respiratory tract. Several pulmonary disease processes have been described. Patients with SS should be routinely screened for respiratory symptoms such as cough and dyspnea, and considerations should be given to the aforementioned pulmonary manifestations in patients who report such complaints.

REFERENCES

1. Helmick CG, Felson DT, Lawrence RC, et al. Estimates of the prevalence of arthritis and other rheumatic conditions in the United States. Part I. Arthritis Rheum 2008;58:15–25.
2. Segal B, Bowman SJ, Fox PC, et al. Primary Sjogren's syndrome: health experiences and predictors of health quality among patients in the United States. Health Qual Life Outcomes 2009;7:46.
3. Strombeck B, Ekdahl C, Manthorpe R, et al. Health-related quality of life in primary Sjogren's syndrome, rheumatoid arthritis and fibromyalgia compared to normal population data using SF-36. Scand J Rheumatol 2000;29:20–8.
4. Nocturne G, Mariette X. Sjogren Syndrome-associated lymphomas: an update on pathogenesis and management. Br J Haematol 2015;168:317–27.
5. Nocturne G, Virone A, Ng WF, et al. Rheumatoid factor and disease activity are independent predictors of lymphoma in primary Sjogren's syndrome. Arthritis Rheumatol 2016;68:977–85.
6. Nishishinya MB, Pereda CA, Munoz-Fernandez S, et al. Identification of lymphoma predictors in patients with primary Sjogren's syndrome: a systematic literature review and meta-analysis. Rheumatol Int 2015;35:17–26.
7. Shiboski CH, Shiboski SC, Seror R, et al. 2016 American College of Rheumatology/European League against Rheumatism classification criteria for primary Sjogren's syndrome: a consensus and data-driven methodology involving three international patient cohorts. Ann Rheum Dis 2017;76:9–16.
8. Shiboski SC, Shiboski CH, Criswell L, et al. American College of Rheumatology classification criteria for Sjogren's syndrome: a data-driven, expert consensus approach in the Sjogren's International Collaborative Clinical Alliance cohort. Arthritis Care Res 2012;64:475–87.
9. Vitali C, Bombardieri S, Jonsson R, et al. Classification criteria for Sjogren's syndrome: a revised version of the European criteria proposed by the American-European Consensus Group. Ann Rheum Dis 2002;61:554–8.
10. Varela Centelles P, Sanchez-Sanchez M, Costa-Bouzas J, et al. Neurological adverse events related to lip biopsy in patients suspicious for Sjogren's syndrome: a systematic review and prevalence meta-analysis. Rheumatology (Oxford) 2014;53:1208–14.
11. Strimlan CV, Rosenow EC 3rd, Divertie MB, et al. Pulmonary manifestations of Sjogren's syndrome. Chest 1976;70:354–61.
12. Uffmann M, Kiener HP, Bankier AA, et al. Lung manifestation in asymptomatic patients with primary Sjogren syndrome: assessment with high resolution CT and pulmonary function tests. J Thorac Imaging 2001;16:282–9.
13. Constantopoulos SH, Papadimitriou CS, Moutsopoulos HM. Respiratory manifestations in primary Sjogren's syndrome. A clinical, functional, and histologic study. Chest 1985;88:226–9.
14. Garcia-Carrasco M, Ramos-Casals M, Rosas J, et al. Primary Sjogren syndrome: clinical and immunologic disease patterns in a cohort of 400 patients. Medicine 2002;81:270–80.
15. Ramos-Casals M, Solans R, Rosas J, et al. Primary Sjogren syndrome in Spain: clinical and immunologic expression in 1010 patients. Medicine 2008;87:210–9.
16. Yazisiz V, Arslan G, Ozbudak IH, et al. Lung involvement in patients with primary Sjogren's

syndrome: what are the predictors? Rheumatol Int 2010;30:1317–24.

17. Palm O, Garen T, Berge Enger T, et al. Clinical pulmonary involvement in primary Sjogren's syndrome: prevalence, quality of life and mortality–a retrospective study based on registry data. Rheumatology (Oxford) 2013;52:173–9.

18. Gardiner P, Ward C, Allison A, et al. Pleuropulmonary abnormalities in primary Sjogren's syndrome. J Rheumatol 1993;20:831–7.

19. Belenguer R, Ramos-Casals M, Brito-Zeron P, et al. Influence of clinical and immunological parameters on the health-related quality of life of patients with primary Sjogren's syndrome. Clin Exp Rheumatol 2005;23:351–6.

20. Wang Y, Hou Z, Qiu M, et al. Risk factors for primary Sjogren syndrome-associated interstitial lung disease. J Thorac Dis 2018;10:2108–17.

21. Ter Borg EJ, Kelder JC. Is extra-glandular organ damage in primary Sjogren's syndrome related to the presence of systemic auto-antibodies and/or hypergammaglobulinemia? A long-term cohort study with 110 patients from The Netherlands. Int J Rheum Dis 2017;20:875–81.

22. Davidson BK, Kelly CA, Griffiths ID. Ten year follow up of pulmonary function in patients with primary Sjogren's syndrome. Ann Rheum Dis 2000;59:709–12.

23. Aerni MR, Vassallo R, Myers JL, et al. Follicular bronchiolitis in surgical lung biopsies: clinical implications in 12 patients. Respir Med 2008;102:307–12.

24. Gao H, Zhang XW, He J, et al. Prevalence, risk factors, and prognosis of interstitial lung disease in a large cohort of Chinese primary Sjogren syndrome patients: a case-control study. Medicine 2018;97:e11003.

25. Papiris SA, Maniati M, Constantopoulos SH, et al. Lung involvement in primary Sjogren's syndrome is mainly related to the small airway disease. Ann Rheum Dis 1999;58:61–4.

26. Mialon P, Barthelemy L, Sebert P, et al. A longitudinal study of lung impairment in patients with primary Sjogren's syndrome. Clin Exp Rheumatol 1997;15:349–54.

27. Bellido-Casado J, Plaza V, Diaz C, et al. Bronchial inflammation, respiratory symptoms and lung function in Primary Sjogren's syndrome. Arch Bronconeumol 2011;47:330–4.

28. Kelly C, Gardiner P, Pal B, et al. Lung function in primary Sjogren's syndrome: a cross sectional and longitudinal study. Thorax 1991;46:180–3.

29. Freeman SR, Sheehan PZ, Thorpe MA, et al. Ear, nose, and throat manifestations of Sjogren's syndrome: retrospective review of a multidisciplinary clinic. J Otolaryngol 2005;34:20–4.

30. Rasmussen N, Brofeldt S, Manthorpe R. Smell and nasal findings in patients with primary Sjogren's syndrome. Scand J Rheumatol Suppl 1986;61:142–5.

31. Oxholm P, Bundgaard A, Birk Madsen E, et al. Pulmonary function in patients with primary Sjogren's syndrome. Rheumatol Int 1982;2:179–81.

32. Chen MH, Chou HP, Lai CC, et al. Lung involvement in primary Sjogren's syndrome: correlation between high-resolution computed tomography score and mortality. J Chin Med Assoc 2014;77:75–82.

33. Papathanasiou MP, Constantopoulos SH, Tsampoulas C, et al. Reappraisal of respiratory abnormalities in primary and secondary Sjogren's syndrome. A controlled study. Chest 1986;90:370–4.

34. Ito I, Nagai S, Kitaichi M, et al. Pulmonary manifestations of primary Sjogren's syndrome: a clinical, radiologic, and pathologic study. Am J Respir Crit Care Med 2005;171:632–8.

35. Dalavanga YA, Constantopoulos SH, Galanopoulou V, et al. Alveolitis correlates with clinical pulmonary involvement in primary Sjogren's syndrome. Chest 1991;99:1394–7.

36. Dalavanga YA, Voulgari PV, Georgiadis AN, et al. Lymphocytic alveolitis: a surprising index of poor prognosis in patients with primary Sjogren's syndrome. Rheumatol Int 2006;26:799–804.

37. Salaffi F, Manganelli P, Carotti M, et al. A longitudinal study of pulmonary involvement in primary Sjogren's syndrome: relationship between alveolitis and subsequent lung changes on high-resolution computed tomography. Br J Rheumatol 1998;37:263–9.

38. Papiris SA, Saetta M, Turato G, et al. CD4-positive T-lymphocytes infiltrate the bronchial mucosa of patients with Sjogren's syndrome. Am J Respir Crit Care Med 1997;156:637–41.

39. Mathieu A, Cauli A, Pala R, et al. Tracheo-bronchial mucociliary clearance in patients with primary and secondary Sjogren's syndrome. Scand J Rheumatol 1995;24:300–4.

40. Shi JH, Liu HR, Xu WB, et al. Pulmonary manifestations of Sjogren's syndrome. Respiration 2009;78:377–86.

41. Nakanishi M, Fukuoka J, Tanaka T, et al. Small airway disease associated with Sjogren's syndrome: clinico-pathological correlations. Respir Med 2011;105:1931–8.

42. Wight EC, Baqir M, Ryu JH. Constrictive bronchiolitis in patients with primary Sjogren syndrome. J Clin Rheumatol 2019;25(2):74–7.

43. Ryu JH, Myers JL, Swensen SJ. Bronchiolar disorders. Am J Respir Crit Care Med 2003;168:1277–92.

44. Yousem SA, Colby TV, Carrington CB. Follicular bronchitis/bronchiolitis. Hum Pathol 1985;16: 700–6.

45. Wells AU, du Bois RM. Bronchiolitis in association with connective tissue disorders. Clin Chest Med 1993;14:655–66.

46. Borie R, Schneider S, Debray MP, et al. Severe chronic bronchiolitis as the presenting feature of primary Sjogren's syndrome. Respir Med 2011; 105:130–6.

47. Gottenberg JE, Cinquetti G, Larroche C, et al. Efficacy of rituximab in systemic manifestations of primary Sjogren's syndrome: results in 78 patients of the AutoImmune and Rituximab registry. Ann Rheum Dis 2013;72:1026–31.

48. Lohrmann C, Uhl M, Warnatz K, et al. High-resolution CT imaging of the lung for patients with primary Sjogren's syndrome. Eur J Radiol 2004;52:137–43.

49. Watanabe M, Naniwa T, Hara M, et al. Pulmonary manifestations in Sjogren's syndrome: correlation analysis between chest computed tomographic findings and clinical subsets with poor prognosis in 80 patients. J Rheumatol 2010;37:365–73.

50. Mandl T, Diaz S, Ekberg O, et al. Frequent development of chronic obstructive pulmonary disease in primary SS–results of a longitudinal follow-up. Rheumatology (Oxford) 2012;51:941–6.

51. Soto-Cardenas MJ, Perez-De-Lis M, Bove A, et al. Bronchiectasis in primary Sjogren's syndrome: prevalence and clinical significance. Clin Exp Rheumatol 2010;28:647–53.

52. Deheinzelin D, Capelozzi VL, Kairalla RA, et al. Interstitial lung disease in primary Sjogren's syndrome. Clinical-pathological evaluation and response to treatment. Am J Respir Crit Care Med 1996;154:794–9.

53. Franquet T, Gimenez A, Monill JM, et al. Primary Sjogren's syndrome and associated lung disease: CT findings in 50 patients. AJR Am J Roentgenol 1997;169:655–8.

54. Taouli B, Brauner MW, Mourey I, et al. Thin-section chest CT findings of primary Sjogren's syndrome: correlation with pulmonary function. Eur Radiol 2002;12:1504–11.

55. Matsuyama N, Ashizawa K, Okimoto T, et al. Pulmonary lesions associated with Sjogren's syndrome: radiographic and CT findings. Br J Radiol 2003;76:880–4.

56. Roca F, Dominique S, Schmidt J, et al. Interstitial lung disease in primary Sjogren's syndrome. Autoimmun Rev 2017;16:48–54.

57. Dong X, Zhou J, Guo X, et al. A retrospective analysis of distinguishing features of chest HRCT and clinical manifestation in primary Sjogren's syndrome-related interstitial lung disease in a Chinese population. Clin Rheumatol 2018;37:2981–8.

58. Li X, Xu B, Ma Y, et al. Clinical and laboratory profiles of primary Sjogren's syndrome in a Chinese population: a retrospective analysis of 315 patients. Int J Rheum Dis 2015;18:439–46.

59. Gao H, Zou YD, Zhang XW, et al. Interstitial lung disease in non-sicca onset primary Sjogren's syndrome: a large-scale case-control study. Int J Rheum Dis 2018;21:1423–9.

60. Liebow AA, Carrington CB. Diffuse pulmonary lymphoreticular infiltrations associated with dysproteinemia. Med Clin North Am 1973;57:809–43.

61. Parambil JG, Myers JL, Lindell RM, et al. Interstitial lung disease in primary Sjogren syndrome. Chest 2006;130:1489–95.

62. Cha SI, Fessler MB, Cool CD, et al. Lymphoid interstitial pneumonia: clinical features, associations and prognosis. Eur Respir J 2006;28:364–9.

63. Johkoh T, Muller NL, Pickford HA, et al. Lymphocytic interstitial pneumonia: thin-section CT findings in 22 patients. Radiology 1999;212:567–72.

64. Johkoh T, Ichikado K, Akira M, et al. Lymphocytic interstitial pneumonia: follow-up CT findings in 14 patients. J Thorac Imaging 2000;15:162–7.

65. Watanabe Y, Koyama S, Miwa C, et al. Pulmonary mucosa-associated lymphoid tissue (MALT) lymphoma in Sjogren's syndrome showing only the LIP pattern radiologically. Intern Med 2012;51: 491–5.

66. Suda T, Kaida Y, Nakamura Y, et al. Acute exacerbation of interstitial pneumonia associated with collagen vascular diseases. Respir Med 2009; 103:846–53.

67. Fischer A, Brown KK, Du Bois RM, et al. Mycophenolate mofetil improves lung function in connective tissue disease-associated interstitial lung disease. J Rheumatol 2013;40:640–6.

68. Isaksen K, Jonsson R, Omdal R. Anti-CD20 treatment in primary Sjogren's syndrome. Scand J Immunol 2008;68:554–64.

69. Martinez-Balzano CD, Touray S, Kopec S. Cystic lung disease among patients with Sjogren syndrome: frequency, natural history, and associated risk factors. Chest 2016;150:631–9.

70. Lechtman S, Debray MP, Crestani B, et al. Cystic lung disease in Sjogren's syndrome: an observational study. Joint Bone Spine 2017;84:317–21.

71. Theander E, Henriksson G, Ljungberg O, et al. Lymphoma and other malignancies in primary Sjogren's syndrome: a cohort study on cancer incidence and lymphoma predictors. Ann Rheum Dis 2006;65:796–803.

72. Tonami H, Matoba M, Kuginuki Y, et al. Clinical and imaging findings of lymphoma in patients with Sjogren syndrome. J Comput Assist Tomogr 2003;27:517–24.

73. Papiris SA, Kalomenidis I, Malagari K, et al. Extranodal marginal zone B-cell lymphoma of the lung in

Sjogren's syndrome patients: reappraisal of clinical, radiological, and pathology findings. Respir Med 2007;101:84–92.

74. Voulgarelis M, Dafni UG, Isenberg DA, et al. Malignant lymphoma in primary Sjogren's syndrome: a multicenter, retrospective, clinical study by the European Concerted Action on Sjogren's Syndrome. Arthritis Rheum 1999;42:1765–72.

75. Kokosi M, Riemer EC, Highland KB. Pulmonary involvement in Sjogren syndrome. Clin Chest Med 2010;31:489–500.

76. Kauppi M, Pukkala E, Isomaki H. Elevated incidence of hematologic malignancies in patients with Sjogren's syndrome compared with patients with rheumatoid arthritis (Finland). Cancer Causes Control 1997;8:201–4.

77. Ioannidis JP, Vassiliou VA, Moutsopoulos HM. Long-term risk of mortality and lymphoproliferative disease and predictive classification of primary Sjogren's syndrome. Arthritis Rheum 2002;46:741–7.

78. Ramos-Casals M, Brito-Zeron P, Yague J, et al. Hypocomplementaemia as an immunological marker of morbidity and mortality in patients with primary Sjogren's syndrome. Rheumatology (Oxford) 2005;44:89–94.

79. Franquet T, Diaz C, Domingo P, et al. Air trapping in primary Sjogren syndrome: correlation of expiratory CT with pulmonary function tests. J Comput Assist Tomogr 1999;23:169–73.

80. Leandro MJ, Isenberg DA. Rheumatic diseases and malignancy–is there an association? Scand J Rheumatol 2001;30:185–8.

81. Kreider M, Highland K. Pulmonary involvement in Sjogren syndrome. Semin Respir Crit Care Med 2014;35:255–64.

82. Sunada K, Hasegawa Y, Kodama T, et al. Thymic and pulmonary mucosa-associated lymphoid tissue lymphomas in a patient with Sjogren's syndrome and literature review. Respirology 2007;12: 144–7.

83. Song MK, Seol YM, Park YE, et al. Pulmonary nodular lymphoid hyperplasia associated with Sjogren's syndrome. Korean J Intern Med 2007; 22:192–6.

84. Rajagopala S, Singh N, Gupta K, et al. Pulmonary amyloidosis in Sjogren's syndrome: a case report and systematic review of the literature. Respirology 2010;15:860–6.

85. Subcutaneous masses and adenopathy in a 77-year-old man with Sjogren's syndrome and amyloidosis. Am J Med 1989;86:585–90.

86. Anderson LG, Talal N. The spectrum of benign to malignant lymphoproliferation in Sjogren's syndrome. Clin Exp Immunol 1972;10:199–221.

87. Bonner H Jr, Ennis RS, Geelhoed GW, et al. Lymphoid infiltration and amyloidosis of lung in Sjogren's syndrome. Arch Pathol 1973;95:42–4.

88. Strimlan CV. Pulmonary involvement in Sjogren's syndrome. Chest 1986;89:901–2.

89. Desai SR, Nicholson AG, Stewart S, et al. Benign pulmonary lymphocytic infiltration and amyloidosis: computed tomographic and pathologic features in three cases. J Thorac Imaging 1997;12:215–20.

90. Jeong YJ, Lee KS, Chung MP, et al. Amyloidosis and lymphoproliferative disease in Sjogren syndrome: thin-section computed tomography findings and histopathologic comparisons. J Comput Assist Tomogr 2004;28:776–81.

91. Fauchais AL, Lambert M, Launay D, et al. Antiphospholipid antibodies in primary Sjogren's syndrome: prevalence and clinical significance in a series of 74 patients. Lupus 2004;13:245–8.

92. Avina-Zubieta JA, Jansz M, Sayre EC, et al. The risk of deep venous thrombosis and pulmonary embolism in primary Sjogren syndrome: a general population-based study. J Rheumatol 2017;44: 1184–9.

93. Naniwa T, Takeda Y. Long-term remission of pulmonary veno-occlusive disease associated with primary Sjogren's syndrome following immunosuppressive therapy. Mod Rheumatol 2011;21: 637–40.

94. Vassiliou VA, Moyssakis I, Boki KA, et al. Is the heart affected in primary Sjogren's syndrome? An echocardiographic study. Clin Exp Rheumatol 2008;26:109–12.

95. Launay D, Hachulla E, Hatron PY, et al. Pulmonary arterial hypertension: a rare complication of primary Sjogren's syndrome: report of 9 new cases and review of the literature. Medicine 2007;86: 299–315.

96. Yan S, Li M, Wang H, et al. Characteristics and risk factors of pulmonary arterial hypertension in patients with primary Sjogren's syndrome. Int J Rheum Dis 2018;21:1068–75.

97. Sato T, Matsubara O, Tanaka Y, et al. Association of Sjogren's syndrome with pulmonary hypertension: report of two cases and review of the literature. Hum Pathol 1993;24:199–205.

98. Bertoni M, Niccoli L, Porciello G, et al. Pulmonary hypertension in primary Sjogren's syndrome: report of a case and review of the literature. Clin Rheumatol 2005;24:431–4.

99. Hedgpeth MT, Boulware DW. Pulmonary hypertension in primary Sjogren's syndrome. Ann Rheum Dis 1988;47:251–3.

100. Teshigawara K, Kakizaki S, Horiya M, et al. Primary Sjogren's syndrome complicated by bilateral pleural effusion. Respirology 2008;13:155–8.

101. Kawamata K, Haraoka H, Hirohata S, et al. Pleurisy in primary Sjogren's syndrome: T cell receptor beta-chain variable region gene bias and local autoantibody production in the pleural effusion. Clin Exp Rheumatol 1997;15:193–6.

102. Langenskiold E, Bonetti A, Fitting JW, et al. Shrinking lung syndrome successfully treated with rituximab and cyclophosphamide. Respiration 2012; 84:144–9.

103. Carmier D, Diot E, Diot P. Shrinking lung syndrome: recognition, pathophysiology and therapeutic strategy. Expert Rev Respir Med 2011;5: 33–9.

104. Reddy KS, Jha V, Nada R, et al. Respiratory paralysis in Sjogren syndrome with normal renal function. Natl Med J India 2003;16:253–4.

105. Ohtani H, Imai H, Kodama T, et al. Severe hypokalaemia and respiratory arrest due to renal tubular acidosis in a patient with Sjogren syndrome. Nephrol Dial Transplant 1999;14:2201–3.

106. Poux JM, Peyronnet P, Le Meur Y, et al. Hypokalemic quadriplegia and respiratory arrest revealing primary Sjogren's syndrome. Clin Nephrol 1992; 37:189–91.

107. Koga T, Kouhisa Y, Nakamura H, et al. A case of primary Sjogren's syndrome complicated with inflammatory myopathy and interstitial lung disease. Rheumatol Int 2012;32:3647–9.

108. Sorajja P, Poirier MK, Bundrick JB, et al. Autonomic failure and proximal skeletal myopathy in a patient with primary Sjogren syndrome. Mayo Clin Proc 1999;74:695–7.

109. Alexander EL. Neurologic disease in Sjogren's syndrome: mononuclear inflammatory vasculopathy affecting central/peripheral nervous system and muscle. A clinical review and update of immunopathogenesis. Rheum Dis Clin North Am 1993;19: 869–908.

110. Gal I, Kovacs J, Zeher M. Case series: coexistence of Sjogren's syndrome and sarcoidosis. J Rheumatol 2000;27:2507–10.

111. Ramos-Casals M, Font J, Garcia-Carrasco M, et al. Primary Sjogren syndrome: hematologic patterns of disease expression. Medicine 2002;81:281–92.

112. Ramos-Casals M, Brito-Zeron P, Garcia-Carrasco M, et al. Sarcoidosis or Sjogren syndrome? Clues to defining mimicry or coexistence in 59 cases. Medicine 2004;83:85–95.

113. Xu Y, Fei Y, Zhong W, et al. The prevalence and clinical characteristics of primary Sjogren's syndrome patients with lung cancer: an analysis of ten cases in China and literature review. Thorac Cancer 2015;6:475–9.

114. Lu J, Ma M, Zhao Q, et al. The clinical characteristics and outcomes of follicular bronchiolitis in Chinese Adult patients. Sci Rep 2018;8:7300.

115. Kim JY, Park SH, Kim SK, et al. Lymphocytic interstitial pneumonia in primary Sjogren's syndrome: a case report. Korean J Intern Med 2011;26:108–11.

Thoracic Manifestations of Rheumatoid Arthritis

Anthony J. Esposito, MD[a], Sarah G. Chu, MD[a], Rachna Madan, MD[b], Tracy J. Doyle, MD[a], Paul F. Dellaripa, MD[c],*

KEYWORDS

- Bronchiectasis • Bronchiolitis • Drug-induced lung toxicity • Rheumatoid arthritis
- Rheumatoid arthritis–associated interstitial lung disease • Rheumatoid nodule

KEY POINTS

- Pulmonary disease is a common extra-articular complication of rheumatoid arthritis and its associated treatment that can affect any anatomic compartment of the thorax.
- The optimal screening, diagnostic, and treatment strategies for rheumatoid arthritis–associated pulmonary disease remain uncertain and are the focus of ongoing investigation.
- Clinicians should regularly assess patients with rheumatoid arthritis for signs and symptoms of pulmonary disease and, reciprocally, consider rheumatoid arthritis and other connective tissue diseases when evaluating a patient with pulmonary disease of unknown etiology.

INTRODUCTION

Rheumatoid arthritis (RA) is a destructive, systemic, inflammatory disorder that characteristically affects small, diarthrodial joints in a progressive, symmetric, and erosive fashion.[1] This rheumatologic disease occurs in approximately 1% of the adult population in developed countries and is associated with decreased quality of life, poor functional status, and increased mortality.[2] It is the 42nd highest etiology of global disability and contributes an estimated $19.3 billion in excess annual US health costs.[3,4] There is evidence that the incidence and prevalence of RA has been increasing over the past 20 years, further increasing the burden of disease.[5]

Although joint disease is the main presentation, RA has a plethora of extra-articular manifestations that contribute to the substantial morbidity and excess mortality observed with this disease.[6]

Although cardiac disease is responsible for most RA-related deaths, pulmonary disease is also a major contributor, accounting for approximately 10% to 20% of all mortality. Pulmonary complications occur in 60% to 80% of patients with RA, many of whom are asymptomatic.[7–10] RA directly affects all anatomic compartments of the thorax, including the lung parenchyma, large and small airways, pleura, and less commonly the vasculature (**Box 1**).[11,12] In addition, pulmonary infection and drug-induced lung disease associated with immunosuppressive agents used for the treatment of RA can occur.

RA-associated lung disease typically occurs within 5 years of RA diagnosis and may even precede joint disease in up to 20% of patients.[13–16] Respiratory symptoms may be masked by the patient's poor functional status from chronic joint and systemic inflammation, which may lead to delays

Disclosure Statement: P.F. Dellaripa participates in clinical trials for Genentech and Bristol-Myers Squibb without income support or fees paid. A.J. Esposito, S.G. Chu, R. Madan, and T.J. Doyle have nothing to disclose.
[a] Division of Pulmonary and Critical Care Medicine, Brigham and Women's Hospital, Harvard Medical School, 75 Francis Street, Boston, MA 02115, USA; [b] Department of Radiology, Brigham and Women's Hospital, Harvard Medical School, 75 Francis Street, Boston, MA 02115, USA; [c] Division of Rheumatology, Immunology and Allergy, Brigham and Women's Hospital, Harvard Medical School, 60 Fenwood Road, Boston, MA 02115, USA
* Corresponding author.
E-mail address: pdellaripa@bwh.harvard.edu

Clin Chest Med 40 (2019) 545–560
https://doi.org/10.1016/j.ccm.2019.05.003

Box 1
Pulmonary manifestations of rheumatoid arthritis

Parenchyma
  Interstitial lung disease
    Usual interstitial pneumonia
    Nonspecific interstitial pneumonia
    Organizing pneumonia
    Diffuse alveolar damage
    Lymphocytic interstitial pneumonitis
    Desquamative interstitial pneumonia
  Necrobiotic nodules
  Caplan syndrome
  Infection
  Drug-induced pneumonitis
Airway
  Cricoarytenoid arthritis
  Bronchiectasis
  Bronchiolitis
    Follicular bronchiolitis
    Bronchiolitis obliterans
    Panbronchiolitis
Pleura
  Pleural effusion
  Pleuritis
  Pneumothorax
  Bronchopleural fistula
Vasculature
  Pulmonary hypertension
  Pulmonary vasculitis
  Venous thromboembolism
  Pulmonary hemorrhage

---

associated lung disease, as patients with RA are approximately 9 times more likely to develop ILD than the general population.[18] Its prevalence, however, has been difficult to estimate due to the extensive heterogeneity among studies that vary by the study population, diagnostic criteria, and imaging method used to establish the diagnosis. The most robust population studies to date estimate the cumulative incidence of clinically significant ILD in the United States to be 5% at 10 years,[19] 6.3% at 15 years,[20] and 6.8% at 30 years of follow-up,[21] with an estimated lifetime risk of 7.7%.[22] Moreover, patients with RA who undergo screening with high-resolution computed tomography (HRCT) regardless of symptoms commonly have pulmonary abnormalities that vary in studies from 19% to 67% depending on the population screened.[8,10,23,24] Despite decreasing mortality rates from RA alone, age-adjusted mortality rates from RA-ILD have been increasing over the past 25 years.[25,26] In one study, patients with RA-ILD had a median survival of 2.6 years after diagnosis, which is a threefold increased risk of death compared with patients with RA without ILD.[22]

HRCT is more sensitive than chest radiograph in the detection of ILD and has led to the identification of subclinical disease in patients with RA.[27] In one study, HRCT abnormalities compatible with ILD were described in 33% of patients with recently diagnosed RA compared with 6% by chest radiograph alone.[28] A significant number of those subjects had mild, subclinical interstitial lung abnormalities (ILAs). Accordingly, ILAs in patients with RA without pulmonary symptoms have been described in up to 44% of subjects.[28–30] Of the patients with ILAs, progression of disease has been described in up to 57% over a 2-year follow-up period.[29,31] These data suggest that although ILD is already known to be a common extra-articular manifestation of RA, it is still underrecognized.

in diagnosis.[17] It is therefore imperative for clinicians to regularly assess patients with RA for signs and symptoms of pulmonary disease and, reciprocally, to consider connective tissue disease, including RA, when evaluating a patient with pulmonary disease of unknown etiology.

INTERSTITIAL LUNG DISEASE
Epidemiology

Interstitial lung disease (ILD) is characterized by fibrosis and inflammation of the pulmonary interstitium. It is the most common manifestation of RA-

Risk Assessment

Risk factors for RA-ILD, which may identify susceptible individuals at risk for poorer outcomes and increased mortality, have been identified that overlap with known risk factors for idiopathic pulmonary fibrosis (IPF). The strongest evidence exists for factors that describe demographics of patients with RA, which include RA disease severity, functional status, and tobacco exposure. Older age and male gender are associated with increased risk of RA-ILD,[32–34] with older age specifically associated with the presence of ILD at the time of RA diagnosis.[22] Although RA is more common in female individuals,[5] RA-ILD is approximately 4 times more common in men,[22,32–34] also similar to the male-predominant disease of IPF.[35] Furthermore, RA disease activity, decreased functional status, and the presence of other non-pulmonary extra-articular disease are risk factors for RA-ILD.[22,36] Smoking is not only a well-established risk factor for RA in general but also for RA-ILD.[24,37,38] The incidence of ILD in an ever-smoker patient with RA has a dose-response relationship, with the highest incidence in those with ≥25 pack-years of cumulative history.[24] Low baseline percentage predicted forced vital capacity (FVC) or diffusion capacity of the lung for carbon monoxide (DLCO) and a significant decline in lung function at follow-up (defined as a >10% decrease in FVC or >15% decrease in DLCO) have all been associated with disease progression and increased mortality.[31–33,39]

Autoantibody profiles as well as genetic variants have also been implicated in the development of RA-ILD. Positive serologies for either rheumatoid factor (RF) or anti-cyclic citrullinated protein (anti-CCP) antibodies are significant predictors for the development of ILD in patients with RA,[33,40,41] with some suggestion that higher anti-CCP titers correlate with extent of disease.[42] Recent evidence has also associated specific genetic mutations implicated in endoplasmic reticulum stress, telomere shortening, and airway microbial defense. In targeted whole exome sequencing of 101 patients with RA-ILD, increased frequency of mutations in several telomere maintenance-associated and surfactant protein genes were identified compared with controls.[43] Furthermore, a gain-of-function promoter variant in the mucin 5B (*MUC5B*) gene was recently associated with RA-ILD and was particularly associated with usual interstitial pneumonia (UIP), the prototypical radiographic and histologic pattern of IPF.[44]

Subtypes of Interstitial Lung Disease

HRCT is the imaging modality of choice for evaluating ILD in patients with RA. RA-ILD has a variety of radiographic and histopathologic subtypes that are well-described and shared with the idiopathic interstitial pneumonias (**Fig. 1**).[45,46] The most frequently encountered are the UIP (see **Fig. 1**A) and nonspecific interstitial pneumonia (NSIP; see **Fig. 1**B) patterns of disease.[47–49] Other less common patterns of disease include organizing pneumonia (see **Fig. 1**C), diffuse alveolar damage, lymphocytic interstitial pneumonia (LIP; see **Fig. 1**D), and desquamative interstitial pneumonia. Most patients with clinically apparent disease have a UIP pattern, which distinguishes RA from

other CTDs in which NSIP is more frequently seen. A UIP pattern on HRCT obviates the need for a surgical lung biopsy to secure the diagnosis, as numerous studies have demonstrated a positive predictive value of 90% to 100% for a pathologic diagnosis of UIP.[50–53] There is increasing evidence that patients with RA with UIP possess a different phenotype, clinical evolution, and prognosis compared with patients with RA with a non-UIP pattern of disease. Notably, UIP pattern is more frequent in older, male patients with RA with a history of smoking and confers a poorer prognosis with survival rates that parallel those seen in IPF.[48–50,54,55] Moreover, patients with RA-ILD with UIP have been reported to have more respiratory-related hospitalizations than other ILD subtypes.[56]

Clinical Presentation

Although ILD is usually diagnosed early in the clinical course of RA,[14] it can develop at any time. It has been described in long-standing RA and has even been shown to precede the onset of articular symptoms.[15,16,57,58] Patients with RA-ILD commonly report nonspecific symptoms of dyspnea (most common), exercise limitation, and/or dry cough, although symptoms can be masked by functional impairment.[16,17,24,59] Less frequent symptoms include chest pain, wheezing, and productive cough.[60] Patients who have abnormal pulmonary function tests (PFTs) are more likely to report symptoms.[60]

As noted previously, up to 44% of patients with RA without pulmonary symptoms may have subclinical ILD or ILA on HRCT.[28–30] These patients are more likely to have lower percent predicted forced expiratory volume in 1 second (FEV1) and FVC than patients without ILA.[34] Some data suggest that ILA progress over time in a subset of patients[28,29,31]; however, the clinical significance of subclinical ILD in RA remains to be determined.

Evaluation and Diagnosis

Development of otherwise unexplained respiratory symptoms in a patient with RA or the presence of articular symptoms in a patient undergoing evaluation for ILD should raise suspicion for RA-ILD, especially if risk factors are present. In patients with known RA, other types of RA lung disease should be considered as well as drug toxicity and opportunistic infections.

Initial evaluation of patients with suspected RA-ILD should include a complete history and physical examination, imaging with HRCT, and PFTs. Patients may report nonspecific respiratory symptoms such as dyspnea, cough, wheeze, or

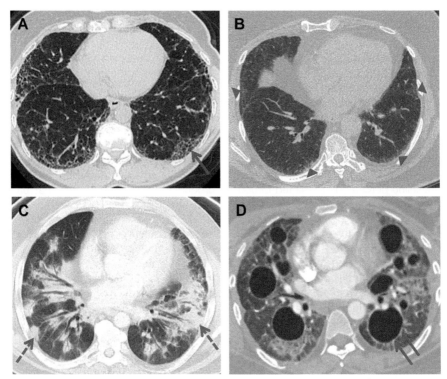

Fig. 1. RA-associated ILD subtypes. (*A*) UIP with characteristic basilar-predominant honeycombing (*solid arrow*) and subpleural reticulation with traction bronchiectasis. (*B*) Nonspecific interstitial pneumonia discernible by relatively symmetric subpleural ground-glass opacities with immediate subpleural sparing (*arrowheads*). (*C*) Cryptogenic organizing pneumonia with bilateral mid to lower lung predominate consolidative opacities in a peripheral and peribronchovascular distribution (*dashed arrows*). (*D*) LIP marked by scattered thin-walled cysts (*double arrow*) and ground-glass opacification.

pleuritic chest pain on history,[16,24,56,59,60] and physical examination may reveal rales, clubbing, wheezing, or signs of right heart failure.[23,29] HRCT is essential to characterize the radiologic pattern and to assess disease severity. The most common findings are ground-glass opacities, honeycombing, and reticulation in the aforementioned disease patterns.[47,61] PFTs assess the physiologic severity of RA-ILD and are useful to monitor disease activity. Up to 30% of patients with RA have abnormal PFTs commonly in the form of restrictive ventilatory deficits and/or a reduced DLCO.[24,34,60]

Other diagnostic studies are rarely indicated for evaluation of RA-ILD. Bronchoscopy with bronchoalveolar lavage adds little value other than to exclude infection when clinically suspected.[62] Surgical lung biopsy is also rarely indicated, as identification of the histopathologic pattern is not currently part of the algorithm to diagnose and treat RA-ILD.[17] Nonetheless, biopsy may be indicated when the etiology of lung disease is unclear. Currently no biomarkers have been identified that are either sensitive or specific for RA-ILD disease

activity or progression; however, emerging biomarkers are being investigated beyond the known demographic and serologic variables and include MMP7, SP-D, and PARC. These may enhance our ability to predict the presence and potential progression of RA-ILD.[40]

Treatment and Disease Monitoring

Treatment of RA has changed dramatically over the past few decades, catalyzed by the introduction of new classification criteria that identify patients with early disease and the expansion of therapeutic options for disease management. Although numerous medications have been described as potential therapies for RA-ILD, there are no large randomized controlled trials (RCTs) to help guide management. Many of the recommendations for treating RA-ILD have been extrapolated from studies of other CTD-associated ILDs, such as scleroderma-ILD.

In general, treatment of RA-ILD consists of supportive measures and anti-inflammatory therapies that target the inflammatory processes putatively responsible for the disease. Supportive treatment is recommended for patients with mild disease or contraindications to pharmacologic therapy. This strategy consists of nonpharmacologic measures that should be implemented in the care of every patient with RA-ILD and include smoking cessation, oxygen supplementation when indicated, age-appropriate vaccinations for pneumonia and influenza, education, exercise rehabilitation, and prophylaxis for *Pneumocystic jirovecii* pneumonia in the profoundly immunosuppressed.[63] In patients with moderate or severe disease, cautious use of immunosuppressive therapy may be considered, although prospective trials are lacking. Features predictive of treatment response include histopathologic patterns other than UIP, younger age, and worsening of symptoms, PFTs, or HRCT findings over the preceding 3 to 6 months.[63–65]

Glucocorticoids are often used as first-line therapy to stabilize and improve the disease course of RA-ILD when the radiographic or histologic pattern suggests a more inflammatory process such as NSIP, LIP, or organizing pneumonia.[63] Treatment of UIP with immunosuppression may be harmful, as it can increase patients' susceptibility to serious infections in a dose-dependent manner.[66,67] This was exemplified by the PANTHER trial in which treatment of IPF with a combination of prednisone, n-acetylcysteine, and azathioprine was associated with increased mortality, hospitalizations, and serious adverse events compared with placebo.[68] The results of this trial raised the concern about use of these agents in patients with RA with UIP though it admittedly did not specifically address UIP in CTD.

Mycophenolate mofetil (MMF) has been used in the management of scleroderma-ILD and other CTDs, with most of the evidence derived from one large prospective trial, small prospective case series, and retrospective reviews.[69–71] In a study of MMF in CTD-ILD that included 18 patients with RA-ILD, MMF was associated with modest improvements in FVC and DLCO and with reduced prednisone dosing[71]; however, it is worth noting that MMF is ineffective for treatment of active articular disease, requiring concomitant use of other immunosuppressive agents that may limit its tolerability. Cyclophosphamide has been commonly used as a second-line agent to treat ILD unresponsive to steroids, although no RCTs have been performed for its use in RA-ILD. Its use in scleroderma-ILD has moderate benefit for those with early disease, although a prior meta-analysis concluded that there was no improvement in pulmonary function following 12 months of treatment.[72,73] Therefore, its use is not recommended for mild/moderate or stable RA-ILD.

Cyclosporine and other calcineurin inhibitors have limited experience for treatment of RA-ILD and are currently not recommended due to their poor safety profile and lack of proven benefit for joint disease.[74,75]

There are limited data to support the use of biologic agents in the treatment of RA-ILD despite small case series/reports and one prospective trial using rituximab in RA-ILD.[76–78] The role of rituximab in UIP-related disease is unknown, although it may play a role in more inflammatory processes such as NSIP or LIP. There is early clinical evidence suggesting that abatacept, an inhibitor of T-cell costimulation, may be an effective treatment for RA-ILD.[79–81] In a large retrospective study, abatacept was associated with stabilization or improvement in symptoms, PFTs, or HRCT findings in up to 12 months of follow-up.[81] Although these studies are promising, current evidence does not support routine switching therapy to a biologic in all patients with RA-ILD regardless of disease severity or active joint disease.

In end-stage RA-ILD, lung transplantation may be considered, although there are limited data on long-term outcomes. Survival at 1 year seems to be similar to IPF lung transplant recipients (67% and 69%, respectively).[82]

Evidence to guide screening strategies, management, and monitoring of treatment of RA-ILD is of low quality or absent. Many practice patterns have been extrapolated from scleroderma-ILD or IPF.[83] Here, we provide a suggested algorithm for identification of ILD in at-risk patients with RA (**Fig. 2**). In patients with RA with symptoms of dyspnea or cough not explained by other causes like infection or heart disease, assessment for underlying RA-ILD with HRCT and pulmonary function testing including ambulatory oximetry is reasonable. Recommendation for baseline screening of all patients with RA for ILD is the subject of ongoing prospective evaluation. For patients with RA with known risk factors for ILD, risk assessment with PFTs may be a sensible and low risk approach. Patients with a history of smoking may be appropriate candidates for low-dose computed tomography (CT) scanning, where surveillance for lung cancer could be coupled with an assessment for ILA or ILD (see **Fig. 2**). Patients at highest risk for progression (those with >10% decrease in FVC or >15% in DLCO) are those that should be considered for therapy and be monitored with serial PFTs every 3 to 6 months.[83]

AIRWAY DISEASE

RA can affect both the upper and lower airways in multiple forms with or without airflow obstruction,

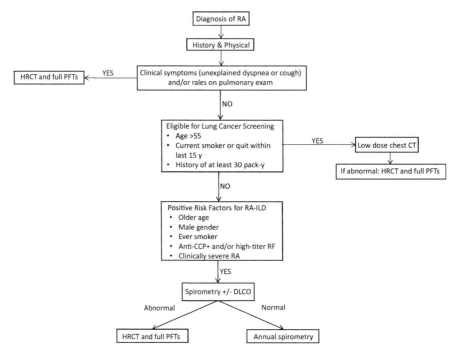

Fig. 2. Suggested algorithm to identify ILD in patients with RA.

including cricoarytenoid arthritis, mucosal edema, myositis, vasculitis, and airway/vocal cord rheumatoid nodules or bamboo nodes.[84–86] Laryngeal involvement is likely underestimated but may involve over 30% of patients with RA[87] and may be the sole manifestation of this disease.[88] In a series of 32 patients with RA, cricoarytenoid joint (CJ) involvement was detected in up to 70% of subjects by direct laryngoscopy and HRCT.[89] CJ arthritis results from accumulation of synovial fluid in the CJ capsule, leading to erosion and subluxation of the cartilage that may ultimately result in fixation.[86] Although laryngeal disease is often clinically silent, patients can present with a globus sensation, hoarseness, dysphagia, odynophonia, dysphonia, which may mistakenly be attributed to laryngopharyngeal reflux or environmental allergies,[86] or with dyspnea and stridor from airway obstruction. Local or systemic corticosteroids as well as nonsteroidal anti-inflammatory drugs have been used for milder cases, although surgical excision of laryngeal nodules or laryngoplasty for fixation may be necessary. Several case reports of acute airway obstruction requiring emergent tracheostomy have also been described.[90,91]

In the lower airways, RA has been associated with airway hyperresponsiveness, small airway disease, and bronchiectasis. The attributable risk of RA has been difficult to define due to confounding factors, particularly smoking. In a series of 50 patients with RA and no ILD, 18% were found to have airway obstruction, 8% had small airway disease (defined by a decreased forced expiratory flow at 25-75% of the pulmonary volume), and 32% had air trapping on PFTs and HRCT.[92] Increased prevalence was noted in women and smokers. Although airflow obstruction is typically diagnosed via PFTs, HRCT abnormalities, particularly with inspiratory/expiratory images (**Fig. 3**), may precede physiologic findings.[92]

The reported prevalence of bronchiolar disease varies widely and includes constrictive bronchiolitis obliterans, follicular bronchiolitis, and, infrequently, diffuse panbronchiolitis. Pathologically, RA-associated bronchiolitis is indistinguishable from other causes. Among 25 nonsmokers with severe fixed airflow obstruction, bronchial wall thickening was the most common radiographic finding, followed by centrilobular emphysema, ground-glass opacification, mosaic attenuation (see **Fig. 3**B), and bronchiectasis. Among the 8 available biopsies in this study, there were 6 cases of constrictive bronchiolitis and 1 case of follicular bronchiolitis. Outcomes were overall poor, with approximately half experiencing progression of their symptoms and acute respiratory failure despite most patients receiving oral corticosteroids.[93] Other immunomodulatory agents, including cyclophosphamide, azathioprine, methotrexate, and tumor necrosis factor (TNF)-alpha inhibitors, have also been used with varying degrees of success.[93–95] Despite unclear efficacy, many

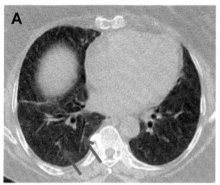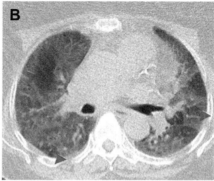

Fig. 3. RA-associated small airway disease. Inspiratory (*A*) and expiratory (*B*) HRCT images of a patient with bronchiolitis. Solid arrows: bronchiectasis. Arrowheads: mosaic attenuation characteristic of air trapping and small airway disease is accentuated on expiratory images.

clinicians will often trial standard treatments for obstructive lung disease such as inhaled and systemic steroids. Macrolide therapy with azithromycin, which has been shown to attenuate lung function decline in post–lung transplant bronchiolitis obliterans,[96] or erythromycin, which may improve symptoms in RA-associated bronchiolitis,[97] is a reasonable option.

Follicular bronchiolitis, characterized by hyperplasia of bronchial associated lymphoid tissue, has been associated with CTDs including RA, Sjögren's syndrome, and systemic lupus erythematosus, as well as immunodeficiency disorders.[98] HRCT may demonstrate centrilobular and peribronchial nodularity in addition to features of small airway disease.[99] It is pathologically related to other lymphoproliferative conditions such as LIP, and immunohistochemistry may be considered to rule out malignancy. Management may involve corticosteroids and in some cases rituximab when there is evidence of exuberant lymphoid aggregates in the airways.[97,98] Outcomes for follicular bronchiolitis are generally more favorable than for constrictive bronchiolitis.

The prevalence of bronchiectasis in RA is higher than the general population, occurring in up to 30% of patients with RA with no ILD[92]; in a series of individuals with RA-associated airflow obstruction, 40% had bronchiectasis.[93] Although often asymptomatic, patients with bronchiectasis and RA have been found to have increased bronchiectasis severity index scores and mortality compared with those with idiopathic bronchiectasis.[100,101] Interestingly, among a group of patients with RA with diffuse bronchiectasis, 15.4% were found to be heterozygous for the CFTR gene delta F508 mutation.[102] In patients with symptomatic disease, management usually consists of standard treatment of bronchiectasis, including bronchodilators, mucus clearance, and

antibiotics. The presence of bronchiectasis may complicate the use of anti-inflammatory therapies for RA, which augment the risk of respiratory infections.

PLEURAL DISEASE

Inflammation of the pleurae, manifesting as pleural thickening and/or effusions (**Fig. 4**A), is a common extra-articular manifestation of RA. In postmortem studies, pleural involvement is described in more than 70% of patients, but less than 3% to 5% of patients are symptomatic.[103–107] In earlier studies, pleural thickening and/or effusion was reported on chest radiograph in 24% of men and 16% of women.[108] Most effusions are unilateral, are more commonly found in male patients older than 35 with rheumatoid nodules, and have been associated with HLA-B8.[103,109] If the patient is symptomatic, the most common presenting complaints are fever and pleuritic chest pain. Cough is uncommon unless parenchymal disease is present.

A "rheumatoid effusion" is classically described as a sterile exudative effusion with a low pH (<7.3), low glucose (<60 mg/dL), and elevated lactate dehydrogenase (as high as >700 IU/L).[103,104] In instances of chronic pleural inflammation, the fluid can appear "pseudochylous" due to the presence of cholesterol crystals in the fluid, which importantly differs from a true chylothorax by the absence of triglycerides and/or chylomicrons.[103] RF is often positive. White cell count and differential is variable but is more commonly lymphocytic predominant; however, neutrophil-predominant and eosinophil-predominant cell counts are also described.[110]

Thoracentesis should be performed for any pleural effusion greater than 1 cm on decubitus imaging. Infection must always be ruled out, as

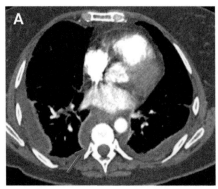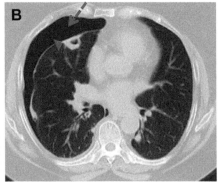

Fig. 4. RA-associated pleural disease. (*A*) Bilateral pleural thickening and hyperenhancement (*solid arrows*) with associated loculated pleural effusions, indicating pleuritis. (*B*) Necrobiotic cavitary nodule (*arrowhead*) resulting in a spontaneous pneumothorax (*dashed arrow*).

low pH, low glucose, and elevated lactate dehydrogenase are also typical of empyema. Tuberculous and malignant effusions can also mimic rheumatoid effusions. Pleural biopsy is rarely indicated but should be performed when the diagnosis is unclear.

Most effusions resolve with management of the underlying RA. If small and asymptomatic, no therapy is indicated; however, long-standing pleural inflammation can result in trapped lung physiology.[103,111]

RHEUMATOID LUNG NODULES

Rheumatoid nodules develop primarily in the subcutaneous tissue over articular joints but can occur in the upper airways, lungs (see **Fig. 4**B), heart, and, rarely, in the sclerae.[84,112–114] Pathologically, they consist of necrobiotic lesions of giant cells within palisaded foci, which produce proinflammatory cytokines similar to those of synovial membrane.[115,116] The presence of nodules is associated with increased severity of RA and an elevated risk of vasculitis, hospitalization, and mortality.[117–119] In a series of 40 patients with RA and open lung biopsy, 32% were found to have rheumatoid nodules,[113] although prevalence varies widely across studies.[120] In the lungs, they often occur in the subpleural regions and fissures,[121] ranging in size from a few millimeters to larger than 7 cm.[122] Infection, particularly with fungal and mycobacterial organisms, and malignancy should be considered in the differential. Although most pulmonary RA nodules are asymptomatic and do not require treatment, larger nodules may cavitate and cause hemoptysis, pleural effusions, spontaneous pneumothoraces (see **Fig. 4**B), or bronchopleural fistulae.[121] B-cell therapies such as rituximab may decrease the size and number of pulmonary rheumatoid

nodules.[123] Disease-modifying antirheumatic drugs (DMARDs), including methotrexate and anti-TNF-alpha inhibitors, have been associated with increased pulmonary nodulosis, although it is unclear that these therapies should be stopped for this reason.[124,125]

The occurrence of multiple, predominantly peripheral pulmonary nodules in a large cohort of coal miners with RA was first described in 1953 and came to be known as Caplan syndrome; as this was later broadened to include exposure to other inorganic dusts, silica in particular, the term rheumatoid pneumoconiosis is also used. Lung nodules may be detected in exposed subjects more than 10 years before the development of arthritis.[126] Radiographically, nodules tend to form rapidly and persist over years, with approximately 10% developing cavitations or calcifications.[127] A causal link between RA and dust exposure has not been established, but it has been hypothesized that the exposure to foreign particles leads to chronic immune activity that might facilitate the formation of autoantibodies. Indeed, pneumoconiosis has been associated with increased immune complexes and RF positivity even without an apparent autoimmune diagnosis.[127,128]

PULMONARY VASCULAR DISEASE

Pulmonary vascular disease is associated with RA but is regarded as a rare manifestation. Pulmonary hypertension in patients with RA can occur as primary pulmonary arterial hypertension, thought to be due to an underlying vasculitis due to concomitant signs of systemic vasculitis that are often present, or secondary to severe parenchymal lung disease. Estimates of the prevalence of asymptomatic, isolated pulmonary hypertension by cross-sectional echocardiography (defined as a pulmonary artery systolic pressure ≥30 mm Hg on echocardiography) in patients with RA are between 21% and 28%, which is significantly higher than age-matched controls (4.5%).[129–132] This finding is especially applicable to older patients, those with longer disease duration, and those with joint deformities.[130,131] However, these echocardiographic studies are limited by the absence of right heart catheterization to confirm imaging observations and by liberal definitions of abnormal right-sided pressures, increasing the false-positive rate and therefore the reported prevalence. Patients with RA are also at slightly increased risk for venous thromboembolism, even when controlling for other risk factors, such as age, sex, comorbid diseases, and recent hospitalization.[133,134] In a Taiwanese study, the risks of deep venous thrombosis and pulmonary embolism were increased approximately 3.5-fold and 2-fold, respectively, in patients with RA compared with healthy age-matched controls.[133]

DRUG-INDUCED LUNG TOXICITY

Drug-induced lung disease should be considered when a patient with RA presents with new respiratory complaints, new findings on HRCT, or unexpected worsening of ILD. Almost all DMARDs and biologic therapies have been associated with lung toxicity in addition to an increased risk of infection.[135] The incidence of drug-induced lung disease in RA is not well characterized, although one systematic review reported a relatively low overall risk of approximately 1% but with high mortality.[136] It is often a diagnosis of exclusion. Empiric drug discontinuation is an important diagnostic step, as noninfectious drug-related toxicity tends to regress on withdrawal of the offending agent and, if disease is significant, treatment with steroids. Other diagnostics include laboratory testing (eg, complete blood count with differential, b-type natriuretic peptide, C-reactive protein, cultures, and serologic studies), imaging, PFTs, and bronchoscopy. Lung biopsy rarely establishes the diagnosis, as there are no pathognomonic findings for drug-induced lung toxicity.[137] The differential includes rheumatoid-associated lung disease, infection, and heart failure, which may be hard to differentiate due to significant overlap of these clinical syndromes.

Methotrexate

Methotrexate (MTX) is the most commonly prescribed DMARD for management of RA. Interstitial pneumonitis is the most common noninfectious pulmonary complication although it is regarded as a rare adverse event in patients with RA. Its incidence, however, is difficult to determine due to diagnostic uncertainty and lack of a gold standard. Estimates vary between 0.43% and 1% of treated patients in up to 3 years of follow-up; however, mortality rates of up to 17% have been reported.[138–140] MTX pneumonitis is thought to represent a unique hypersensitivity reaction. Onset typically occurs early in the course of MTX therapy (often within the first year),[141] resolves after discontinuation of the drug and administration of corticosteroids,[142] and has been reported in other conditions treated with MTX, such as psoriatic arthritis.[143] It is unclear if preexisting RA-ILD increases the risk of MTX pneumonitis, as some studies have found up to 7.5 times increased risk,[144,145] whereas others suggest no association.[146,147] There is currently no conclusive evidence that pulmonary disease progresses in patients with RA-ILD on MTX who do not develop pneumonitis.[140,148] Less commonly, rheumatoid lung nodulosis, asthma, or air trapping can occur with MTX treatment, but it is unclear if these manifestations are drug-related or are due to underlying RA.[140] Given data that show a clear mortality benefit with use of MTX for RA in general,[149] the decision to withhold or withdraw MTX in patients with RA with underlying lung disease can be difficult. Nonetheless, it may be justified to continue MTX in some cases in the face of stable joint disease and suppression of systemic inflammation.

Biologic Agents/Synthetic Disease-modifying Antirheumatic Drugs

TNF-alpha inhibitors, anakinra, rituximab, abatacept, and now Janus kinase inhibitors improve symptoms, joint disease, and possibly pulmonary disease in patients with RA[150]; however, rare cases of pulmonary toxicity, including provocation or exacerbation of ILD, have been described.[83,151] A systematic review estimated the overall risk of drug-induced ILD with biologic agents to be 1% in patients with RA.[136] Data regarding morbidity and mortality associated with ILD due to anti-TNF-alpha therapy is conflicted and is most often associated with infliximab.[136,152,153] However, a study of post marketing surveillance of TNF-alpha inhibitors failed to identify any significant difference in the risk of ILD or its related complications compared with other biologics.[80] Drug-induced ILD has been reported with TNF-alpha inhibitors and anakinra, though not abatacept, and is more common in patients with preexisting ILD or who are aged 65 or older.[154,155] Only a few cases of ILD have been described for rituximab therapy in patients with RA.[78,156] Several of these agents have also been associated with granulomatous lung disease and an increased risk of serious infections, particularly with TNF-alpha inhibitors.[125,157] Although the frequency is thought to be low, development of new or worsening cough, dyspnea, or radiographic abnormalities in patients with RA on biologic therapies should alert the physician to the possibility of drug-induced ILD.

Sulfasalazine

Sulfasalazine has been associated with pneumonitis, with nearly half of affected patients presenting with pulmonary infiltrates and eosinophilia.[136,158] Clinical improvement usually occurs with cessation of the drug although respiratory failure and death have been described. Other disorders associated with sulfasalazine include NSIP, organizing pneumonia, granulomatous disease, bronchiolitis obliterans, and pleural effusion.[158–160]

EMERGING DIAGNOSTIC APPROACHES AND TREATMENT MODALITIES

Our understanding of pulmonary complications in RA, especially RA-ILD, is still hampered by limited data regarding the natural history of disease and by imperfect diagnostic tools that are not sufficiently precise to identify which patients are at the greatest risk for progressive disease. There is promise, however, that emerging biomarkers, genomics, and computer-generated quantified CT assessments, among other newer technologies, may offer better tools to identify high-risk patients and thus candidates for treatment and clinical trials.[161,162]

At this time, there are no formalized recommendations regarding screening for lung disease in RA. In light of potential therapeutic options that may become available, early assessment for ILD either with baseline physiologic testing or by CT in the context of lung cancer screening for high-risk patients may be reasonable to identify ILD or early airway changes that are associated with RA (see **Fig. 2**).[13]

Therapeutically, efforts to attenuate the development of fibrosis via the many identified pathways leading to fibrosis are being used in clinical trials of IPF and may offer promise for RA-associated disease, though it is unclear whether these approaches may be equally applicable to RA-ILD. As of this publication, there are 2 trials in progress using antifibrotic therapy approved by the Food and Drug Administration in RA and other CTD-ILD. Newer insights into the mechanisms of RA, including the role of specific cytokines like interleukin-17, may demonstrate

that the mechanisms important in the development of articular disease also play a role in lung disease and fibrosis.[163] In summary, our understanding of lung disease in RA and its treatment is at an inflection point of discovery and potential therapy, making lung health a priority in the care of patients with RA.

REFERENCES

1. Firestein GS. Evolving concepts of rheumatoid arthritis. Nature 2003;423(6937):356–61.
2. Gabriel SE, Crowson CS, O'Fallon WM. The epidemiology of rheumatoid arthritis in Rochester, Minnesota, 1955-1985. Arthritis Rheum 1999;42(3): 415–20.
3. Birnbaum H, Pike C, Kaufman R, et al. Societal cost of rheumatoid arthritis patients in the US. Curr Med Res Opin 2010;26(1):77–90.
4. Cross M, Smith E, Hoy D, et al. The global burden of rheumatoid arthritis: estimates from the global burden of disease 2010 study. Ann Rheum Dis 2014;73(7):1316–22.
5. Myasoedova E, Crowson CS, Kremers HM, et al. Is the incidence of rheumatoid arthritis rising? Results from Olmsted County, Minnesota, 1955-2007. Arthritis Rheum 2010;62(6):1576–82.
6. Turesson C, O'Fallon WM, Crowson CS, et al. Extra-articular disease manifestations in rheumatoid arthritis: incidence trends and risk factors over 46 years. Ann Rheum Dis 2003;62(8):722–7.
7. Cortet B, Perez T, Roux N, et al. Pulmonary function tests and high resolution computed tomography of the lungs in patients with rheumatoid arthritis. Ann Rheum Dis 1997;56(10):596–600.
8. Bilgici A, Ulusoy H, Kuru O, et al. Pulmonary involvement in rheumatoid arthritis. Rheumatol Int 2005;25(6):429–35.
9. Demir R, Bodur H, Tokoglu F, et al. High resolution computed tomography of the lungs in patients with rheumatoid arthritis. Rheumatol Int 1999;19(1–2): 19–22.
10. Kanat F, Levendoglu F, Teke T. Radiological and functional assessment of pulmonary involvement in the rheumatoid arthritis patients. Rheumatol Int 2007;27(5):459–66.
11. Brown KK. Rheumatoid lung disease. Proc Am Thorac Soc 2007;4(5):443–8.
12. Yunt ZX, Solomon JJ. Lung disease in rheumatoid arthritis. Rheum Dis Clin North Am 2015;41(2): 225–36.
13. Demoruelle MK, Weisman MH, Simonian PL, et al. Brief report: airways abnormalities and rheumatoid arthritis-related autoantibodies in subjects without arthritis: early injury or initiating site of autoimmunity? Arthritis Rheum 2012;64(6):1756–61.

14. Wilsher M, Voight L, Milne D, et al. Prevalence of airway and parenchymal abnormalities in newly diagnosed rheumatoid arthritis. Respir Med 2012; 106(10):1441–6.

15. Fischer A, Solomon JJ, du Bois RM, et al. Lung disease with anti-CCP antibodies but not rheumatoid arthritis or connective tissue disease. Respir Med 2012;106(7):1040–7.

16. Gizinski AM, Mascolo M, Loucks JL, et al. Rheumatoid arthritis (RA)-specific autoantibodies in patients with interstitial lung disease and absence of clinically apparent articular RA. Clin Rheumatol 2009;28(5):611–3.

17. Hamblin MJ, Horton MR. Rheumatoid arthritis-associated interstitial lung disease: diagnostic dilemma. Pulm Med 2011;2011:872120.

18. Saag KG, Teng GG, Patkar NM, et al. American College of Rheumatology 2008 recommendations for the use of nonbiologic and biologic disease-modifying antirheumatic drugs in rheumatoid arthritis. Arthritis Rheum 2008;59(6):762–84.

19. Myasoedova E, Crowson CS, Turesson C, et al. Incidence of extraarticular rheumatoid arthritis in Olmsted County, Minnesota, in 1995-2007 versus 1985-1994: a population-based study. J Rheumatol 2011;38(6):983–9.

20. Koduri G, Norton S, Young A, et al. Interstitial lung disease has a poor prognosis in rheumatoid arthritis: results from an inception cohort. Rheumatology (Oxford) 2010;49(8):1483–9.

21. Turesson C, O'Fallon WM, Crowson CS, et al. Occurrence of extraarticular disease manifestations is associated with excess mortality in a community based cohort of patients with rheumatoid arthritis. J Rheumatol 2002;29(1):62–7.

22. Bongartz T, Nannini C, Medina-Velasquez YF, et al. Incidence and mortality of interstitial lung disease in rheumatoid arthritis: a population-based study. Arthritis Rheum 2010;62(6):1583–91.

23. Dawson JK, Fewins HE, Desmond J, et al. Fibrosing alveolitis in patients with rheumatoid arthritis as assessed by high resolution computed tomography, chest radiography, and pulmonary function tests. Thorax 2001;56(8):622–7.

24. Saag KG, Kolluri S, Koehnke RK, et al. Rheumatoid arthritis lung disease. Determinants of radiographic and physiologic abnormalities. Arthritis Rheum 1996;39(10):1711–9.

25. Olson AL, Swigris JJ, Sprunger DB, et al. Rheumatoid arthritis-interstitial lung disease-associated mortality. Am J Respir Crit Care Med 2011;183(3): 372–8.

26. Raimundo K, Solomon JJ, Olson AL, et al. Rheumatoid arthritis-interstitial lung disease in the United States: prevalence, incidence, and healthcare costs and mortality. J Rheumatol 2019;46(2):218.

27. Padley SP, Hansell DM, Flower CD, et al. Comparative accuracy of high resolution computed tomography and chest radiography in the diagnosis of chronic diffuse infiltrative lung disease. Clin Radiol 1991;44(4):222–6.

28. Gabbay E, Tarala R, Will R, et al. Interstitial lung disease in recent onset rheumatoid arthritis. Am J Respir Crit Care Med 1997;156(2 Pt 1):528–35.

29. Gochuico BR, Avila NA, Chow CK, et al. Progressive preclinical interstitial lung disease in rheumatoid arthritis. Arch Intern Med 2008;168(2):159–66.

30. Chen J, Shi Y, Wang X, et al. Asymptomatic preclinical rheumatoid arthritis-associated interstitial lung disease. Clin Dev Immunol 2013;2013:406927.

31. Dawson JK, Fewins HE, Desmond J, et al. Predictors of progression of HRCT diagnosed fibrosing alveolitis in patients with rheumatoid arthritis. Ann Rheum Dis 2002;61(6):517–21.

32. Assayag D, Elicker BM, Urbania TH, et al. Rheumatoid arthritis-associated interstitial lung disease: radiologic identification of usual interstitial pneumonia pattern. Radiology 2014;270(2):583–8.

33. Kelly CA, Saravanan V, Nisar M, et al. Rheumatoid arthritis-related interstitial lung disease: associations, prognostic factors and physiological and radiological characteristics–a large multicentre UK study. Rheumatology (Oxford) 2014;53(9): 1676–82.

34. Doyle TJ, Dellaripa PF, Batra K, et al. Functional impact of a spectrum of interstitial lung abnormalities in rheumatoid arthritis. Chest 2014;146(1): 41–50.

35. Esposito DB, Lanes S, Donneyong M, et al. Idiopathic pulmonary fibrosis in United States automated claims. Incidence, prevalence, and algorithm validation. Am J Respir Crit Care Med 2015;192(10):1200–7.

36. Turesson C. Extra-articular rheumatoid arthritis. Curr Opin Rheumatol 2013;25(3):360–6.

37. Bergstrom U, Jacobsson LT, Nilsson JA, et al. Pulmonary dysfunction, smoking, socioeconomic status and the risk of developing rheumatoid arthritis. Rheumatology (Oxford) 2011;50(11): 2005–13.

38. Hassan WU, Keaney NP, Holland CD, et al. High resolution computed tomography of the lung in lifelong non-smoking patients with rheumatoid arthritis. Ann Rheum Dis 1995;54(4):308–10.

39. Solomon JJ, Chung JH, Cosgrove GP, et al. Predictors of mortality in rheumatoid arthritis-associated interstitial lung disease. Eur Respir J 2016;47(2): 588–96.

40. Doyle TJ, Patel AS, Hatabu H, et al. Detection of rheumatoid arthritis-interstitial lung disease is enhanced by serum biomarkers. Am J Respir Crit Care Med 2015;191(12):1403–12.

41. Mori S, Koga Y, Sugimoto M. Different risk factors between interstitial lung disease and airway disease in rheumatoid arthritis. Respir Med 2012; 106(11):1591–9.

42. Giles JT, Danoff SK, Sokolove J, et al. Association of fine specificity and repertoire expansion of anticitrullinated peptide antibodies with rheumatoid arthritis associated interstitial lung disease. Ann Rheum Dis 2014;73(8):1487–94.

43. Juge PA, Borie R, Kannengiesser C, et al. Shared genetic predisposition in rheumatoid arthritis-interstitial lung disease and familial pulmonary fibrosis. Eur Respir J 2017;49(5) [pii:1602314].

44. Seibold MA, Wise AL, Speer MC, et al. A common MUC5B promoter polymorphism and pulmonary fibrosis. N Engl J Med 2011;364(16): 1503–12.

45. American Thoracic Society, European Respiratory Society. American Thoracic Society/European Respiratory Society International Multidisciplinary consensus classification of the idiopathic interstitial pneumonias. This joint statement of the American Thoracic Society (ATS), and the European Respiratory Society (ERS) was adopted by the ATS board of directors, June 2001 and by the ERS Executive Committee, June 2001. Am J Respir Crit Care Med 2002;165(2):277–304.

46. Raghu G, Collard HR, Egan JJ, et al. An official ATS/ERS/JRS/ALAT statement: idiopathic pulmonary fibrosis: evidence-based guidelines for diagnosis and management. Am J Respir Crit Care Med 2011;183(6):788–824.

47. Tanaka N, Kim JS, Newell JD, et al. Rheumatoid arthritis-related lung diseases: CT findings. Radiology 2004;232(1):81–91.

48. Lee HK, Kim DS, Yoo B, et al. Histopathologic pattern and clinical features of rheumatoid arthritis-associated interstitial lung disease. Chest 2005;127(6):2019–27.

49. Solomon JJ, Ryu JH, Tazelaar HD, et al. Fibrosing interstitial pneumonia predicts survival in patients with rheumatoid arthritis-associated interstitial lung disease (RA-ILD). Respir Med 2013;107(8): 1247–52.

50. Swensen SJ, Aughenbaugh GL, Myers JL. Diffuse lung disease: diagnostic accuracy of CT in patients undergoing surgical biopsy of the lung. Radiology 1997;205(1):229–34.

51. Raghu G, Mageto YN, Lockhart D, et al. The accuracy of the clinical diagnosis of new-onset idiopathic pulmonary fibrosis and other interstitial lung disease: a prospective study. Chest 1999; 116(5):1168–74.

52. Hunninghake GW, Zimmerman MB, Schwartz DA, et al. Utility of a lung biopsy for the diagnosis of idiopathic pulmonary fibrosis. Am J Respir Crit Care Med 2001;164(2):193–6.

53. Mathieson JR, Mayo JR, Staples CA, et al. Chronic diffuse infiltrative lung disease: comparison of diagnostic accuracy of CT and chest radiography. Radiology 1989;171(1):111–6.

54. Assayag D, Lee JS, King TE Jr. Rheumatoid arthritis associated interstitial lung disease: a review. Medicina (B Aires) 2014;74(2):158–65.

55. Kim EJ, Elicker BM, Maldonado F, et al. Usual interstitial pneumonia in rheumatoid arthritis-associated interstitial lung disease. Eur Respir J 2010;35(6):1322–8.

56. Nurmi HM, Purokivi MK, Karkkainen MS, et al. Variable course of disease of rheumatoid arthritis-associated usual interstitial pneumonia compared to other subtypes. BMC Pulm Med 2016;16(1):107.

57. Mori S, Cho I, Koga Y, et al. A simultaneous onset of organizing pneumonia and rheumatoid arthritis, along with a review of the literature. Mod Rheumatol 2008;18(1):60–6.

58. Brannan HM, Good CA, Divertie MB, et al. Pulmonary disease associated with rheumatoid arthritis. JAMA 1964;189:914–8.

59. Mohd Noor N, Mohd Shahrir MS, Shahid MS, et al. Clinical and high resolution computed tomography characteristics of patients with rheumatoid arthritis lung disease. Int J Rheum Dis 2009;12(2):136–44.

60. Pappas DA, Giles JT, Connors G, et al. Respiratory symptoms and disease characteristics as predictors of pulmonary function abnormalities in patients with rheumatoid arthritis: an observational cohort study. Arthritis Res Ther 2010;12(3):R104.

61. Skare TL, Nakano I, Escuissiato DL, et al. Pulmonary changes on high-resolution computed tomography of patients with rheumatoid arthritis and their association with clinical, demographic, serological and therapeutic variables. Rev Bras Reumatol 2011;51(4):325–30, 336-327.

62. Biederer J, Schnabel A, Muhle C, et al. Correlation between HRCT findings, pulmonary function tests and bronchoalveolar lavage cytology in interstitial lung disease associated with rheumatoid arthritis. Eur Radiol 2004;14(2):272–80.

63. Krause ML, Zamora AC, Vassallo R, et al. The lung disease of rheumatoid arthritis. Curr Respir Med Rev 2015;11(2):119–29.

64. Lake F, Proudman S. Rheumatoid arthritis and lung disease: from mechanisms to a practical approach. Semin Respir Crit Care Med 2014; 35(2):222–38.

65. Raghu G, Rochwerg B, Zhang Y, et al. An official ATS/ERS/JRS/ALAT clinical practice guideline: treatment of idiopathic pulmonary fibrosis. An update of the 2011 clinical practice guideline. Am J Respir Crit Care Med 2015;192(2):e3–19.

66. Zamora-Legoff JA, Krause ML, Crowson CS, et al. Risk of serious infection in patients with rheumatoid arthritis-associated interstitial lung disease. Clin Rheumatol 2016;35(10):2585–9.

67. Dixon WG, Abrahamowicz M, Beauchamp ME, et al. Immediate and delayed impact of oral glucocorticoid therapy on risk of serious infection in older patients with rheumatoid arthritis: a nested case-control analysis. Ann Rheum Dis 2012;71(7): 1128–33.

68. Idiopathic Pulmonary Fibrosis Clinical Research Network, Raghu G, Anstrom KJ, King TE Jr, et al. Prednisone, azathioprine, and N-acetylcysteine for pulmonary fibrosis. N Engl J Med 2012; 366(21):1968–77.

69. Mendoza FA, Nagle SJ, Lee JB, et al. A prospective observational study of mycophenolate mofetil treatment in progressive diffuse cutaneous systemic sclerosis of recent onset. J Rheumatol 2012;39(6):1241–7.

70. Shenoy PD, Bavaliya M, Sashidharan S, et al. Cyclophosphamide versus mycophenolate mofetil in scleroderma interstitial lung disease (SSc-ILD) as induction therapy: a single-centre, retrospective analysis. Arthritis Res Ther 2016;18(1):123.

71. Fischer A, Brown KK, Du Bois RM, et al. Mycophenolate mofetil improves lung function in connective tissue disease-associated interstitial lung disease. J Rheumatol 2013;40(5):640–6.

72. Nannini C, West CP, Erwin PJ, et al. Effects of cyclophosphamide on pulmonary function in patients with scleroderma and interstitial lung disease: a systematic review and meta-analysis of randomized controlled trials and observational prospective cohort studies. Arthritis Res Ther 2008; 10(5):R124.

73. Tashkin DP, Elashoff R, Clements PJ, et al. Cyclophosphamide versus placebo in scleroderma lung disease. N Engl J Med 2006;354(25):2655–66.

74. Ogawa D, Hashimoto H, Wada J, et al. Successful use of cyclosporin A for the treatment of acute interstitial pneumonitis associated with rheumatoid arthritis. Rheumatology (Oxford) 2000;39(12): 1422–4.

75. Chang HK, Park W, Ryu DS. Successful treatment of progressive rheumatoid interstitial lung disease with cyclosporine: a case report. J Korean Med Sci 2002;17(2):270–3.

76. Eissa K, Palomino J. B-cell depletion salvage therapy in rapidly progressive dermatomyositis related interstitial lung disease. J La State Med Soc 2016; 168(3):99–100.

77. Keir GJ, Maher TM, Hansell DM, et al. Severe interstitial lung disease in connective tissue disease: rituximab as rescue therapy. Eur Respir J 2012;40(3): 641–8.

78. Matteson EL, Bongartz T, Ryu JH, et al. Open-label, pilot study of the safety and clinical effects of rituximab in patients with rheumatoid arthritis associated interstitial pneumonia. Open J Rheumatol Autoimmune Dis 2012;2:53–8.

79. Mera-Varela A, Perez-Pampin E. Abatacept therapy in rheumatoid arthritis with interstitial lung disease. J Clin Rheumatol 2014;20(8):445–6.

80. Curtis JR, Sarsour K, Napalkov P, et al. Incidence and complications of interstitial lung disease in users of tocilizumab, rituximab, abatacept and anti-tumor necrosis factor alpha agents, a retrospective cohort study. Arthritis Res Ther 2015;17:319.

81. Fernandez-Diaz C, Loricera J, Castaneda S, et al. Abatacept in patients with rheumatoid arthritis and interstitial lung disease: a national multicenter study of 63 patients. Semin Arthritis Rheum 2018; 48(1):22–7.

82. Yazdani A, Singer LG, Strand V, et al. Survival and quality of life in rheumatoid arthritis-associated interstitial lung disease after lung transplantation. J Heart Lung Transplant 2014;33(5):514–20.

83. Jani M, Hirani N, Matteson EL, et al. The safety of biologic therapies in RA-associated interstitial lung disease. Nat Rev Rheumatol 2014;10(5):284–94.

84. Friedman BA. Rheumatoid nodules of the larynx. Arch Otolaryngol 1975;101(6):361–3.

85. Webb J, Payne WH. Rheumatoid nodules of the vocal folds. Ann Rheum Dis 1972;31(2):122–5.

86. Hamdan AL, Sarieddine D. Laryngeal manifestations of rheumatoid arthritis. Autoimmune Dis 2013;2013:103081.

87. Lawry GV, Finerman ML, Hanafee WN, et al. Laryngeal involvement in rheumatoid arthritis. A clinical, laryngoscopic, and computerized tomographic study. Arthritis Rheum 1984;27(8):873–82.

88. Guerra LG, Lau KY, Marwah R. Upper airway obstruction as the sole manifestation of rheumatoid arthritis. J Rheumatol 1992;19(6):974–6.

89. Brazeau-Lamontagne L, Charlin B, Levesque RY, et al. Cricoarytenoiditis: CT assessment in rheumatoid arthritis. Radiology 1986;158(2):463–6.

90. Chen JJ, Branstetter BF, Myers EN. Cricoarytenoid rheumatoid arthritis: an important consideration in aggressive lesions of the larynx. AJNR Am J Neuroradiol 2005;26(4):970–2.

91. Erb N, Pace AV, Delamere JP, et al. Control of unremitting rheumatoid arthritis by the prolactin antagonist cabergoline. Rheumatology (Oxford) 2001; 40(2):237–9.

92. Perez T, Remy-Jardin M, Cortet B. Airways involvement in rheumatoid arthritis: clinical, functional, and HRCT findings. Am J Respir Crit Care Med 1998;157(5 Pt 1):1658–65.

93. Devouassoux G, Cottin V, Liote H, et al. Characterisation of severe obliterative bronchiolitis in rheumatoid arthritis. Eur Respir J 2009;33(5):1053–61.

94. Pommepuy I, Farny M, Billey T, et al. Bronchiolitis obliterans organizing pneumonia in a patient with rheumatoid arthritis. Rev Rhum Engl Ed 1998; 65(1):65–7.

95. Cortot AB, Cottin V, Miossec P, et al. Improvement of refractory rheumatoid arthritis-associated constrictive bronchiolitis with etanercept. Respir Med 2005;99(4):511–4.

96. Vos R, Vanaudenaerde BM, Verleden SE, et al. Azithromycin in posttransplant bronchiolitis obliterans syndrome. Chest 2011;139(5):1246.

97. Hayakawa H, Sato A, Imokawa S, et al. Bronchiolar disease in rheumatoid arthritis. Am J Respir Crit Care Med 1996;154(5):1531–6.

98. Tashtoush B, Okafor NC, Ramirez JF, et al. Follicular bronchiolitis: a literature review. J Clin Diagn Res 2015;9(9):OE01–5.

99. Howling SJ, Hansell DM, Wells AU, et al. Follicular bronchiolitis: thin-section CT and histologic findings. Radiology 1999;212(3):637–42.

100. De Soyza A, McDonnell MJ, Goeminne PC, et al. Bronchiectasis rheumatoid overlap syndrome is an independent risk factor for mortality in patients with bronchiectasis: a multicenter cohort study. Chest 2017;151(6):1247–54.

101. Swinson DR, Symmons D, Suresh U, et al. Decreased survival in patients with co-existent rheumatoid arthritis and bronchiectasis. Br J Rheumatol 1997;36(6):689–91.

102. Puechal X, Fajac I, Bienvenu T, et al. Increased frequency of cystic fibrosis deltaF508 mutation in bronchiectasis associated with rheumatoid arthritis. Eur Respir J 1999;13(6):1281–7.

103. Balbir-Gurman A, Yigla M, Nahir AM, et al. Rheumatoid pleural effusion. Semin Arthritis Rheum 2006;35(6):368–78.

104. Corcoran JP, Ahmad M, Mukherjee R, et al. Pleuro-pulmonary complications of rheumatoid arthritis. Respir Care 2014;59(4):e55–9.

105. Fingerman DL, Andrus FC. Visceral lesions associated with rheumatoid arthritis. Ann Rheum Dis 1943;3(3):168–81.

106. Horler AR, Thompson M. The pleural and pulmonary complications of rheumatoid arthritis. Ann Intern Med 1959;51:1179–203.

107. Hyland RH, Gordon DA, Broder I, et al. A systematic controlled study of pulmonary abnormalities in rheumatoid arthritis. J Rheumatol 1983;10(3):395–405.

108. Jurik AG, Davidsen D, Graudal H. Prevalence of pulmonary involvement in rheumatoid arthritis and its relationship to some characteristics of the patients. A radiological and clinical study. Scand J Rheumatol 1982;11(4):217–24.

109. Hakala M, Tiilikainen A, Hameenkorpi R, et al. Rheumatoid arthritis with pleural effusion includes a subgroup with autoimmune features and HLA-B8, Dw3 association. Scand J Rheumatol 1986;15(3):290–6.

110. Avnon LS, Abu-Shakra M, Flusser D, et al. Pleural effusion associated with rheumatoid arthritis: what cell predominance to anticipate? Rheumatol Int 2007;27(10):919–25.

111. Walker WC, Wright V. Rheumatoid pleuritis. Ann Rheum Dis 1967;26(6):467–74.

112. Ojeda VJ, Stuckey BG, Owen ET, et al. Cardiac rheumatoid nodules. Med J Aust 1986;144(2):92–3.

113. Yousem SA, Colby TV, Carrington CB. Lung biopsy in rheumatoid arthritis. Am Rev Respir Dis 1985;131(5):770–7.

114. Lyne AJ, Rosen ES. Still's disease and rheumatoid nodule of the sclera. Br J Ophthalmol 1968;52(11):853–6.

115. Patterson JW. Rheumatoid nodule and subcutaneous granuloma annulare. A comparative histologic study. Am J Dermatopathol 1988;10(1):1–8.

116. Wikaningrum R, Highton J, Parker A, et al. Pathogenic mechanisms in the rheumatoid nodule: comparison of proinflammatory cytokine production and cell adhesion molecule expression in rheumatoid nodules and synovial membranes from the same patient. Arthritis Rheum 1998;41(10):1783–97.

117. Nyhall-Wahlin BM, Turesson C, Jacobsson LT, et al. The presence of rheumatoid nodules at early rheumatoid arthritis diagnosis is a sign of extra-articular disease and predicts radiographic progression of joint destruction over 5 years. Scand J Rheumatol 2011;40(2):81–7.

118. Turesson C, McClelland RL, Christianson T, et al. Clustering of extraarticular manifestations in patients with rheumatoid arthritis. J Rheumatol 2008;35(1):179–80.

119. Voskuyl AE, Zwinderman AH, Westedt ML, et al. Factors associated with the development of vasculitis in rheumatoid arthritis: results of a case-control study. Ann Rheum Dis 1996;55(3):190–2.

120. Walker WC, Wright V. Pulmonary lesions and rheumatoid arthritis. Medicine (Baltimore) 1968;47(6):501–20.

121. Chansakul T, Dellaripa PF, Doyle TJ, et al. Intrathoracic rheumatoid arthritis: imaging spectrum of typical findings and treatment related complications. Eur J Radiol 2015;84(10):1981–91.

122. Sargin G, Senturk T. Multiple pulmonary rheumatoid nodules. Reumatologia 2015;53(5):276–8.

123. Glace B, Gottenberg JE, Mariette X, et al. Efficacy of rituximab in the treatment of pulmonary rheumatoid nodules: findings in 10 patients from the French AutoImmunity and Rituximab/Rheumatoid Arthritis registry (AIR/PR registry). Ann Rheum Dis 2012;71(8):1429–31.

124. Akiyama M, Mawatari T, Nakashima Y, et al. Prevalence of dyslipidemia in Japanese patients with rheumatoid arthritis and effects of atorvastatin treatment. Clin Rheumatol 2015;34(11):1867–75.

125. Toussirot E, Berthelot JM, Pertuiset E, et al. Pulmonary nodulosis and aseptic granulomatous

lung disease occurring in patients with rheumatoid arthritis receiving tumor necrosis factor-alpha-blocking agent: a case series. J Rheumatol 2009;36(11):2421–7.

126. Caplan A. Certain unusual radiological appearances in the chest of coal-miners suffering from rheumatoid arthritis. Thorax 1953;8(1):29–37.

127. Schreiber J, Koschel D, Kekow J, et al. Rheumatoid pneumoconiosis (Caplan's syndrome). Eur J Intern Med 2010;21(3):168–72.

128. Jones RN, Turner-Warwick M, Ziskind M, et al. High prevalence of antinuclear antibodies in sand-blasters' silicosis. Am Rev Respir Dis 1976; 113(3):393–5.

129. Shahane A. Pulmonary hypertension in rheumatic diseases: epidemiology and pathogenesis. Rheumatol Int 2013;33(7):1655–67.

130. Udayakumar N, Venkatesan S, Rajendiran C. Pulmonary hypertension in rheumatoid arthritis–relation with the duration of the disease. Int J Cardiol 2008;127(3):410–2.

131. Keser G, Capar I, Aksu K, et al. Pulmonary hypertension in rheumatoid arthritis. Scand J Rheumatol 2004;33(4):244–5.

132. Dawson JK, Goodson NG, Graham DR, et al. Raised pulmonary artery pressures measured with Doppler echocardiography in rheumatoid arthritis patients. Rheumatology (Oxford) 2000; 39(12):1320–5.

133. Chung WS, Peng CL, Lin CL, et al. Rheumatoid arthritis increases the risk of deep vein thrombosis and pulmonary thromboembolism: a nationwide cohort study. Ann Rheum Dis 2014;73(10): 1774–80.

134. Bacani AK, Gabriel SE, Crowson CS, et al. Noncardiac vascular disease in rheumatoid arthritis: increase in venous thromboembolic events? Arthritis Rheum 2012;64(1):53–61.

135. Singh JA, Cameron C, Noorbaloochi S, et al. Risk of serious infection in biological treatment of patients with rheumatoid arthritis: a systematic review and meta-analysis. Lancet 2015;386(9990): 258–65.

136. Roubille C, Haraoui B. Interstitial lung diseases induced or exacerbated by DMARDS and biologic agents in rheumatoid arthritis: a systematic literature review. Semin Arthritis Rheum 2014;43(5): 613–26.

137. Flieder DB, Travis WD. Pathologic characteristics of drug-induced lung disease. Clin Chest Med 2004;25(1):37–45.

138. Salliot C, van der Heijde D. Long-term safety of methotrexate monotherapy in patients with rheumatoid arthritis: a systematic literature research. Ann Rheum Dis 2009;68(7):1100–4.

139. Sathi N, Chikura B, Kaushik VV, et al. How common is methotrexate pneumonitis? A large prospective study investigates. Clin Rheumatol 2012;31(1): 79–83.

140. Dawson JK, Graham DR, Desmond J, et al. Investigation of the chronic pulmonary effects of low-dose oral methotrexate in patients with rheumatoid arthritis: a prospective study incorporating HRCT scanning and pulmonary function tests. Rheumatology (Oxford) 2002;41(3):262–7.

141. Carroll GJ, Thomas R, Phatouros CC, et al. Incidence, prevalence and possible risk factors for pneumonitis in patients with rheumatoid arthritis receiving methotrexate. J Rheumatol 1994;21(1): 51–4.

142. Imokawa S, Colby TV, Leslie KO, et al. Methotrexate pneumonitis: review of the literature and histopathological findings in nine patients. Eur Respir J 2000;15(2):373–81.

143. Ameen M, Taylor DA, Williams IP, et al. Pneumonitis complicating methotrexate therapy for pustular psoriasis. J Eur Acad Dermatol Venereol 2001; 15(3):247–9.

144. Alarcon GS, Kremer JM, Macaluso M, et al. Risk factors for methotrexate-induced lung injury in patients with rheumatoid arthritis. A multicenter, case-control study. Methotrexate-Lung Study Group. Ann Intern Med 1997;127(5):356–64.

145. Saravanan V, Kelly CA. Reducing the risk of methotrexate pneumonitis in rheumatoid arthritis. Rheumatology (Oxford) 2004;43(2):143–7.

146. Cottin V, Tebib J, Massonnet B, et al. Pulmonary function in patients receiving long-term low-dose methotrexate. Chest 1996;109(4):933–8.

147. Carson CW, Cannon GW, Egger MJ, et al. Pulmonary disease during the treatment of rheumatoid arthritis with low dose pulse methotrexate. Semin Arthritis Rheum 1987;16(3):186–95.

148. Rojas-Serrano J, Gonzalez-Velasquez E, Mejia M, et al. Interstitial lung disease related to rheumatoid arthritis: evolution after treatment. Reumatol Clin 2012;8(2):68–71.

149. Wasko MC, Dasgupta A, Hubert H, et al. Propensity-adjusted association of methotrexate with overall survival in rheumatoid arthritis. Arthritis Rheum 2013;65(2):334–42.

150. Furst DE, Keystone EC, So AK, et al. Updated consensus statement on biological agents for the treatment of rheumatic diseases, 2012. Ann Rheum Dis 2013;72(Suppl 2):ii2–34.

151. Ramos-Casals M, Perez-Alvarez R, Perez-de-Lis M, et al. Pulmonary disorders induced by monoclonal antibodies in patients with rheumatologic autoimmune diseases. Am J Med 2011; 124(5):386–94.

152. Dixon WG, Hyrich KL, Watson KD, et al. Influence of anti-TNF therapy on mortality in patients with rheumatoid arthritis-associated interstitial lung disease: results from the British Society for

Rheumatology Biologics Register. Ann Rheum Dis 2010;69(6):1086–91.

153. Watson K, Symmons D, Griffiths I, et al. The British Society for Rheumatology biologics register. Ann Rheum Dis 2005;64(Suppl 4):iv42–3.

154. Perez-Alvarez R, Perez-de-Lis M, Diaz-Lagares C, et al. Interstitial lung disease induced or exacerbated by TNF-targeted therapies: analysis of 122 cases. Semin Arthritis Rheum 2011;41(2): 256–64.

155. Weinblatt ME, Moreland LW, Westhovens R, et al. Safety of abatacept administered intravenously in treatment of rheumatoid arthritis: integrated analyses of up to 8 years of treatment from the abatacept clinical trial program. J Rheumatol 2013;40(6): 787–97.

156. Naqibullah M, Shaker SB, Bach KS, et al. Rituximab-induced interstitial lung disease: five case reports. Eur Clin Respir J 2015;2:27178.

157. Leon L, Gomez A, Vadillo C, et al. Severe adverse drug reactions to biological disease-modifying anti-rheumatic drugs in elderly patients with rheumatoid arthritis in clinical practice. Clin Exp Rheumatol 2018;36(1):29–35.

158. Parry SD, Barbatzas C, Peel ET, et al. Sulphasalazine and lung toxicity. Eur Respir J 2002;19(4): 756–64.

159. Boyd O, Gibbs AR, Smith AP. Fibrosing alveolitis due to sulphasalazine in a patient with rheumatoid arthritis. Br J Rheumatol 1990;29(3):222–4.

160. Ulubas B, Sahin G, Ozer C, et al. Bronchiolitis obliterans organizing pneumonia associated with sulfasalazine in a patient with rheumatoid arthritis. Clin Rheumatol 2004;23(3):249–51.

161. Jacob J, Hirani N, van Moorsel CHM, et al. Predicting outcomes in rheumatoid arthritis related interstitial lung disease. Eur Respir J 2019;53(1) [pii: 1800869].

162. Inchingolo R, Varone F, Sgalla G, et al. Existing and emerging biomarkers for disease progression in idiopathic pulmonary fibrosis. Expert Rev Respir Med 2019;13(1):39–51.

163. Zhang J, Wang D, Wang L, et al. Pro-fibrotic effects of IL-17A and elevated IL-17RA in IPF and RA-ILD support a direct role for IL-17A/IL-17RA in human fibrotic interstitial lung disease. Am J Physiol Lung Cell Mol Physiol 2019;316(3):L487–97.

Interstitial Lung Disease in Polymyositis and Dermatomyositis

Kathryn Long, MD[a], Sonye K. Danoff, MD, PhD[b],*

KEYWORDS

• Interstitial lung disease • Myositis • Dermatomyositis • Polymyositis

KEY POINTS

• Interstitial lung disease (ILD) is a major complication of the idiopathic interstitial myopathies and is associated with increased mortality.
• Antisynthetase syndrome is a unique subset of patients with myositis with anti-aminoacyl-tRNA antibodies, ILD, mechanic's hands, fever, and arthritis.
• Anti-melanoma differentiation factor 5 antibodies are associated with rapidly progressive ILD and overall poor prognosis.
• Corticosteroids are first-line therapy for myositis-associated ILD, but addition of other immunosuppressive therapy is typically necessary to achieve disease control.

IDIOPATHIC INFLAMMATORY MYOPATHIES

The idiopathic inflammatory myopathies (IIMs) are a diverse group of connective tissue diseases characterized by varying degrees of muscle inflammation and systemic involvement. In adults they include polymyositis (PM), dermatomyositis (DM), and inclusion body myositis (IBM). Criteria for the diagnosis of the IIMs was first proposed by Bohan and Peter[1,2] and included 5 clinical criteria: symmetric proximal muscle weakness, muscle biopsy with evidence of necrosis, serum elevation of the skeletal muscle enzymes creatinine kinase (CK) and aldolase, characteristic triad of electromyography findings, and distinctive skin manifestations, including violaceous discoloration and edema of the upper eyelids (heliotrope rash), scaly and erythematous raised rash on the dorsum of the hands (Gottron papules), and involvement of the face and upper back and chest (**Fig. 1**). More recently, it has been recognized that some patients with the classic skin manifestations of DM have minimal (hypomyopathic) or no muscle involvement (amyopathic), termed clinically amyopathic DM (CADM).[3] Patients with IIMs, with the exception of IBM, can have a broad range of systemic manifestations involving the joints, skin, heart, and the lungs.

Patients with IIMs fall under the broad class of autoimmune connective tissue diseases (CTDs) and can have overlapping features with other CTDs. Autoantibodies are thought to play a key role in the pathogenesis of myositis and have been identified in more than 50% of patients with IIM. These can be divided into 2 subsets: myositis-specific antibodies (MSAs), which are generally specific for myositis and mutually exclusive, and myositis-associated antibodies (MAAs),

Disclosure Statement: The authors have no financial interests to disclose.
[a] Johns Hopkins Hospital, 600 N Wolfe Street, Osler 292-A, Baltimore, MD 21287, USA; [b] Department of Medicine, Division of Pulmonary and Critical Care Medicine, Johns Hopkins School of Medicine, 1830 East Monument Street, 5th Floor, Baltimore, MD 212015, USA
* Corresponding author.
E-mail address: sdanoff@jhmi.edu

chestmed.theclinics.com

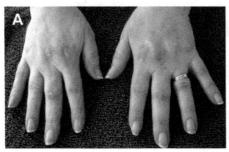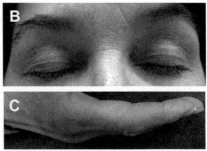

Fig. 1. DM. Classic skin findings in DM include (*A*) Gottron papules and (*B*) heliotrope rash. (*C*) Mechanic hands are frequently seen in AS.

which are found in other CTDs as well.[4] Although MSAs and MAAs as a whole are not part of the current diagnostic and classification criteria for myositis, it is well recognized that specific autoantibodies confer distinct clinical phenotypes (**Table 1**). Several MSAs, notably the anti-aminoacyl-tRNA (ARS) antibodies and anti-melanoma differentiation factor 5 (MDA5), are characterized by a high prevalence of interstitial lung disease (ILD), whereas others, such as anti-TIF1-γ and anti-NXP2, are associated with an increased risk of malignancy.[4–8]

ILD has been recognized as one of the most common systemic complications of the IIMs.[9] Pulmonary involvement has been associated with worse outcomes and increased mortality.[10,11] Although other pulmonary complications, such as pulmonary hypertension and pneumomediastinum, have been described in patients with myositis,[9,12] this review will focus on ILD as a major complication of PM/DM, used here interchangeably with IIM. Although ILD has been described in multiple myositis subtypes, including those without identifiable autoantibodies, the anti-ARS antibodies and anti-MDA5 antibodies are more significantly associated with the development of ILD compared with other MSAs.[6,13–16] This review describes the distinct clinical phenotypes of myositis-associated ILD (MA-ILD) depending on the specific class of MSA/MAA, and discusses the clinical course, prognosis, and management of these patients.

ANTISYNTHETASE SYNDROME

Antibodies directed against aminoacyl-tRNA synthetase enzymes (ARS antibodies) have collectively come to define a distinct subtype of myositis known as the antisynthetase syndrome (AS). First described in a case series of patients with myositis and ILD,[17] AS is now classified by the presence of anti-ARS antibodies and a group of clinical manifestations including myositis, ILD,

polyarthritis, Raynaud phenomenon, fever, and mechanic's hands (see **Fig. 1**).[18] The autoantigen for ARS antibodies are the cytoplasmic synthetase enzymes responsible for attaching specific amino acids to tRNA to make aminoacyl-tRNAs, which are used in the assembly of polypeptide chains at the ribosome level.[4,9] At least 8 specific anti-aminoacyl-tRNA synthetase antibodies have been described including anti-Jo-1 (histadyl), anti-PL7 (threonyl), anti-PL12 (alanyl), anti-EJ (glycyl), anti-OJ (isoleucyl), anti-KS (asparaginyl), anti-Zo (phenylalanyl), and anti-Ha/YRS (tyrosyl) (**Table 2**).[4,19] Although the anti-ARS antibodies were once thought to be associated with a characteristic clinical phenotype, newer studies have found that the different antisynthetase antibodies can have distinct clinical manifestations leading to considerable clinical heterogeneity within the syndrome.[16,20–23] In fact, the heterogeneity within the syndrome has led some to question whether the ARS antibodies define a distinct clinical syndrome or whether some of the distinctive autoimmune features, such as arthralgias, mechanic's hands, and Raynaud phenomenon, could be explained by the presence of other MAAs, such as anti-PM/SCL or anti-SSA/Ro.[24] The clinical associations of the MAAs are described elsewhere.

Among the antisynthetase antibodies, and in fact among all MSAs, the most common is anti-Jo-1, accounting for 26% to 88% of ARS antibodies and found in 9% to 24% of all patients with IIM.[4,7,21] Anti-Jo-1 was the first antisynthetase antibody described,[25] and perhaps for this reason best aligns with the clinical phenotype most commonly ascribed to AS. Compared with other MSAs, anti-Jo-1 is significantly associated with ILD and mechanic's hands.[8] Patient's with anti-Jo-1 antibodies also have higher frequencies of polyarthralgia and mechanic's hands compared with patients with other anti-ARS antibodies.[16,24] Anti-Jo-1 is more frequently detected in white patients and tends to have a female predominance.[21,25] In terms of the myositis phenotype,

Table 1
Myositis-specific and myositis-associated antibodies

Myositis Antibodies	Target Antigen	Prevalence in IIMs	Clinical Phenotype
Myositis-specific antibodies (MSAs)			
Anti-aminoacyl-tRNA synthetase antibodies (ARS) (Anti-Jo, Anti-PL7, Anti-PL12, Anti-EJ, Anti-OJ)	Cytoplasmic aminoacyl-tRNA synthetase enzymes	Anti-Jo: 9%–24% Other ARS antibodies: <5%	Antisynthetase syndrome: ILD, myositis, arthritis, Raynaud phenomenon, mechanic hand
Anti-MDA-5 (Anti-CADM-140)	Melanoma differentiation–associated gene-5	10%–48% (East Asia)[a] 0%–13% (United States and Europe)[a]	Skin ulcerations, CADM, RP-ILD
Anti-Mi2	Nucleosome-remodeling deacetylase complex	11%–59%[a]	Classic DM skin findings (heliotrope rash, Gottron sign, shawl sign), <ILD
Anti-SRP	Cytoplasmic signal recognition particle	5%–13%	Decreased cutaneous involvement, severe necrotizing myopathy, no increased ILD risk
Anti-TIF1-γ	Transcriptional intermediary factor 1-gamma	13%–31%[a]	Malignancy, <ILD
Anti-NXP2	Nuclear matric protein 2	1%–17%	Malignancy, <ILD
Myositis-associated antibodies (MAAs)			
Anti-Ro52	52-kDa ribonuclear protein complex	9%–46%	ILD, arthritis, mechanic hands, overlaps with pSS, SLE, SSc
Anti-PM/Scl-75/100	Nuclear exome complex (70-kDa and 100-kDa subunits)	4%–11%	Inflammatory joint disease, Raynaud, mechanic hands, ILD. Polymyositis-SSc overlap
Anti-Ku	70-kDa and 80-kDa Ku heterodimers	1%–3%	Arthralgia, Raynaud, mechanics hands, ILD, overlaps with SSc, SLE

Abbreviations: CADM, clinically amyopathic dermatomyositis; DM, dermatomyositis; IIM, idiopathic inflammatory myopathy; ILD, interstitial lung disease; PM, polymyositis; pSS, primary Sjogren's syndrome; RP-ILD, rapidly progressive interstitial lung disease; SLE, systemic lupus erythematosus; SSc, systemic sclerosis/scleroderma.
[a] Prevalence reported in DM/CADM only.
Data from Refs.[4–8,43,48]

anti-Jo-1 commonly presents as PM ,[16,26] and may have a more severe myositis course compared with the other anti-ARS antibodies, with higher rates of myalgias, muscle weakness, elevated CK at diagnosis, and lower rates of remission of myositis symptoms.[23] Development of ILD is common in patients with anti-Jo-1, although they are less likely to present with ILD alone at initial diagnosis[16] and more likely to have asymptomatic ILD at diagnosis.[23] Some studies suggest that patients who are positive for anti-Jo-1 have improved survival rates compared with patients who are non-anti-Jo-1 ARS positive, although,

notably, patients with non Jo-1 ARS were found to have significant delays in diagnosis.[26,27]

The other antisynthetase antibodies implicated in MA-ILD, anti-PL7, anti-PL12, anti-EJ, anti-OJ, and anti-KS, are less common and tend to have different clinical characteristics than anti-Jo-1 (see **Table 2**). Anti-PL7 and anti-PL12 antibodies are detected in 2% to 34% patients with anti-ARS antibodies. These antibodies are detected more commonly in African American patients and more frequently present with ILD alone than patients with anti-Jo-1.[21] Compared with patients who are anti-Jo-1 positive, patients with

Table 2
Antisynthetase antibodies

Antisynthetase Antibody (ARS)	Target Antigen	% of ARS Antibodies	Clinical Features
Anti-Jo-1	Histadyl-tRNA synthetase	26%–88%	PM, classic DM, ILD
Anti-PL7	Threonyl-tRNA synthetase	9.5%–34.0%	Classic DM, ILD, RP-ILD
Anti-PL12	Alanyl-tRNA synthetase	2.3%–15.3%	CADM, ILD alone
Anti-EJ	Glycyl-tRNA synthetase	1.8%–23.0%	Classic DM, CADM, ILD alone
Anti-OJ	Isoleucyl-tRNA synthetase	1.8%–5.0%	ILD alone
Anti-KS	Asparaginyl-tRNA synthetase	3.8%–8.0%	ILD alone
Anti-Zo	Phenylalanyl-tRNA synthetase	<1	unknown
Anti-Ha/YRS	Tyrosyl-tRNA synthetase	<1	unknown

Abbreviations: CADM, clinically amyopathic dermatomyositis; DM, dermatomyositis; ILD, interstitial lung disease; PM, polymyositis; RP-ILD, rapidly progressive interstitial lung disease.
Data from Refs.[7,16,19–23]

anti-PL7/anti-PL12 had less joint involvement, higher prevalence of ILD (90% vs 68%), and more frequently presented with symptoms of cough and dyspnea.[23] Patients with anti-PL12 have been noted to have more severe ILD, based on forced vital capacity (FVC) and diffusing capacity of carbon monoxide (DLCO) at diagnosis,[21] whereas patients with anti-PL7 have been noted to have higher rates of rapidly progressive ILD (RP-ILD).[20] Anti-EJ has been described in patients with ILD alone,[28] although myositis and muscle weakness are often present initially.[16] In contrast, anti-OJ and anti-KS generally present with ILD alone and are not associated with clinical myositis.[16,29]

Despite these differences between the anti-ARS antibody subtypes, the detection of any anti-ARS antibody has significant clinical implications for patients with myositis. As already mentioned, presence of anti-ARS antibodies increases the likelihood of development of ILD,[14–16] which can be asymptomatic. Therefore, screening for ILD with pulmonary function tests (PFTs) and high-resolution chest computed tomography (HRCT) in patients with myositis with anti-ARS antibodies is important for the detection and management of ILD.[18] Although rates of ILD are high in anti-ARS patients, these patients tend to have better overall prognosis than other MA-ILD patients. Patients with anti-ARS antibodies have been shown to have better responses to therapy, lower death rates, and overall increased survival rates compared with MA-ILD patients without anti-ARS antibodies.[7,30,31] The anti-ARS antibodies are also frequently associated with other MAAs, most notably anti-Ro52,[14,22,32] the clinical implications of which are discussed later in this article.

ANTI-MELANOMA DIFFERENTIATION FACTOR 5

Apart from anti-ARS antibodies, anti-MDA5 antibodies have also been shown to be highly associated with ILD in patients with myositis. These antibodies were originally discovered against a 140-kDa polypeptide in patients with CADM, and thus previously termed anti-CADM-140.[33] The autoantigen was later determined to be an RNA-helicase encoded by the MDA5 gene, which plays an important role in the innate immune response to intracellular viral infection.[34] Although originally identified in patients with CADM, anti-MDA5 autoantibodies are also present in patients with DM with active muscle disease; however, they are not present in patients with PM .[7,31] The prevalence of anti-MDA5 antibodies is much higher in East Asian DM cohorts than in US and European cohorts.[4] The presence of anti-MDA5 antibodies has been shown to be highly specific for the development of ILD[6,13,35] and more frequently associated with acute-onset lung disease and RP-ILD.[7,13,31,35–37] Patients with anti-MDA5 antibody also are more likely to exhibit characteristic DM skin findings, such as heliotrope rash and Gottron papules.[7,38]

Both the presence of anti-MDA5 antibodies and the antibody titer have been shown to have prognostic implications for patients with DM-ILD. Presence of anti-MDA5 antibodies has been associated with increased 90-day mortality and is a marker for poor overall survival.[7,31,35,36,38,39] Among patients with anti-MDA5 antibodies, those with higher initial titers were less likely to respond to therapy and had increased risk of acute death.[40,41] Interestingly, one study showed that titers of anti-MDA5 decreased with treatment, whereas recurrent increases in titers correlated with relapse of disease, indicating its potential use as a marker for monitoring disease status.[42]

MYOSITIS-ASSOCIATED ANTIBODIES

Antibodies to anti-SSA/Ro, specifically the 52-kDA protein complex (anti-Ro52), are the most frequently detected MAA, occurring in 31% to 46% of all patients with PM/DM.[6,8,14] Anti-Ro52 has been shown to be highly associated with anti-ARS antibodies, especially anti-Jo-1.[8,14,32,43,44] Several studies have demonstrated that anti-Ro52–positive patients with PM/DM have higher rates of ILD, even after correcting for anti-Jo-1 positivity.[6,8,43] In patients with anti-synthetase syndrome, anti-Ro52 positivity seems to be associated with a more severe course. Patients with anti-Ro52 positivity have higher rates of mechanic hands, arthritis, and joint deterioration, and myositis deterioration.[8,45] Pulmonary symptoms of ILD, such as dyspnea and cough, are more frequent in antisynthetase patients with anti-Ro52 along with higher fibrosis scores on HRCT.[45–47] One study found that antisynthetase patients with anti-Ro52 antibody had higher rates of RP-ILD than those without anti-Ro52.[20] Another found that anti-SSA/Ro was associated with higher rates of pulmonary relapse in all patients with PM/DM-ILD.[44]

Anti-PM/Scl antibodies (75 kDa and 100 kDa) are frequently found in patients with overlap myositis.[24] Patients with anti-PM/Scl antibodies can present with a similar clinical phenotype to AS, with high rates of ILD, arthritis, and mechanic hands.[24,48] Compared with anti-ARS patients, patients with anti-PM/Scl antibodies have higher rates of sclerodactyly and Raynaud phenomenon.[8,24]

OTHER MYOSITIS-SPECIFIC ANTIBODIES

Most other MSAs have not been shown to be associated with increased risk of ILD. Antibodies to signal recognition particle (anti-SRP) are associated with severe necrotizing myopathy with high rates of profound muscle weakness and dysphagia; however, rates of ILD are similar to that of myositis controls.[49] Anti-Mi2 antibody is specific to DM and is associated with classic DM skin findings and low rates of ILD.[8,43] Patients with antibodies to transcriptional intermediate factor 1-gamma, TIF1-γ (previously called anti-p155/140), and to nuclear matrix protein 2, NXP-2, have high rates of malignancy, but low rates of ILD.[4–6]

PATHOLOGY

Surgical lung biopsy is not routinely performed in patients with MA-ILD, as it is not necessary to confirm the diagnosis and has limited utility for changing management decisions. Many studies report only a limited sample of biopsy data, and the results are highly variable. Nonspecific interstitial pneumonia (NSIP) appears to be the most common pattern identified in MA-ILD patients.[30,50,51] Organizing pneumonia (OP) and usual interstitial pneumonia are also frequently reported.[19,25,50–52] Diffuse alveolar damage and unclassifiable patterns are less frequently seen.[25,51] Given the relative paucity of data, there has been no clear association identified between antibody type and pathologic classification.

PULMONARY FUNCTION TESTS

Pulmonary function testing of patients with PM/DM is important both for the diagnosis of ILD and for monitoring disease progression over time. The interpretation of PFTs in patients with myositis has unique challenges, as diaphragmatic weakness can result in changes in FVC and DLCO and intrapatient testing can vary significantly as muscle strength improves with treatment.[18] For this reason, concurrent HRCT is needed for the definitive diagnosis of ILD. PFTs in patients with MA-ILD typically show a moderate restrictive pattern with decreased FVC and total lung capacity, and moderate decreases in DLCO.[19,25] Most studies have not shown significant differences in PFT findings based on antibody type.[7,19,23,31] A 2017 Japanese study found that patients with anti-ARS antibodies had significantly lower FVC and forced expiratory volume in 1 second (FEV1) compared with patients with antibody-negative idiopathic pulmonary fibrosis, although patients with anti-ARS antibodies had better overall survival.[53] Among patients with MA-ILD, lower baseline FVC and DLCO have been associated with disease progression and decreased survival.[27,50,51,54]

RADIOGRAPHIC MANIFESTATIONS

HRCT is a useful tool in the diagnosis and management of ILD. The computed tomography (CT) findings of patients with PM/DM-associated ILD can be highly variable depending on the severity and acuity of the pulmonary process (**Fig. 2**). In patients with anti-ARS antibody ILD, the most frequent findings are ground glass opacities (GGOs) and reticulations, although consolidations are also common.[55] In fact, patients with PM/DM-associated ILD are much more likely to present with consolidations than patients with other CTD-ILDs.[56] As the disease progresses, consolidations typically resolve, whereas honeycombing and

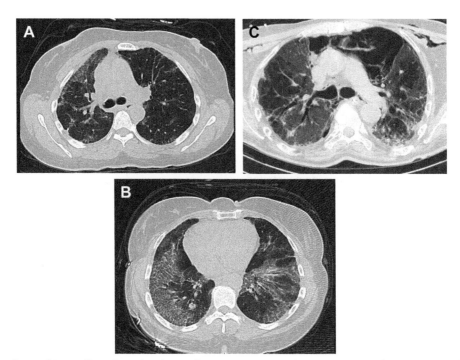

Fig. 2. Radiographic manifestations. (*A, B*) Two thin-section CT scans from a patient with NSIP pattern show predominant basal reticulations. (*C*) Thin-section CT scan from a patient with RP-ILD shows diffuse ground glass attenuation and pneumomediastinum.

fibrosis become more common.[52] The anatomic distribution in anti-ARS ILD is typically basal, peripheral, and peribronchovascular.[52,55,56] The CT pattern most frequently ascribed to patients with anti-ARS ILD falls under NSIP or NSIP with OP.[7,25,52,55] As might be expected, the CT findings of patients with anti-MDA5 antibody ILD, which is more often associated with RP-ILD and fatal disease, differ from patients with anti-ARS ILD. Patients with anti-MDA5 ILD have frequent GGOs and consolidation and less reticulation. Anatomic distribution is more variable with lower lobe consolidation and GGOs being most common, followed by random distribution.[57,58] These patients more frequently had CT patterns that were unclassifiable, which was more commonly associated with acute death in RP-ILD.[40,58]

TREATMENT

There is no standard treatment regimen for the management of MA-ILD and practices vary considerably. Most of the data to support the use of various immunosuppressive agents are based on retrospective reviews and case series, and there are few prospective or randomized controlled trials. Corticosteroids are the mainstay of therapy for myositis-associated ILD, although this is generally based on historical precedent.[59]

Patients with severe exacerbations or RP-ILD are typically treated with pulse dose intravenous (IV) methylprednisolone 1000 mg/d for 3 days, whereas stable patients with severe ILD are typically treated with 0.75 to 1 mg/kg per day of oral prednisone.[59–61] Unfortunately, many patients do not respond to initial corticosteroid treatment or have progressive disease when treated with corticosteroids alone,[60,62,63] especially among patients with RP-ILD.[61,64] There have been several studies that have shown survival benefit to early addition of a second immunosuppressive agent,[61,62,65] and it is common practice to add an additional immunosuppressive agent with initial corticosteroid treatment.

Many immunosuppressive (IS) agents have been used for the treatment of MA-ILD (**Table 3**). Azathioprine (AZA) is commonly used in MA-ILD, although there are relatively few studies to support its use. Mira-Avendano and colleagues[63] showed in a retrospective review that 13 patients treated with AZA and prednisone had reduction in dyspnea and stabilization in PFTs along with decreased daily steroid dose at 12 months. Typical dosages are 2 mg/kg per day, and it is generally well tolerated with potential side effects, including leukopenia, elevation of liver enzymes, and opportunistic infections.[59] Mycophenolate mofetil (MMF) is another commonly used IS agent

Table 3
Treatment of myositis-associated interstitial lung disease

Medication	Dosing	Side Effects	Outcomes
Prednisone	Severe ILD 0.75–1 mg/kg po daily, consider pulse 1 g/d IV ×3 days for AE or RP-ILD	Weight gain, osteoporosis, diabetes	Improvement in ILD in 50%–89% of patients
Azathioprine	2 mg/kg per day po	Cytopenias, infection, skin cancer, LFT elevation	Stabilization of PFTs, decreased dyspnea
Mycophenolate mofetil	2000–3000 mg/d po	Diarrhea, cytopenias, recurrent infection	Stabilization of PFTs, decreased dyspnea
Tacrolimus	1–3.5 mg/d po	Nephrotoxicity, tremors, HTN, hypomagnesemia	Improved FVC, DLCO, improved muscle strength, lowers CK
Cyclosporine A	Varies po, goal trough 100–200 ng/mL	Nephrotoxicity, HTN, neurotoxicity, hyperkalemia, hypomagnesemia	Improvement in PFTs, early initiation may increase survival
Cyclophosphamide	0.3–1.5 g/m^2 or 10–15 mg/kg, IV pulse (weekly vs monthly)	Nausea, opportunistic infection, cytopenias, alopecia	Improvement in PFTs and HRCT, improvement in muscle strength
Rituximab	1000 mg IV at day 0 and day 14	Opportunistic infection	Improvement in PFTs, improvement in HRCT, improvement in myositis in antisynthetase patients
Intravenous immunoglobulin	0.4 g/kg IV daily for 5 d	Headache, malaise, fever, chills, anaphylaxis	Case reports with improvement of ILD, randomized trials showing improvement in muscle strength

Abbreviations: AE, acute exacerbation; CK, creatinine kinase; DLCO, diffusing capacity of carbon monoxide; FVC, forced vital capacity; HRCT, high-resolution chest CT; HTN, hypertension; ILD, interstitial lung disease; IV, intravenous; po, by mouth; PFT, pulmonary function test; RP-ILD, rapidly progressive ILD.
Data from Refs.[59,63,65,67,68,71–73,76,77]

in CTD-associated ILD. Several studies of patients with CTD-ILD, including patients with PM/DM, have shown stabilization or improvement of PFTs, along with decreased daily steroid dosages with addition of 2000 to 3000 mg/d of MMF.[63,66,67] Potential side effects include gastrointestinal intolerance, cytopenias, and recurrent infections.[67]

The use of calcineurin inhibitors, including cyclosporine A (CsA) and tacrolimus, is becoming more common in the management of MA-ILD. A meta-analysis by Ge and colleagues[68] showed that patients treated with tacrolimus generally had improvement in muscle strength, decreased CK levels, and improvement in FVC and DLCO. In patients who failed conventional therapy with corticosteroids and another immunosuppressive agent, Sharma and colleagues[69] found that 94% of patients treated with tacrolimus had improvement in their lung function, with PM-ILD being more likely

to respond than patients with DM-ILD. Kurita and colleagues[70] showed in a retrospective study that patients who received tacrolimus as part of their initial treatment regimen had longer event-free survival. In another retrospective study, Go and colleagues[65] found that patients who received CsA early in their ILD course had improved survival and stabilization of their HRCT scores compared with those who received CsA after failure of conventional treatment. In a prospective trial comparing a new protocol using early IV CsA along with high-dose corticosteroids compared with historical controls treated with corticosteroids alone initially, Shimojima and colleagues[61] showed increased total survival and longer event-free survival in the early CsA protocol compared with historical controls. In a recent meta-analysis comparing treatment outcomes of patients with MA-ILD, Barba and colleagues[64] showed that patients with RP-ILD treated with CsA had improved survival compared with corticosteroids alone (69.2% vs 54%). In patients with chronic-ILD, patients treated with either corticosteroids alone or corticosteroids with a calcineurin inhibitor had high overall rates of improvement in ILD.

Cyclophosphamide (CYC) has been used in patients with severe MA-ILD and has been shown to improve both overall muscle strength and FVC and DLCO.[71] It has also been used in triple therapy along with corticosteroids and calcineurin inhibitor in patients with RP-ILD, or as a rescue therapy when patients fail initial management.[61,63,70] Rituximab has recently shown promising results for the treatment of MA-ILD, specifically in patients with AS. Several retrospective studies have shown that most patients with AS treated with rituximab had improvement of their ILD,[72,73] with some patients having greater than 30% improvement in FVC, FEV1, and DLCO.[73] A recent prospective phase II trial of 10 patients with AS and ILD found that 40% had improvement in FVC and 50% had stabilization of their disease following rituximab therapy.[74] Intravenous immunoglobulin (IVIG) also has been used as a salvage therapy in a few case series and case reports and it has had increasing off-label use in patients with refractory MA-ILD[75–77] but data regarding its efficacy remain limited.

The choice of which immunosuppressive agent to add to conventional corticosteroid therapy depends on the severity of ILD presentation along with other comorbidities for each patient. In a recent review, Morisset and colleagues[59] offers a proposed treatment algorithm for patients presenting with MA-ILD. Patients presenting with chronic or mild to moderate ILD are treated with steroids and a well-tolerated oral immunosuppressive agent, such as AZA or MMF, and are followed at regular intervals. Those with improvement or stabilization undergo steroid tapering with maintenance of the steroid-sparing agent, whereas those with deterioration change to a different immunosuppressive therapy. Patients presenting initially with severe ILD or RP-ILD are treated with high-dose corticosteroids combined with either cyclophosphamide, rituximab, or a calcineurin inhibitor (CsA or tacrolimus) and treatments tapered or intensified based on response to therapy.

CLINICAL COURSE AND PROGNOSIS

Despite these advances in therapy, the development of ILD is associated with increased mortality in patients with myositis.[10,11] For this reason, it is important to determine which patients with myositis are at risk for developing ILD over the course of their disease. As stated previously, anti-MDA5 antibodies, anti-Jo-1 antibodies, and anti-Ro52 antibodies are all associated with increased risk of ILD in patients with myositis.[6,15] Other studies have found that older age, presence of arthritis, mechanic hands, ulcerations, and elevated levels of erythrocyte sedimentation rate and C-reactive protein also increase the risk of ILD.[15,78] Serum levels of KL-6, used to monitor disease activity in MA-ILD,[79] have also been shown to be a predictive factor for the development of ILD.[80]

The overall clinical course in patients with MA-ILD can be quite variable. Marie and colleagues[50] followed a cohort of 107 patients with PM/DM-ILD and found ILD resolution in 32%, improvement or stabilization in 51%, and deterioration in 16%. Johnson and colleagues[19] described a similar cohort of 77 patients with PM/DM-ILD and found

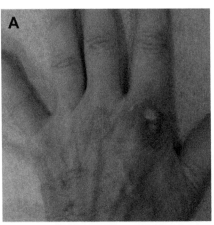
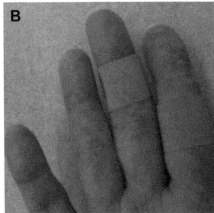

Fig. 3. Skin ulcerations from 2 patients (*A*, *B*) with anti-MDA5 antibody. Presence of skin ulcerations is associated with the development of RP-ILD.

improvement of disease in 44%, stable disease in 16%, and progression of disease in 40%. Zamora and colleagues[25] followed a cohort of patients positive for anti-Jo-1 and observed improvement of ILD in 11%, stable disease in 36%, and progression of disease in 53%. Disease progression is more likely in patients with lower %FVC and who present with symptomatic disease.[50,51,54] Pinal-Fernandez and colleagues[21] showed that African American patients with AS tend to have more severe ILD independent of age or autoantibody status. Other studies have shown that older age, increasing levels of KL-6, and presence of ARS antibodies are risk factors for disease progression or recurrence of disease.[50,80,81] Risk factors for the development of RP-ILD include positive anti-MDA5 antibody, peripheral lymphocyte count less than 500, skin ulcerations, and ferritin greater than 5000 (**Fig. 3**).[37]

In terms of overall survival in MA-ILD, patients with anti-MDA5 antibodies have the lowest survival, whereas anti-ARS patients have higher overall survival and a greater improvement rate in response to therapy.[7,30,31] Other factors associated with poor prognosis are elevated ferritin, RP-ILD, acute/subacute onset, complications with severe infections, and higher HRCT scores.[7,20,78,82,83] Development of malignancy also is a major contributor to poor prognosis in patients with myositis; however, patients with ILD are much less likely to develop malignancy, and in fact malignancy is associated with decreased risk of ILD.[15,84] Good prognostic indicators are presence of anti-ARS antibodies, higher %FVC at diagnosis, and higher Pao_2.[7]

SUMMARY

The IIMs, including PM and DM, are autoimmune CTDs with variable degrees of muscle inflammation and systemic involvement. ILD is a common complication of the IIMs and is associated with increased mortality. Many patients with PM/DM have MSA/MAAs that result in distinct clinical phenotypes. Among these MSAs, anti-ARS antibodies and anti-MDA5 antibodies have high rates of ILD. Corticosteroids are the mainstay of treatment, although the addition of other immunosuppressive therapy is typically necessary to achieve disease control.

REFERENCES

1. Bohan A, Peter J. Polymyositis and dermatomyositis (first of two parts). N Engl J Med 1975;292(7):344–7.
2. Bohan A, Peter J. Polymyositis and dermatomyositis (second of two parts). N Engl J Med 1975;292(8):403–7.
3. Sontheimer RD. Would a new name hasten the acceptance of amyopathic dermatomyositis (dermatomyositis siné myositis) as a distinctive subset within the idiopathic inflammatory dermatomyopathies spectrum of clinical illness? J Am Acad Dermatol 2002;46(4):626–36.
4. Betteridge Z, Mchugh N. Myositis-specific autoantibodies: an important tool to support diagnosis of myositis. J Intern Med 2016;280(1):8–23.
5. Hoshino K, Muro Y, Sugiura K, et al. Anti-MDA5 and anti-TIF1-γ antibodies have clinical significance for patients with dermatomyositis. Rheumatology 2010;49(9):1726–33.
6. Li L, Wang H, Wang Q, et al. Myositis-specific autoantibodies in dermatomyositis/polymyositis in patients with interstitial lung disease. J Neurol Sci 2019;397:123–8.
7. Hozumi H, Fujisawa T, Nakashima R, et al. Comprehensive assessment of myositis-specific autoantibodies in polymyositis/dermatomyositis-associated interstitial lung disease. Respir Med 2016;121:91–9.
8. Srivastava P, Dwivedi S, Lawrence A, et al. Myositis-specific and myositis associated autoantibodies in Indian patients with inflammatory myositis. Indian J Rheumatol 2014;9:935–43.
9. Hallowell R, Ascherman D, Danoff S. Pulmonary manifestations of polymyositis/dermatomyositis. Semin Respir Crit Care Med 2014;35(02):239–48.
10. Johnson C, Pinal-Fernandez I, Parikh R, et al. Assessment of mortality in autoimmune myositis with and without associated interstitial lung disease. Lung 2016;194(5):733–7.
11. Chen IJ, Jan Wu YJ, Lin CW, et al. Interstitial lung disease in polymyositis and dermatomyositis. Clin Rheumatol 2009;28(6):639–46.
12. Kalluri M, Oddis CV. Pulmonary manifestations of the idiopathic inflammatory myopathies. Clin Chest Med 2010;31(3):501–12.
13. Li L, Wang Q, Wen X, et al. Assessment of anti-MDA5 antibody as a diagnostic biomarker in patients with dermatomyositis-associated interstitial lung disease or rapidly progressive interstitial lung disease. Oncotarget 2017;8(44):76129–40.
14. Zampeli E, Venetsanopoulou A, Argyropoulou OD, et al. Myositis autoantibody profiles and their clinical associations in Greek patients with inflammatory myopathies. Clin Rheumatol 2018;38(1):125–32.
15. Zhang L, Wu G, Gao D, et al. Factors associated with interstitial lung disease in patients with polymyositis and dermatomyositis: a systematic review and meta-analysis. Plos One 2016;11(5):e0155381.
16. Hamaguchi Y, Fujimoto M, Matsushita T, et al. Common and distinct clinical features in adult patients with anti-aminoacyl-tRNA synthetase antibodies: heterogeneity within the syndrome. PLoS One 2013;8(4):e60442.

17. Marguerie C, Bunn CC, Beynon HLC, et al. Polymyositis, pulmonary fibrosis and autoantibodies to aminoacyl-tRNA synthetase enzymes. QJM 1990; 77(1):1019–38.

18. Connors GR, Christopher-Stine L, Oddis CV, et al. Interstitial lung disease associated with the idiopathic inflammatory myopathies. Chest 2010; 138(6):1464–74.

19. Johnson C, Connors G, Oaks J, et al. Clinical and pathologic differences in interstitial lung disease based on antisynthetase antibody type. Respir Med 2014;108(10):1542–8.

20. Shi J, Li S, Yang H, et al. Clinical profiles and prognosis of patients with distinct antisynthetase antibodies. J Rheumatol 2017;44(7):1051–7.

21. Dugar M, Cox S, Limaye V, et al. Clinical heterogeneity and prognostic features of South Australian patients with anti-synthetase autoantibodies. Intern Med J 2011;41(9):674–9.

22. Pinal-Fernandez I, Casal-Dominguez M, Huapaya JA, et al. A longitudinal cohort study of the anti-synthetase syndrome: increased severity of interstitial lung disease in black patients and patients with anti-PL7 and anti-PL12 autoantibodies. Rheumatology 2017;56(6):999–1007.

23. Marie I, Josse S, Decaux O, et al. Comparison of long-term outcome between anti-Jo1- and anti-PL7/PL12 positive patients with antisynthetase syndrome. Autoimmun Rev 2012;11(10):739–45.

24. Lega J-C, Fabien N, Reynaud Q, et al. The clinical phenotype associated with myositis-specific and associated autoantibodies: a meta-analysis revisiting the so-called antisynthetase syndrome. Autoimmun Rev 2014;13(9):883–91.

25. Zamora AC, Hoskote SS, Abascal-Bolado B, et al. Clinical features and outcomes of interstitial lung disease in anti-Jo-1 positive antisynthetase syndrome. Respir Med 2016;118:39–45.

26. Aggarwal R, Cassidy E, Fertig N, et al. Patients with non-Jo-1 anti-tRNA-synthetase autoantibodies have worse survival than Jo-1 positive patients. Ann Rheum Dis 2014;73(1):227–32.

27. Rojas-Serrano J, Herrera-Bringas D, Mejía M, et al. Prognostic factors in a cohort of antisynthetase syndrome (ASS): serologic profile is associated with mortality in patients with interstitial lung disease (ILD). Clin Rheumatol 2015;34(9):1563–9.

28. Schneider F, Yousem SA, Bi D, et al. Pulmonary pathologic manifestations of anti-glycyl-tRNA synthetase (anti-EJ)-related inflammatory myopathy. J Clin Pathol 2014;67(8):678–83.

29. Hirakata M, Suwa A, Nagai S, et al. Anti-KS: identification of autoantibodies to asparaginyl-transfer RNA synthetase associated with interstitial lung disease. J Immunol 1999;162:2315–20.

30. Hozumi H, Enomoto N, Kono M, et al. Prognostic significance of anti-aminoacyl-tRNA synthetase antibodies in polymyositis/dermatomyositis-associated interstitial lung disease: a retrospective case control study. Plos One 2015;10(3):e0120313.

31. Chen F, Li S, Wang T, et al. Clinical heterogeneity of interstitial lung disease in polymyositis and dermatomyositis patients with or without specific autoantibodies. Am J Med Sci 2018;355(1):48–53.

32. Yamasaki Y, Satoh M, Mizushima M, et al. Clinical subsets associated with different anti-aminoacyl transfer RNA synthetase antibodies and their association with coexisting anti-Ro52. Mod Rheumatol 2015;26(3):403–9.

33. Sato S, Hirakata M, Kuwana M, et al. Autoantibodies to a 140-kd polypeptide, CADM-140, in Japanese patients with clinically amyopathic dermatomyositis. Arthritis Rheum 2005;52(5):1571–6.

34. Sato S, Hoshino K, Satoh T, et al. RNA helicase encoded by melanoma differentiation-associated gene 5 is a major autoantigen in patients with clinically amyopathic dermatomyositis: association with rapidly progressive interstitial lung disease. Arthritis Rheum 2009;60(7):2193–200.

35. Moghadam-Kia S, Oddis CV, Sato S, et al. Anti-melanoma differentiation-associated gene 5 is associated with rapidly progressive lung disease and poor survival in US patients with amyopathic and myopathic dermatomyositis. Arthritis Care Res 2016;68(5):689–94.

36. Yoshida N, Okamoto M, Kaieda S, et al. Association of anti-aminoacyl-transfer RNA synthetase antibody and anti-melanoma differentiation-associated gene 5 antibody with the therapeutic response of polymyositis/dermatomyositis-associated interstitial lung disease. Respir Investig 2017;55(1):24–32.

37. Xu Y, Yang CS, Li YJ, et al. Predictive factors of rapidly progressive-interstitial lung disease in patients with clinically amyopathic dermatomyositis. Clin Rheumatol 2016;35(1):113–6.

38. Kishaba T, Mcgill R, Nei Y, et al. Clinical characteristics of dermatomyositis/polymyositis associated interstitial lung disease according to the autoantibody. J Med Invest 2018;65(3.4):251–7.

39. Ikeda S, Arita M, Morita M, et al. Interstitial lung disease in clinically amyopathic dermatomyositis with and without anti-MDA-5 antibody: to lump or split? BMC Pulm Med 2015;15(1):159.

40. Sakamoto S, Okamoto M, Kaieda S, et al. Low positive titer of anti-melanoma differentiation-associated gene 5 antibody is not associated with a poor long-term outcome of interstitial lung disease in patients with dermatomyositis. Respir Invest 2018;56(6):464–72.

41. Sato S, Kuwana M, Fujita T, et al. Anti-CADM-140/MDA5 autoantibody titer correlates with disease activity and predicts disease outcome in patients with dermatomyositis and rapidly progressive interstitial lung disease. Mod Rheumatol 2013;23(3):496–502.

42. Matsushita T, Mizumaki K, Kano M, et al. Antimela-noma differentiation-associated protein 5 antibody level is a novel tool for monitoring disease activity in rapidly progressive interstitial lung disease with dermatomyositis. Br J Dermatol 2017;176(2): 395–402.

43. Cruellas M, Viana V, Levy-Neto M, et al. Myositis-specific and myositis-associated autoantibody pro-files and their clinical associations in a large series of patients with polymyositis and dermatomyositis. Clinics (Sao Paulo) 2013;68(7):909–14.

44. Tatebe N, Sada K-E, Asano Y, et al. Anti-SS-A/Ro antibody positivity as a risk factor for relapse in pa-tients with polymyositis/dermatomyositis. Mod Rheu-matol 2018;28(1):141–6.

45. Marie I, Hatron PY, Dominique S, et al. Short-term and long-term outcome of anti-Jo1-positive patients with anti-Ro52 antibody. Semin Arthritis Rheum 2012;41(6):890–9.

46. Váncsa A, Csípő I, Németh J, et al. Characteristics of interstitial lung disease in SS-A positive/Jo-1 positive inflammatory myopathy patients. Rheumatol Int 2009;29(9):989–94.

47. La Corte R, Naco ALM, Locaputo A, et al. In patients with antisynthetase syndrome the occurrence of anti-Ro/SSA antibodies causes a more severe inter-stitial lung disease. Autoimmunity 2006;39(3): 249–53.

48. Marie I, Lahaxe L, Benveniste O, et al. Long-term outcome of patients with polymyositis/dermatomyo-sitis and anti-PM-Scl antibody. Br J Dermatol 2010; 162(2):337–44.

49. Hengstman GJD, Laak HJT, Egberts WTMV, et al. Anti-signal recognition particle autoantibodies: marker of a necrotizing myopathy. Ann Rheum Dis 2006;65(12):1635–8.

50. Marie I, Hatron PY, Dominique S, et al. Short-term and long-term outcomes of interstitial lung dis-ease in polymyositis and dermatomyositis: a se-ries of 107 patients. Arthritis Rheum 2011;63(11): 3439–47.

51. Obert J, Freynet O, Nunes H, et al. Outcome and prognostic factors in a French cohort of patients with myositis-associated interstitial lung disease. Rheumatol Int 2016;36(12):1727–35.

52. Debray M-P, Borie R, Revel M-P, et al. Interstitial lung disease in anti-synthetase syndrome: initial and follow-up CT findings. Eur J Radiol 2015;84(3): 516–23.

53. Tanizawa K, Handa T, Nakashima R, et al. The long-term outcome of interstitial lung disease with anti-aminoacyl-tRNA synthetase antibodies. Respir Med 2017;127:57–64.

54. Fujisawa T, Hozumi H, Kono M, et al. Predictive fac-tors for long-term outcome in polymyositis/dermatomyositis-associated interstitial lung dis-eases. Respir Invest 2017;55(2):130–7.

55. Waseda Y, Johkoh T, Egashira R, et al. Antisynthe-tase syndrome: pulmonary computed tomography findings of adult patients with antibodies to aminoacyl-tRNA synthetases. Eur J Radiol 2016; 85(8):1421–6.

56. Yamanaka Y, Baba T, Hagiwara E, et al. Radiological images of interstitial pneumonia in mixed connective tissue disease compared with scleroderma and polymyositis/dermatomyositis. Eur J Radiol 2018; 107:26–32.

57. Tanizawa K, Handa T, Nakashima R, et al. High-res-olution computed tomography (HRCT) features of interstitial lung disease in dermatomyositis with anti-CADM-140 antibody. Respir Med 2011;105(9): 1380–7.

58. Tanizawa K, Handa T, Nakashima R, et al. The prog-nostic value of HRCT in myositis-associated intersti-tial lung disease. Respir Med 2013;107(5):745–52.

59. Morisset J, Johnson C, Rich E, et al. Management of myositis-related interstitial lung disease. Chest 2016;150(5):1118–28.

60. Takada T, Suzuki E, Nakano M, et al. Clinical features of polymyositis/dermatomyositis with steroid-resistant interstitial lung disease. Intern Med 1998; 37(8):669–73.

61. Shimojima Y, Ishii W, Matsuda M, et al. Effective use of calcineurin inhibitor in combination therapy for interstitial lung disease in patients with dermatomyo-sitis and polymyositis. J Clin Rheumatol 2017;23(2): 87–93.

62. Takada K, Kishi J, Miyasaka N. Step-up versus pri-mary intensive approach to the treatment of intersti-tial pneumonia associated with dermatomyositis/polymyositis: a retrospective study. Mod Rheumatol 2007;17(2):123–30.

63. Mira-Avendano IC, Parambil JG, Yadav R, et al. A retrospective review of clinical features and treat-ment outcomes in steroid-resistant interstitial lung disease from polymyositis/dermatomyositis. Respir Med 2013;107(6):890–6.

64. Barba T, Fort R, Cottin V, et al. Treatment of idio-pathic inflammatory myositis associated interstitial lung disease: a systematic review and meta-anal-ysis. Autoimmun Rev 2019;18(2):113–22.

65. Go DJ, Park JK, Kang EH, et al. Survival benefit associated with early cyclosporine treatment for dermatomyositis-associated interstitial lung disease. Rheumatol Int 2015;36(1):125–31.

66. Swigris JJ, Olson AL, Fischer A, et al. Mycopheno-late mofetil is safe, well tolerated, and preserves lung function in patients with connective tissue disease-related interstitial lung disease. Chest 2006;130(1):30–6.

67. Fischer A, Brown KK, Du Bois RM, et al. Mycophe-nolate mofetil improves lung function in connective tissue disease-associated interstitial lung disease. J Rheumatol 2013;40(5):640–6.

68. Ge Y, Zhou H, Shi J, et al. The efficacy of tacrolimus in patients with refractory dermatomyositis/polymyositis: a systematic review. Clin Rheumatol 2015; 34(12):2097–103.

69. Sharma N, Putman MS, Vij R, et al. Myositis-associated interstitial lung disease: predictors of failure of conventional treatment and response to tacrolimus in a US cohort. J Rheumatol 2017;44(11):1612–8.

70. Kurita T, Yasuda S, Oba K, et al. The efficacy of tacrolimus in patients with interstitial lung diseases complicated with polymyositis or dermatomyositis. Rheumatology 2014;54(1):39–44.

71. Ge Y, Peng Q, Zhang S, et al. Cyclophosphamide treatment for idiopathic inflammatory myopathies and related interstitial lung disease: a systematic review. Clin Rheumatol 2014;34(1):99–105.

72. Bauhammer J, Blank N, Max R, et al. Rituximab in the treatment of Jo1 antibody–associated antisynthetase syndrome: anti-Ro52 positivity as a marker for severity and treatment response. J Rheumatol 2016;43(8):1566–74.

73. Andersson H, Sem M, Lund MB, et al. Long-term experience with rituximab in anti-synthetase syndrome-related interstitial lung disease. Rheumatology 2015;54(8):1420–8.

74. Allenbach Y, Guiguet M, Rigolet A, et al. Efficacy of rituximab in refractory inflammatory myopathies associated with anti- synthetase auto-antibodies: an open-label, phase II trial. PLoS One 2015; 10(11):e0133702.

75. Suzuki Y, Hayakawa H, Miwa S, et al. Intravenous immunoglobulin therapy for refractory interstitial lung disease associated with polymyositis/dermatomyositis. Lung 2009;187(3):201–6.

76. Bakewell CJ, Raghu G. Polymyositis associated with severe interstitial lung disease. Chest 2011;139(2): 441–3.

77. Hallowell RW, Amariei D, Danoff SK. Intravenous immunoglobulin as potential adjunct therapy for interstitial lung disease. Ann Am Thorac Soc 2016; 13(10):1682–8.

78. Cobo-Ibáñez T, López-Longo F-J, Joven B, et al. Long-term pulmonary outcomes and mortality in idiopathic inflammatory myopathies associated with interstitial lung disease. Clin Rheumatol 2019; 38(3):803–15.

79. Fathi M, Helmers SB, Lundberg IE. KL-6: a serological biomarker for interstitial lung disease in patients with polymyositis and dermatomyositis. J Intern Med 2011;271(6):589–97.

80. Chen F, Lu X, Shu X, et al. Predictive value of serum markers for the development of interstitial lung disease in patients with polymyositis and dermatomyositis: a comparative and prospective study. Intern Med J 2015;45(6):641–7.

81. Nakazawa M, Kaneko Y, Takeuchi T. Risk factors for the recurrence of interstitial lung disease in patients with polymyositis and dermatomyositis: a retrospective cohort study. Clin Rheumatol 2017;37(3): 765–71.

82. Sugiyama Y, Yoshimi R, Tamura M, et al. The predictive prognostic factors for polymyositis/dermatomyositis associated interstitial lung disease. Arthritis Res Ther 2018;20:7.

83. Zou J, Guo Q, Chi J, et al. HRCT score and serum ferritin level are factors associated to the 1-year mortality of acute interstitial lung disease in clinically amyopathic dermatomyositis patients. Clin Rheumatol 2015;34(4):707–14.

84. Ikeda S, Arita M, Misaki K, et al. Incidence and impact of interstitial lung disease and malignancy in patients with polymyositis, dermatomyositis, and clinically amyopathic dermatomyositis: a retrospective cohort study. Springerplus 2015;4(1):240.

Update on the Management of Respiratory Manifestations of the Antineutrophil Cytoplasmic Antibodies-Associated Vasculitides

Gwen E. Thompson, MD, MPH, Ulrich Specks, MD*

KEYWORDS

- Antineutrophil cytoplasmic antibodies • ANCA • Vasculitis • Granulomatosis with polyangiitis
- Microscopic polyangiitis • Eosinophilic granulomatosis with polyangiitis • Interstitial lung disease
- Alveolar hemorrhage

KEY POINTS

- Necrotizing granulomatous inflammation is the disease-defining pathologic feature separating granulomatosis with polyangiitis (GPA) from microscopic polyangiitis (MPA).
- Tracheobronchial involvement is more common in GPA than MPA and can cause airway obstruction. Management requires an individualized approach.
- Rituximab has replaced cyclophosphamide in the management of most patients with GPA and MPA, including those presenting with diffuse alveolar hemorrhage.
- An association between MPA and interstitial lung disease has recently been recognized.
- Targeting interleukin-5 with mepolizumab has significant and clinically important glucocorticoid-sparing effects in the management of eosinophilic ganulomatosis with polyangiitis (EGPA).

INTRODUCTION

Antineutrophil cytoplasmic antibody-associated vasculitis (AAV) is an umbrella term for the 3 small vessel vasculitis syndromes, granulomatosis with polyangiitis (GPA), microscopic polyangiitis (MPA), and eosinophilic polyangiitis (EGPA).[1] The designation AAV was chosen because antineutrophil cytoplasmic antibodies (ANCA) are common and thought to contribute materially to the pathogenesis of the small vessel vasculitis.[1] However, the diagnosis of an AAV does not require the presence of ANCA.[1] In GPA and MPA, the prevalence of ANCA is greater than 85%, whereas ANCA occur only in about 30% to 70% of patients with newly diagnosed untreated EGPA.[2–5] ANCA encountered in AAV are autoantibodies that are either directed against the neutrophil serine protease, proteinase 3 (PR3), or against the neutrophil enzyme, myeloperoxidase (MPO).[2] PR3-ANCA are the prevailing ANCA type in GPA, whereas most patients with MPA have MPO-ANCA.[2] Patients with EGPA are either ANCA-negative or have MPO-ANCA.[2–5]

In this article we describe the main clinical features and differential diagnosis of large airway

Disclosures: None for all authors.
Thoracic Disease Research Unit, Division of Pulmonary and Critical Care Medicine, Mayo Clinic, 200 First Street Southwest, Rochester, MN 55905, USA
* Corresponding author.
E-mail address: specks.ulrich@mayo.edu

Clin Chest Med 40 (2019) 573–582
https://doi.org/10.1016/j.ccm.2019.05.012

involvement and pulmonary parenchymal mani-festations of GPA and MPA. The pulmonologist's perspective is emphasized. General treatment recommendations for GPA and MPA are referred to briefly, as we focus on recent practice-changing developments in the field. We also pro-vide a brief overview of EGPA with particular emphasis on the rationale and emerging role of biologic therapy.

NECROTIZING GRANULOMATOUS INFLAMMATION OF THE LUNG

Necrotizing granulomatous inflammation is the disease-defining histopathologic hallmark of GPA, setting it apart from MPA and EGPA.[1] Accordingly, clinical disease manifestations including radiographic findings caused by necro-tizing granulomatous inflammation allow the distinction of GPA from MPA.[1] Most patients with GPA have PR3-ANCA rather than MPO-ANCA (**Fig. 1**). Pathognomonic histopathologic pulmo-nary features associated with GPA include neutro-philic microabscesses, fibrinoid necrosis, palisading histiocytes, and giant cells forming a pattern that is, often called "geographic necro-sis."[6] Areas involved with this type of necrotizing granulomatous inflammation may encroach on vessel walls or contain focal vasculitis, throm-bosis, and fibrous obliteration of the lumen of ves-sels.[6] Less-specific histopathologic features including organizing pneumonia, bronchocentric inflammation, and occasionally prominent eosino-phils within inflammatory infiltrates have also been reported to occur.[7,8]

Solitary or multiple pulmonary nodules or mass lesions with or without cavitation or nonspecific pulmonary infiltrates that are radiographically indistinguishable from pneumonia represent the radiographic correlates of the necrotizing granulo-matous inflammation (**Fig. 2**). The inflammatory le-sions often have a peribronchial distribution that is detectable by computed tomography (CT).[9] As nodules or mass lesions shrink and ultimately disappear under appropriate medical therapy,

fibrotic strands may be left behind as residual scars. These are not to be confused with the inter-stitial lung disease associated with MPO-ANCA or MPA (see later discussion). The differential diag-nosis of these lesions includes infections, orga-nizing pneumonia, and malignancies.[9] Fungal infections such as histoplasmosis, coccidioidomy-cosis, or blastomycosis are endemic in certain defined areas of the world. *Nocardia* infections, which can affect both immunocompetent and immunocompromised patients have been re-ported as mimickers of GPA.[10,11] Organizing pneumonia may represent a particularly difficult differential diagnostic challenge for several rea-sons: cryptogenic organizing pneumonia can be radiographically indistinguishable from GPA limited to the lung, organizing pneumonia can occur in GPA,[8] and cryptogenic organizing pneu-monia responds to glucocorticoid therapy. Multi-ple bilateral pulmonary nodules should also prompt consideration of metastatic disease and lymphoproliferative disorders in the differential diagnosis. Lymphomatoid granulomatosis is a rare angiocentric and angiodestructive, Epstein-Barr virus-related T-cell-rich B-cell lymphoma that can also mimic GPA because, like GPA, it often affects different extrapulmonary organs.[12,13]

The pulmonary lesions caused by the necro-tizing granulomatous inflammation may be asymp-tomatic and result in little or no measurable impairment of lung function. In fact, in newly diag-nosed patients lung nodules and mass lesions may represent incidental radiographic findings. For the same reason, chest imaging needs to be an integral component of the diagnostic evaluation when patients with GPA are screened for disease activity during follow-up, even in the absence of respiratory symptoms.

Such lesions may cause cough and minor he-moptysis when the lesions have access to subseg-mental bronchi. Cavitation develops when the central necrosis of the granulomatous inflamma-tory lesion feeds into a draining airway. When cav-ities become infected, air-fluid levels may appear;

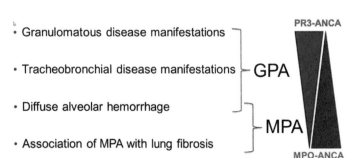

- Granulomatous disease manifestations
- Tracheobronchial disease manifestations
- Diffuse alveolar hemorrhage
- Association of MPA with lung fibrosis

GPA

MPA

PR3-ANCA

MPO-ANCA

Fig. 1. Schematic of tracheobronchial and pulmonary disease manifestations of GPA and MPA and their relation-ship with clinical diagnosis and ANCA serology.

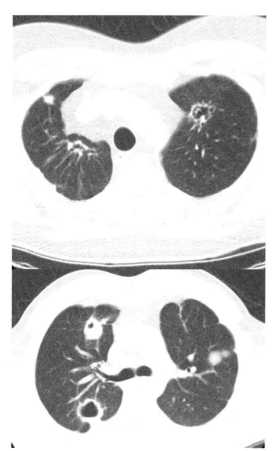

Fig. 2. Examples of necrotizing granulomatous lung lesions of GPA.

this should lead to a careful microbiologic evaluation with subsequent targeted antibiotic therapy.

Bronchoscopically obtained samples for cytology and mirobiologic studies should be part of the differential diagnostic evaluation of lung nodules or masses. Transbronchoscopically obtained tissue samples support the diagnosis of GPA in about 50% of patients with other supportive clinical features or positive ANCA test results.[14] In up to 25% of patients such tissue samples were found to be diagnostic by themselves.[14] Depending on the location of the lesions, CT-guided core needle biopsy or transbronchial biopsies may be preferred. The highest diagnostic yield is achieved with a video-assisted thoracoscopic (VATS) lung biopsy, but because of the associated higher morbidity, and even some mortality, its risk benefit ratio should be weighed carefully. VATS biopsy is usually only necessary in patients who present with isolated pulmonary involvement.

The disease manifestations caused by necrotizing granulomatous inflammation are rarely life threatening or organ threatening, and they progress more slowly than capillaritis-related disease manifestations (see later discussion). Therefore, they are classified as "non-severe" disease manifestations for the purpose of treatment stratification. Patients who have only non-severe disease manifestations, but no "severe" disease manifestations, should receive glucocorticoids in combination with methotrexate as first-line remission induction therapy.[15] Patients who fail this regimen usually respond well to the combination of glucocorticoids and rituximab.[16,17] If the overall pulmonary disease burden is deemed extensive, treatment following the recommendations for severe disease (defined as either life threatening or organ threatening) consisting of the combination of glucocorticoids with either cyclophosphamide or rituximab may be appropriate.[15] Most of the patients with such severe disease are PR3-ANCA positive. Rituximab has been shown to be superior to cyclophosphamide for relapsing patients with GPA and for patients who are PR3-ANCA positive and, consequently, is the preferred choice for initial therapy.[18]

TRACHEOBRONCHIAL INFLAMMATION

Tracheobronchial involvement has been reported in 15% to 55% of patients with GPA, but it is not a frequent disease manifestation of MPA.[19] Women are more frequently affected (76%) than men.[20] PR3-ANCA is the most common ANCA type encountered in patients with tracheobronchial inflammation, including subglottic inflammation and subsequent stenosis.[20] However, MPO-ANCA has also been reported with less frequency, and patients may be ANCA negative.[20] The tracheobronchial inflammation is interpreted as a sign of necrotizing granulomatous inflammation, but the classic histopathologic features of GPA can rarely be found on endobronchial biopsy specimens. Consequently, whether tracheobronchial involvement is reported as a feature of GPA or MPA in cohort reports depends on the clinician's acceptance and application of different disease definitions, as well as of clinical surrogates for GPA-defining necrotizing granulomatous inflammation.[21–23]

The tracheobronchial inflammation of GPA is usually localized or patchy in distribution throughout the airway with affected areas adjacent to normal appearing airways. This distribution pattern sets it apart from tracheobronchial inflammation encountered in the context of relapsing polychondritis.[24] The airway inflammation may affect any level of the tracheobronchial tree from the trachea down to the subsegmental airways, with the subglottic region being most commonly involved. The bronchoscopic appearance of airways affected by tracheobronchial inflammation can include mucosal erythema, edematous swelling, friability, and ulcerations or so-called "cobble-stoning" (**Fig. 3**A). The inflammation is often circumferential, which predisposes to the development of subsequent cicatricial stenosis or complete occlusion during otherwise successful immunosuppressive therapy (**Fig. 3**B). If the inflammation is transmural it is detectable by CT imaging of the chest. When the inflammation affects tracheobronchial cartilages, significant expiratory dynamic airway collapse may ensue from tracheomalacia or bronchomalacia.

In the absence of other typical organ manifestations of GPA or typical PR3- or MPO-ANCA, the differential diagnosis of the tracheobronchial inflammation of GPA may be difficult. Relapsing polychondritis,[24] inflammatory bowel disease,[25,26] sarcoidosis,[27] and infections, particularly with fungal organisms, should be considered as alternative causes. The differential diagnostic reasoning is further complicated because patients with relapsing polychondritis, inflammatory bowel disease, or bacterial infections, all may have nonspecific ANCA.[2]

Symptoms related to the airway inflammation of GPA are nonspecific. Early inflammatory lesions without significant airway stenosis may be completely asymptomatic or cause cough with or without hemoptysis. Localized large airway obstruction can result in localized wheezes heard on careful auscultation, whereas stridor is a feature of subglottic stenosis.

If airway lesions are suspected, the diagnostic approach should include pulmonary function testing, flexible fiberoptic bronchoscopy, and, in selected cases, CT for 3-dimensional reconstruction images of the airways.[19] Pulmonary function testing should be performed in any patient with GPA with respiratory symptoms or with radiographic abnormalities of the pulmonary parenchyma or the airways. Abnormalities of the shapes of the inspiratory or expiratory flow-volume tracings are sensitive, but not specific, indicators of the presence of airway stenoses, and may provide an estimate of their functional severity. Measurements of the maximum voluntary ventilation during pulmonary function testing or of the peak expiratory flow using a peak flow meter are useful for the functional assessment of airflow limitation. Repeated measurements over time provide valuable information about the effect of medical therapy or bronchoscopic interventions on airway patency (see later discussion).

Flexible fiberoptic bronchoscopy is indicated for patients who have respiratory symptoms, abnormalities on pulmonary function testing, or abnormal findings on chest imaging studies. Bronchoscopy is useful to assess and map inflammatory lesions of the large airways, to obtain

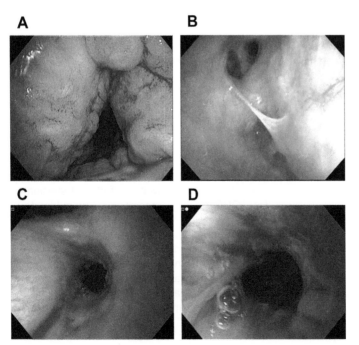

A **B** **C** **D**

Fig. 3. Examples of tracheobronchial lesions and intervention. (A) Inflammatory lesions of GPA in the subglottic region of a patient causing a "cobblestone" appearance. (B) Complete occlusion of the bronchus intermedius as well as a nonobstructing synechial band just distal to the RC1 carina without any sign of active inflammation in a patient with longstanding history of GPA with tracheobronchial involvement. (C) Recurrent stenosis at the right mainstem orifice. (D) Same right mainstem stenosis after balloon dilation.

specimens for microbiologic studies, and to plan therapeutic interventions and monitor their outcomes. When patients are evaluated for dilation procedures or stent placement it is important to know the length of airway stenoses and the patency of airways distal to stenoses that cannot accommodate a pediatric bronchoscope. This information can often be provided by "virtual bronchoscopy" or 3-dimensional reconstruction of CT images of the airways.[28]

The management of tracheobronchial involvement of GPA is often complex and challenging as it requires an individualized approach to each patient and often goes beyond standard immunosuppressive therapy. Tracheobronchial inflammatory lesions may be more resistant to systemic immunosuppressive therapy compared with other disease manifestations. Progressive airway obstruction sometimes occurs during systemic immunosuppressive therapy as a consequence of scarring or damage, which may explain their resistance to immunosuppressive therapy. Fixed airway obstructions may be amenable to dilation procedures or stent placements (**Fig. 3**C, D). Dynamic airway collapse resulting from tracheo- or bronchomalacia may benefit from continuous positive airway pressure treatment. Persistent or recurrent airway infections with *Staphylococcus aureus* or *Pseudomonas aeruginosa* are common, and may represent "antigenic drivers" of the autoimmune inflammation. Therefore, positive culture results of specimens obtained from the airways of patients with GPA should not be dismissed as "colonization" but should rather be treated according to antimicrobial susceptibility results. As silent gastro-esophageal reflux may also aggravate airway inflammation, particularly subglottic inflammation, we advocate for dietary and behavioral reflux precautions, in addition to acid-blocking therapy, for patients with GPA and airway involvement. Lastly, to suppress airway inflammation while minimizing cumulative systemic glucocorticoid exposure, we also advocate for the use of high-dose inhaled glucocorticoids in patients with tracheobronchial disease.

DIFFUSE ALVEOLAR HEMORRHAGE AND PULMONARY CAPILLARITIS

ANCA-associated vasculitis is the leading cause of capillaritis causing diffuse alveolar hemorrhage (DAH).[29] DAH is a severe disease manifestation of GPA or MPA occurring in about a quarter of patients.[17,30] By contrast, DAH is a rare occurrence (0%–10%) in EGPA.[3–5] Symptoms of DAH are nonspecific, consisting of various degrees of dyspnea, hypoxemia, diffuse alveolar filling defects detectable by chest imaging studies (**Fig. 4**), and anemia.

Up to 50% of patients with DAH do not present with hemoptysis.[31,32] Therefore, DAH should be suspected in patients with GPA or MPA who have alveolar filling defects on chest imaging and need to be confirmed or ruled out by bronchoscopy with bronchoalveolar lavage (BAL). Hemorrhage originating in the alveolar spaces results in progressively bloodier BAL returns, whereas returned aliquots gradually clear if the blood is aspirated, or the bleeding source is in the tracheobronchial tree.[33] BAL also offers the opportunity to obtain specimens for microbiologic studies to identify or exclude infection. The BAL return may be clear if bleeding has ceased by the time the procedure is performed. In that case at least 20% of alveolar macrophages should be laden with hemosiderin. Unfortunately, the finding of greater than 20% hemosiderin-laden macrophages on the differential cell count of the BAL fluid is not specific for DAH,

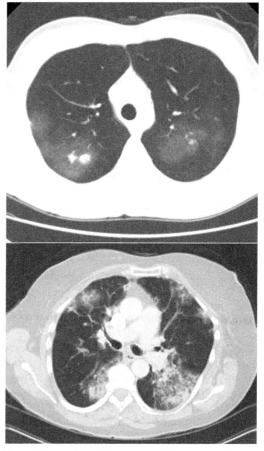

Fig. 4. Examples of radiographic appearance of diffuse alveolar hemorrhage in patients with GPA. Alveolar hemorrhage was documented by bronchoalveolar lavage in both cases.

because up to 30% of patients with diffuse alveolar damage may also fulfill this criterion.[34] It is not entirely clear how long it takes for iron-laden alveolar macrophages to become detectable after the onset of intra-alveolar bleeding in humans. Based on a study performed in mice, in which hemosiderin was first detectable in alveolar macrophages on day 3 following intranasal blood instillation, it is assumed to take a minimum of 24 to 48 hours for the macrophages to engulf the hemoglobin and turn positive on iron stains.[35] The percentage of BAL hemosiderin-laden alveolar macrophages has not been associated with the severity of DAH, but the presence of greater than 30% neutrophils on the BAL differential cell count has been identified as an independent risk factor for development of respiratory failure, probably because it is an indirect marker for the severity of the interstitial inflammation.[31] Although bronchoscopy with BAL is indispensable for the unequivocal diagnosis of DAH, it cannot be emphasized enough that the procedure itself may result in the temporary acute worsening of the patient's respiratory status. Therefore, it should only be performed in a setting that allows for an escalation of the level of care that assures the needed respiratory support including intubation and mechanical ventilation.

A lung biopsy is usually not necessary for the diagnosis of GPA or MPA in patients with DAH. In fact, it is associated with a very unfavorable risk-to-benefit ratio. A tissue confirmation of GPA or MPA, if necessary, can usually be obtained more safely from other organs including skin, nose and sinuses, or kidneys. In contrast to a lung biopsy, a kidney biopsy may not only provide a diagnosis, but also valuable prognostic information.[36–38]

DAH may be part of the initial presentation of GPA or MPA or occur as part of a disease relapse. Consequently, in patients who receive immunosuppressive therapy for the underlying disease, the development of dyspnea, hypoxemia, and radiographic alveolar filling defects should prompt a bronchoscopic evaluation with BAL to look for DAH and to rule out an immunocompromised host infection.

Any degree of DAH needs to be categorized as a severe disease manifestation of GPA and MPA because it can rapidly progress to respiratory failure threatening the patient's life. Mortality rates of 10% to 25% have been reported for large patient cohorts.[31,39] Three independent risk factors for the progression to respiratory failure have recently been identified by multivariate analysis in DAH caused by GPA or MPA.[31] These include (i) an oxygen saturation measured by pulse oximetry (SpO_2) to fraction of inspired oxygen (Fio_2) ratio

of less than 450 (odds ratio [OR] = 74, 95% CI, 9–180) measured at the time of first presentation, (ii) a C-reactive protein level >25 mg/dL (OR = 7.4, 95% CI, 1.7–48), and (iii) the presence of greater than 30% neutrophils on the differential cell count of the BAL fluid (OR = 6.4, 95% CI, 1.6–34).[31] These data emphasize that the SpO_2:-Fio_2 ratio should be determined in any patient with GPA or MPA presenting with dyspnea or with a pulmonary infiltrate, even if dyspnea or hemoptysis are absent, so that the appropriate level of care can be chosen for the implementation of further diagnostic and therapeutic interventions.

If patients survive the original episode of DAH, their response to immunosuppressive therapy following the standard recommendations for treatment of patients severe disease manifestation of GPA or MPA is similar to patients with all other disease manifestations of GPA and MPA in aggregate.[17,31] Moreover, the lung parenchyma usually recovers without significant loss in lung function provided that effective therapy can be implemented early and before the development of diffuse alveolar damage.[40]

If implemented in a timely fashion, patients with DAH caused by GPA or MPA respond well to standard therapy for severe disease manifestations. In the Rituximab for ANCA-Associated Vasculitis (RAVE) trial the response of patients with DAH to the application of 1 to 3 daily pulses of 1 g of intravenous methyl-prednisolone followed by oral prednisone in combination with either rituximab (RTX) or cyclophosphamide (CYC) was equivalent to that of the entire trial cohort.[17] A detailed analysis of the largest single center cohort (n = 73) revealed that patients with DAH caused by GPA or MPA had similar early response rates and hospital survival whether treated with RTX or CYC. Complete remission, defined as a Birmingham Vasculitis Activity score of 0 and complete discontinuation of prednisone by 6 months, was superior in patients treated with RTX compared with those who received CYC (89% vs 68%, P = .02). This was also the case for the subset of patients who required mechanical ventilation (n = 31, 83% with RTX vs 42% with CYC, P = .02), a group of patients who were excluded from enrollment into the RAVE trial.[31]

A single report of 20 patients with DAH caused by MPA who received treatment with plasma exchange (PLEX) in addition to standard immunosuppressive therapy raised enthusiasm for PLEX as an adjuvant with potential to curb the early mortality associated with DAH in the setting of AAV.[41] However, a larger single-center cohort analysis of 73 patients, 32 of which were treated with PLEX, did not identify any benefit derived from PLEX after adjustment for the disease severity and treatment (RTX vs CYC).[31] More importantly, the results from the largest multicenter randomized controlled trial (RCT) ever conducted in AAV, which was designed to compare the efficacy of PLEX versus no PLEX also showed no benefit of PLEX in the entire cohort or in the subset of patients with DAH.[42] Consequently, the use of PLEX in addition to standard immunosuppressive therapy can no longer be advocated for patients with DAH caused by GPA or MPA.

INTERSTITIAL LUNG DISEASE AND ANTINEUTROPHIL CYTOPLASMIC ANTIBODIES WITH OR WITHOUT MICROSCOPIC POLYANGIITIS

Case reports and case series from all over the world have recently documented interstitial lung disease in patients who are ANCA positive, and an association between fibrotic interstitial lung disease (ILD) and MPO-ANCA and MPA is increasingly recognized.[43–45] However, it remains unclear whether there is a pathogenic relationship between MPO-ANCA and pulmonary fibrosis, or whether lung fibrosis is a disease manifestation of AAV versus an independent comorbidity. Based on careful review and analysis of available reports the following theme emerges.

For most cases the ILD either has radiographic and histopathologic features of usual interstitial pneumonia (UIP) or nonspecific interstitial pneumonitis (NSIP) (**Fig. 5**).[44] In addition, atypical features including follicular bronchiolitis have also been reported.[44] MPO-ANCA is the predominant ANCA type encountered in the context of ILD. In contrast, PR3-ANCA occur rarely. These patients may or may not have abnormal markers of inflammation or typical signs of vasculitis (MPA) in other organs. Patients who are MPO-ANCA positive with ILD have a 25% chance of subsequently developing clinical features of MPA.[46,47] This progression to MPA has been documented for MPO-ANCA, but not for PR3-ANCA.[46]

The lung disease seems to precede the development of frank MPA. This is most clearly documented for lung fibrosis with radiographic patterns of UIP.[44] Patients who present with a radiographic pattern of NSIP show a response to immunosuppressive therapy for their ILD, whereas patients with UIP seem unresponsive to immunosuppressive therapy, and lung function continues to decline as expected for idiopathic pulmonary fibrosis.

Patients with overt manifestations of MPA, with or without DAH superimposed on their ILD, show

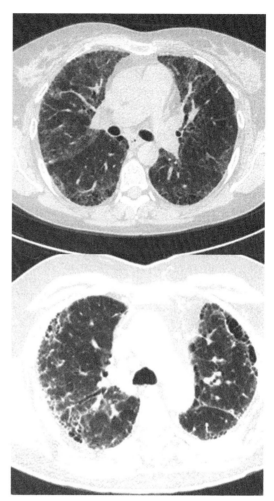

Fig. 5. Interstitial lung disease in patients with microscopic polyangiitis. The upper panel shows a computed tomography section obtained from a patient with MPO-ANCA and pauci-immune glomerulonephritis. Prominent ground glass infiltrates as well as traction bronchiectasis are seen. Alveolar hemorrhage and infection were ruled out by bronchoscopy with BAL. The findings are consistent with a predominant NSIP pattern even though some peripheral honeycombing was also noted. The lower panel shows a typical UIP pattern by high-resolution computed tomography.

a clinical response to immunosuppressive therapy for the vasculitis disease manifestations as expected for MPA. If overt MPA is present, the ILD may respond to immunosuppressive therapy if the fibrosis has features of cellular NSIP. However, if the patient's lung fibrosis pattern is consistent with UIP, a response of the lung fibrosis to immunosuppression should not be expected. It remains unclear whether such patients with UIP would benefit from treatment with antifibrotic agents.

Based on these observations, pulmonologists at Mayo Clinic have adopted an empiric clinical management approach to patients with MPO-ANCA and ILD, which is summarized in **Fig. 6**. This clinical approach assures that patients with unequivocal disease manifestations attributable to MPA receive appropriate therapy for severe disease manifestations of MPA in the form of remission induction therapy with glucocorticoids and cyclophosphamide or rituximab following the principles and guidelines of therapy for AAV.[15] Also, patients who present with an NSIP pattern will receive a trial of immunosuppressive therapy, even in the absence of other organ disease manifestations of MPA. Because this immunosuppressive therapy is generally regarded as effective remission maintenance therapy for AAV, it may prevent the development of overt MPA in other organs and prevent progression of the lung disease to irreversible fibrosis. At present, no beneficial effect of immunosuppressive therapy on the lung fibrosis of the UIP pattern has been reported in patients with MPO-ANCA, with or without features of MPA. Therefore, we do not believe that immunosuppressive therapy is beneficial or indicated in such patients in the absence of other overt features of MPA. However, because up to 25% of such patients will subsequently develop MPA, and the development of renal disease can be slow and indolent, yet cause irreversible renal insufficiency, we monitor patients for the development of glomerulonephritis by screening the urine for microhematuria (Hemastix) at least on a monthly basis. By doing so, the development of glomerulonephritis can be detected early, and effective therapy can be initiated before severe renal damage occurs. At the same time, such patients with UIP are not exposed to immunosuppressive therapy that may be detrimental as documented by a RCT of idiopathic pulmonary fibrosis.[48] As the UIP seems to precede disease manifestations of MPA in most patients, we do not consider the lung fibrosis a priori a disease manifestation of MPA, but rather a preexisting comorbidity, and

antifibrotic therapy may be an appropriate option for such patients with UIP.

BRIEF UPDATE ON THE MANAGEMENT OF EOSINOPHILIC GRANULOMATOSIS WITH POLYANGIITIS

EGPA is 1 of the 3 AAV syndromes despite the presence of ANCA, usually of the MPO-ANCA type, reported only for 30% to 70% of patients with newly diagnosed and untreated EGPA.[3–5] The disease is distinguished from MPA and GPA by an allergic background consisting of various degrees of atopy, nose and sinus disease, including nasal polyposis, as well as asthma, peripheral blood, and tissue eosinophilia, which usually precede the development of small vessel vasculitis.[1,3–5] Because of these differences, patients with EGPA have been excluded from most RCTs conducted in AAV, and only 1 recent RCT dedicated to EGPA has been completed.[49] Nevertheless, treatment recommendations for the vasculitis disease manifestations of EGPA are extrapolated from studies completed in the MPA and GPA patient populations.[50] Glucocorticoids are the mainstay of therapy in EGPA and are used as primary remission induction agent for all patients. In patients without life-threatening or organ-threatening disease manifestations, such as cardiac, gastrointestinal or renal involvement, or mononeuritis multiplex, additional immunosuppression is considered if the prednisone dose cannot be effectively tapered below a stable prednisone dose of 10 mg per day.[50] For patients with life-threatening or organ-threatening disease manifestations, CYC has been most frequently used for induction of remission in conjunction with glucocorticoids, and once remission has been induced CYC is replaced by other glucocorticoid-sparing agents such as azathioprine for maintenance of remission.[50]

RTX has also been used for induction of remission in EGPA. However, no RCTs have been completed to date, and the existing evidence from small pilot studies and retrospective reviews

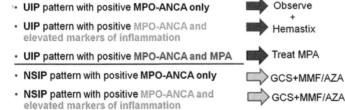

- • **UIP** pattern with positive **MPO-ANCA only** ➡ Observe + Hemastix
- • **UIP** pattern with positive MPO-ANCA and elevated markers of inflammation ➡
- • **UIP** pattern with positive **MPO-ANCA and MPA** ➡ Treat MPA
- • **NSIP** pattern with positive **MPO-ANCA only** ⇨ GCS+MMF/AZA
- • **NSIP** pattern with positive MPO-ANCA and elevated markers of inflammation ⇨ GCS+MMF/AZA
- • **NSIP** pattern with positive **MPO-ANCA and MPA** ➡ Treat MPA

Fig. 6. Proposed management approach for patients with interstitial lung disease and positive MPO-ANCA test result.

suggests that patients who are positive for MPO-ANCA benefit the most.[51,52] Two RCTs currently being conducted in France are designed to further characterize the role of RTX for induction and maintenance of remission in EGPA.

The most significant advance in the management of EGPA has been achieved with the introduction of mepolizumab, a humanized monoclonal antibody targeting interleukin-5 (IL-5), a cytokine that regulates the proliferation and maturation of eosinophils, and which has been found to be increased in patients with EGPA.[53] Results from a large randomized double-blind placebo-controlled trial have shown significant and clinically relevant glucocorticoid-sparing effects of mepolizumab in most patients with EGPA.[49] Unfortunately, the effect of IL-5 targeted therapy on severe eosinophil-driven or vasculitic disease manifestations remains unclear, because patients with such disease manifestations were excluded from the trial.[49,54]

REFERENCES

1. Jennette JC, Falk RJ, Bacon PA, et al. 2012 Revised international Chapel Hill consensus conference nomenclature of vasculitides. Arthritis Rheum 2013; 65(1):1–11.

2. Hoffman GS, Specks U. Antineutrophil cytoplasmic antibodies. Arthritis Rheum 1998;41(9):1521–37.

3. Keogh KA, Specks U. Churg-Strauss syndrome: clinical presentation, antineutrophil cytoplasmic antibodies, and leukotriene receptor antagonists. Am J Med 2003;115(4):284–90.

4. Sinico RA, Di Toma L, Maggiore U, et al. Prevalence and clinical significance of antineutrophil cytoplasmic antibodies in Churg-Strauss syndrome. Arthritis Rheum 2005;52(9):2926–35.

5. Comarmond C, Pagnoux C, Khellaf M, et al. Eosinophilic granulomatosis with polyangiitis (Churg-Strauss): clinical characteristics and long-term followup of the 383 patients enrolled in the French Vasculitis Study Group cohort. Arthritis Rheum 2013;65(1):270–81.

6. Colby TV, Specks U. Wegener's granulomatosis in the 1990s–a pulmonary pathologist's perspective. Monogr Pathol 1993;(36):195–218.

7. Travis WD, Hoffman GS, Leavitt RY, et al. Surgical pathology of the lung in Wegener's granulomatosis. Review of 87 open lung biopsies from 67 patients. Am J Surg Pathol 1991;15(4):315–33.

8. Travis WD. Common and uncommon manifestations of Wegener's granulomatosis. Cardiovasc Pathol 1994;3(3):217–25.

9. Martinez F, Chung JH, Digumarthy SR, et al. Common and uncommon manifestations of Wegener granulomatosis at chest CT: radiologic-pathologic correlation. Radiographics 2012;32(1):51–69.

10. Gibb W, Williams A. Nocardiosis mimicking Wegener's granulomatosis. Scand J Infect Dis 1986; 18(6):583–5.

11. Singh A, Chhina D, Soni RK, et al. Clinical spectrum and outcome of pulmonary nocardiosis: 5-year experience. Lung India 2016;33(4):398–403.

12. Wechsler RJ, Steiner RM, Israel HL, et al. Chest radiograph in lymphomatoid granulomatosis: comparison with Wegener granulomatosis. AJR Am J Roentgenol 1984;142(1):79–83.

13. Roschewski M, Wilson WH. Lymphomatoid granulomatosis. Cancer J 2012;18(5):469–74.

14. Daum TE, Specks U, Colby TV, et al. Tracheobronchial involvement in Wegener's granulomatosis. Am J Respir Crit Care Med 1995;151(2 Pt 1):522–6.

15. Yates M, Watts RA, Bajema IM, et al. EULAR/ERA-EDTA recommendations for the management of ANCA-associated vasculitis. Ann Rheum Dis 2016;75(9): 1583–94.

16. Seo P, Specks U, Keogh KA. Efficacy of rituximab in limited Wegener's granulomatosis with refractory granulomatous manifestations. J Rheumatol 2008; 35(10):2017–23.

17. Stone JH, Merkel PA, Spiera R, et al. Rituximab versus cyclophosphamide for ANCA-associated vasculitis. N Engl J Med 2010;363(3):221–32.

18. Unizony S, Villarreal M, Miloslavsky EM, et al. Clinical outcomes of treatment of anti-neutrophil cytoplasmic antibody (ANCA)-associated vasculitis based on ANCA type. Ann Rheum Dis 2016;75(6):1166–9.

19. Polychronopoulos VS, Prakash UB, Golbin JM, et al. Airway involvement in Wegener's granulomatosis. Rheum Dis Clin North Am 2007;33(4):755–75, vi.

20. Marroquin-Fabian E, Ruiz N, Mena-Zuniga J, et al. Frequency, treatment, evolution, and factors associated with the presence of tracheobronchial stenoses in granulomatosis with polyangiitis. Retrospective analysis of a case series from a single respiratory referral center. Semin Arthritis Rheum 2019;48(4):714–9.

21. Jennette JC, Falk RJ, Andrassy K, et al. Nomenclature of systemic vasculitides. Proposal of an international consensus conference. Arthritis Rheum 1994; 37(2):187–92.

22. Watts R, Lane S, Hanslik T, et al. Development and validation of a consensus methodology for the classification of the ANCA-associated vasculitides and polyarteritis nodosa for epidemiological studies. Ann Rheum Dis 2007;66(2):222–7.

23. Lionaki S, Blyth ER, Hogan SL, et al. Classification of antineutrophil cytoplasmic autoantibody vasculitides: the role of antineutrophil cytoplasmic autoantibody specificity for myeloperoxidase or proteinase 3 in disease recognition and prognosis. Arthritis Rheum 2012;64(10):3452–62.

24. Ernst A, Rafeq S, Boiselle P, et al. Relapsing polychondritis and airway involvement. Chest 2009; 135(4):1024–30.

25. Chiu K, Wright JL. Large and small airway disease related to inflammatory bowel disease. Arch Pathol Lab Med 2017;141(3):470–3.

26. Camus P, Colby TV. The lung in inflammatory bowel disease. Eur Respir J 2000;15(1):5–10.

27. Polychronopoulos VS, Prakash UBS. Airway involvement in sarcoidosis. Chest 2009;136(5):1371–80.

28. Summers RM, Aggarwal NR, Sneller MC, et al. CT virtual bronchoscopy of the central airways in patients with Wegener's granulomatosis. Chest 2002;121(1):242–50.

29. Niles JL, Bottinger EP, Saurina GR, et al. The syndrome of lung hemorrhage and nephritis is usually an ANCA-associated condition. Arch Intern Med 1996;156(4):440–5.

30. Hoffman GS, Kerr GS, Leavitt RY, et al. Wegener granulomatosis: an analysis of 158 patients. Ann Intern Med 1992;116(6):488–98.

31. Cartin-Ceba R, Diaz-Caballero L, Al-Qadi MO, et al. Diffuse alveolar hemorrhage secondary to antineutrophil cytoplasmic antibody-associated vasculitis: predictors of respiratory failure and clinical outcomes. Arthritis Rheumatol 2016;68(6):1467–76.

32. Lara AR, Schwarz MI. Diffuse alveolar hemorrhage. Chest 2010;137(5):1164–71.

33. Robbins RA, Linder J, Stahl MG, et al. Diffuse alveolar hemorrhage in autologous bone marrow transplant recipients. Am J Med 1989;87(5):511–8.

34. Maldonado F, Parambil JG, Yi ES, et al. Haemosiderin-laden macrophages in the bronchoalveolar lavage fluid of patients with diffuse alveolar damage. Eur Respir J 2009;33(6):1361–6.

35. Epstein CE, Elidemir O, Colasurdo GN, et al. Time course of hemosiderin production by alveolar macrophages in a murine model. Chest 2001;120(6):2013–20.

36. Berden AE, Ferrario F, Hagen EC, et al. Histopathologic classification of ANCA-associated glomerulonephritis. J Am Soc Nephrol 2010;21(10):1628–36.

37. Berti A, Cornec-Le Gall E, Cornec D, et al. Incidence, prevalence, mortality and chronic renal damage of anti-neutrophil cytoplasmic antibody-associated glomerulonephritis in a 20-year population-based cohort. Nephrol Dial Transplant 2018. https://doi.org/10.1093/ndt/gfy250.

38. Sethi S, Zand L, De Vriese AS, et al. Complement activation in pauci-immune necrotizing and crescentic glomerulonephritis: results of a proteomic analysis. Nephrol Dial Transplant 2017;32(suppl_1):i139–45.

39. de Prost N, Parrot A, Picard C, et al. Diffuse alveolar haemorrhage: factors associated with in-hospital and long-term mortality. Eur Respir J 2010;35(6):1303–11.

40. Lauque D, Cadranel J, Lazor R, et al. Microscopic polyangiitis with alveolar hemorrhage. A study of 29 cases and review of the literature. Groupe d'Etudes et de Recherche sur les Maladies "Orphelines" Pulmonaires (GERM"O"P). Medicine (Baltimore) 2000;79(4):222–33.

41. Klemmer PJ, Chalermskulrat W, Reif MS, et al. Plasmapheresis therapy for diffuse alveolar hemorrhage in patients with small-vessel vasculitis. Am J Kidney Dis 2003;42(6):1149–53.

42. Walsh M, Merkel PA, Jayne D. The effects of plasma exchange and reduced-dose glucocorticoids during remission-induction for treatment of severe ANCA-associated vasculitis [abstract]. Arthritis Rheumatol 2018;70(suppl 10).

43. Katsumata Y, Kawaguchi Y, Yamanaka H. Interstitial lung disease with ANCA-associated vasculitis. Clin Med Insights Circ Respir Pulm Med 2015;9(Suppl 1):51–6.

44. Alba MA, Flores-Suarez LF, Henderson AG, et al. Interstitial lung disease in ANCA vasculitis. Autoimmun Rev 2017;16(7):722–9.

45. Borie R, Crestani B. Antineutrophil cytoplasmic antibody-associated lung fibrosis. Semin Respir Crit Care Med 2018;39(4):465–70.

46. Kagiyama N, Takayanagi N, Kanauchi T, et al. Antineutrophil cytoplasmic antibody-positive conversion and microscopic polyangiitis development in patients with idiopathic pulmonary fibrosis. BMJ Open Respir Res 2015;2(1):e000058.

47. Hozumi H, Oyama Y, Yasui H, et al. Clinical significance of myeloperoxidase-anti-neutrophil cytoplasmic antibody in idiopathic interstitial pneumonias. PLoS One 2018;13(6):e0199659.

48. Idiopathic Pulmonary Fibrosis Clinical Research Network, Raghu G, Anstrom KJ, King TE, et al. Prednisone, azathioprine, and N-acetylcysteine for pulmonary fibrosis. N Engl J Med 2012;366(21):1968–77.

49. Wechsler ME, Akuthota P, Jayne D, et al. Mepolizumab or placebo for eosinophilic granulomatosis with polyangiitis. N Engl J Med 2017;376(20):1921–32.

50. Groh M, Pagnoux C, Baldini C, et al. Eosinophilic granulomatosis with polyangiitis (Churg-Strauss) (EGPA) Consensus Task Force recommendations for evaluation and management. Eur J Intern Med 2015;26(7):545–53.

51. Cartin-Ceba R, Keogh KA, Specks U, et al. Rituximab for the treatment of Churg-Strauss syndrome with renal involvement. Nephrol Dial Transplant 2011;26(9):2865–71.

52. Mohammad AJ, Hot A, Arndt F, et al. Rituximab for the treatment of eosinophilic granulomatosis with polyangiitis (Churg-Strauss). Ann Rheum Dis 2016;75(2):396–401.

53. Kim S, Marigowda G, Oren E, et al. Mepolizumab as a steroid-sparing treatment option in patients with Churg-Strauss syndrome. J Allergy Clin Immunol 2010;125(6):1336–43.

54. Steinfeld J, Bradford ES, Brown J, et al. Evaluation of clinical benefit from treatment with mepolizumab for patients with eosinophilic granulomatosis with polyangiitis. J Allergy Clin Immunol 2019;143(6):2170–7.

Immunoglobulin G4–related Disease

Zachary S. Wallace, MD, MSc[a,b,*], Cory Perugino, DO[b], Mark Matza, MD, MBA[c], Vikram Deshpande, MBBS[d], Amita Sharma, MBBS[e], John H. Stone, MD, MPH[b]

KEYWORDS

- IgG4-related disease • Pulmonary • Chest

KEY POINTS

- Thoracic manifestations of immunoglobulin G4–related disease (IgG4-RD) include lung nodules, pleural thickening, aortitis, and lymphadenopathy.
- Thoracic manifestations of IgG4-RD are often detected incidentally on imaging but can present with nonspecific symptoms such as dyspnea or cough.
- Biopsies of pulmonary lesions can distinguish IgG4-RD from common mimickers, including sarcoidosis, antineutrophil cytoplasmic antibody–associated vasculitis, and malignancy.

INTRODUCTION

Immunoglobulin G4 (IgG4)–related disease (IgG4-RD) is an immune-mediated condition that can cause fibroinflammatory lesions in nearly any organ.[1] The cause remains unknown. Common manifestations include dacryoadenitis (lacrimal gland inflammation), sclerosing sialoadenitis of the major salivary glands (submandibular, parotid, and sublingual), autoimmune pancreatitis, sclerosing cholangitis, and retroperitoneal fibrosis (RPF). Although variable across cohorts, up to 35% of patients with IgG4-RD[2] have manifestations in the chest. These manifestations include lung nodules, pleural thickening, pleural effusions, aortitis, sclerosing pericarditis, lymphadenopathy, and paravertebral masses. Patients with thoracic disease often present with nonspecific symptoms, including dyspnea or cough, but asymptomatic thoracic involvement is detected incidentally in many if not most IgG4-RD cases involving the chest.[2] The differential diagnosis of thoracic IgG4-RD is broad and includes infections (eg, tuberculosis), other autoimmune conditions (eg, antineutrophil cytoplasmic antibody [ANCA]–associated vasculitis), and malignancy, (eg, lymphoma, lung cancer). This article reviews IgG4-RD with an emphasis on thoracic disease, including its epidemiology, common presentations, diagnostic approach, and management.

EPIDEMIOLOGY

Because of its recent recognition, the incidence and prevalence of IgG4-RD are difficult to estimate. Knowledge of IgG4-RD and recognition of

Conflicts of interest: None.
Disclosure: Dr Z.S. Wallace received grant support through a Scientist Development Award from the Rheumatology Research Foundation and from the National Institute of Arthritis and Musculoskeletal and Skin Diseases (NIAMS/NIH; Loan Repayment Award and K23 AR073334).
[a] Clinical Epidemiology Program, Massachusetts General Hospital, Harvard Medical School, 55 Fruit Street, Boston, MA 02114, USA; [b] Rheumatology Unit, Division of Rheumatology, Allergy, and Immunology, Massachusetts General Hospital, Harvard Medical School, 55 Fruit Street, Boston, MA 02114, USA; [c] Rheumatology Unit, Division of Rheumatology, Allergy, and Immunology, Massachusetts General Hospital, 55 Fruit Street, Boston, MA 02114, USA; [d] Department of Pathology, Massachusetts General Hospital, Harvard Medical School, 55 Fruit Street, Boston, MA 02114, USA; [e] Department of Radiology, Massachusetts General Hospital, Harvard Medical School, 55 Fruit Street, Boston, MA 02114, USA
* Corresponding author. Rheumatology Unit, Division of Rheumatology, Allergy, and Immunology, Massachusetts General Hospital, 100 Cambridge Street, 16th Floor, Boston, MA 02114.
E-mail address: zswallace@mgh.harvard.edu

Clin Chest Med 40 (2019) 583–597
https://doi.org/10.1016/j.ccm.2019.05.005

its manifestations has improved in recent years, but persistent delays in diagnosis underscore the problem of under-recognition of this disease.[3]

Demographics

Much of the understanding of the epidemiology of IgG4-RD derives from single-center case series from around the world[4–7] as well as a large, international cohort assembled to derive and validate the forthcoming American College of Rheumatology/European League Against Rheumatism IgG4-RD Classification Criteria.[3] Across cohorts, men tend to be affected more often than women and patients typically present in their fifth, sixth, and seventh decades of life. However, patients of all ages, including children, have been diagnosed with IgG4-RD. Although it was originally described in a cohort of Japanese patients with autoimmune pancreatitis, IgG4-RD has now been reported in patients of nearly all racial backgrounds. A recent cluster analysis suggests that Asian patients and women are at increased risk for head and neck disease, but the cause of this organ predilection in these disease subsets is unclear.[3]

Risk Factors

Risk factors for IgG4-RD are poorly understood. Tobacco and asbestos exposure have been found to be risk factors for idiopathic retroperitoneal fibrosis in multiple studies conducted before IgG4-RD was recognized as a common cause of RPF.[8,9] In a recent case-control study including patients with diverse manifestations, tobacco exposure was found to be a risk factor for IgG4-RD but much of this association was driven by a very strong association observed among the subset of patients with RPF.[10] Potential associations between tobacco exposure and the risk of IgG4-RD in the chest, particularly pulmonary manifestations, require further evaluation. Antecedent malignancy has been identified as a risk factor for the subsequent development of IgG4-RD but this observation requires further study.[11] The association between malignancy and IgG4-RD is especially relevant in the chest, where the differential of IgG4-RD includes lung cancer and lymphoma. Other environmental exposures, especially occupational antigens (eg, solvents), have also been suggested as risk factors for IgG4-RD.[12]

ETIOPATHOGENESIS

Understanding of the pathogenesis of IgG4-RD has expanded rapidly in recent years. Although

genetic (eg, human leukocyte antigen DR4 in autoimmune pancreatitis) and other risk factors (eg, cigarette smoking, as discussed earlier) have been proposed, precise inciting mechanisms have not been identified.[13,14]

Plasmablasts

In IgG4-RD, IgG4-expressing and oligoclonally expanded plasmablasts (ie, short-lived antibody-producing cells, often defined as being $CD20^-19^+38^+27^+$) have been described in affected tissue and found to be increased in the circulation compared with controls.[15] Circulating plasmablast levels correlate with disease activity and the number of organs involved, regardless of serum IgG4 concentration, suggesting a pathogenic role.[16,17] Moreover, B-cell depletion, which eliminates the progenitors of plasmablasts, consistently results in clinical improvement.[18–23]

Autoantibodies

At least 11 autoantigens have been reported in IgG4-RD but their pathogenic significance remains undefined.[24] Their identification supports the hypothesis that IgG4-RD is an autoimmune condition. One of the identified autoantigens, galectin-3, was shown to be an antigenic target of dominantly expanded plasmablasts and present in 28% of a diverse, multiorgan cohort.[25] Another, a human protein named laminin-511, was detected in 50% of subjects with IgG4-related pancreatitis. Immunization of mice with laminin-511 resulted in antibody responses and pancreatic injury.[26]

T Follicular Helper Cells

T follicular helper (TFH) cells are essential to B-cell maturation and Ig class switching. In IgG4-RD, activated type 2 TFH cells are expanded in the circulation, accumulate in affected organs, and correlate with serum IgG4 concentrations, plasmablast levels, and the number of affected organs.[27] In addition, type 2 TFH cells can induce naive B-cell differentiation into IgG4-producing plasmablasts in vitro, implicating them in a key feature of pathophysiology.[27] The mechanism through which type 2 TFH cells drive naive B-cell differentiation seems to be through interleukin (IL)-4 secretion.

Immunoglobulin G4 Molecule

The precise role of the IgG4 molecule in IgG4-RD remains surprisingly unclear.[28] The phenomenon of IgG4 class switching is nonspecific and occurs in the setting of any chronic antigen exposure (eg, allergic disease). Furthermore, in contrast with other IgG subclasses, IgG4 is not very effective at activating complement or binding to Fc receptors on immune cells.[29] There are therefore several reasons for believing that IgG4 is not central to the disease bearing IgG4 in its name. However, recent experimental data[30–32] have suggested a possible pathologic role for IgG4. For instance, IgG4 derived from the serum of patients with IgG4-RD has been found to bind C1q with enhanced affinity compared with IgG4 from healthy controls.[30] Moreover, in an adoptive transfer model of purified human IgG4, the recipient mice showed acute pancreatitis, with demonstrable deposition of human IgG4 within the pancreas.[33]

CD4+ Cytotoxic T Lymphocytes

Even though B cells are clearly important in the pathogenesis of IgG4-RD, the tissue infiltrate is dominated by T cells,[34] particularly CD4+ cytotoxic T lymphocytes (CD4+CTLs).[35] CD4+CTLs are clonally expanded in the circulation of patients with IgG4-RD, decline in conjunction with treatment-induced remission, and correlate with the number of affected organs.[35,36] In addition to driving cytotoxicity via expression of perforin and granzymes, CD4+CTLs also secrete a collection of profibrotic molecules such as IL-1β and transforming growth factor beta.[35] The precise contributions of these CD4+CTLs to the fibrosis that characterizes IgG4-RD remains a focus of investigation, with potential relevance to other conditions associated with fibrosis.

CLINICAL MANIFESTATIONS
Overview

IgG4-RD can affect nearly any organ (**Box 1**).[37] Patients may present with involvement isolated to a single organ or with multiple organs involved at the same time. In untreated patients, manifestations in different organs may accumulate over time in a pattern that is termed metachronous. In contrast with the acute presentation that typically characterizes conditions such as infections, IgG4-RD typically presents in an indolent fashion and is sometimes discovered incidentally. When present, symptoms are typically attributable to mass effect caused by the tumefactive lesions or injury caused by the inflammatory lesions. For instance, patients with sclerosing sialoadenitis often come to medical attention because of the appearance of a painless lump or mass. In contrast, patients with aortitis may present with acute pain related to dissection.

Constitutional symptoms such as fatigue and arthralgias may occur in IgG4-RD but are

---

Box 1
Manifestations of immunoglobulin G4–related disease

Head and neck
Hypertrophic pachymeningitis
Hypophysitis
Orbital pseudotumor and/or orbital myositis
Lacrimal gland enlargement (dacryoadenitis)
Sinusitis
Submandibular, parotid, and/or sublingual gland enlargement (sialoadenitis)
Fibrosing thyroiditis

Pulmonary
Airway
　Tracheobronchial stenosis
Lung parenchyma
　Pulmonary nodules and/or infiltrates
　Interstitial lung disease
　Mediastinal and/or hilar lymphadenopathy
Pleura
　Pleural thickening and nodules
　Pleural effusion

Cardiac/mediastinum
Thoracic periaortitis with or without aneurysm
Fibrosing pericarditis and/or mediastinitis
Paravertebral mass

Pancreatohepatobiliary
Autoimmune pancreatitis (type 1)
Sclerosing cholangitis
Hepatic pseudotumors

Renal
Tubulointerstitial nephritis
Membranous glomerulonephritis

Abdominal aorta and iliac arteries
Retroperitoneal fibrosis
Periaortitis

Lymphadenopathy (any region)
Other
　Sclerosing mesenteritis
　Breast (mastitis)
　Prostate (prostatitis)

generally subtle and insidious rather than profound and sudden in onset.[37] Substantial weight loss can occur in patients with IgG4-related autoimmune pancreatitis because of exocrine pancreatic failure. Such patients simply cannot absorb the requisite nutrition from ingested food and weight loss of up to 9 to 23 kg (20–50 pounds) over a period of months may be reported. Fever is atypical but has been reported in cases of thoracic IgG4-RD.[2,38] The presence of prominent fevers should prompt a search for an alternative explanation, such as ascending cholangitis complicating biliary disease.

Symptoms Related to Immunoglobulin G4–Related Disease in the Chest

Respiratory symptoms are sometimes unimpressive even in patients with substantial thoracic involvement by IgG4-RD.[2] However, in one study, approximately 25% of patients presented with what would eventually be diagnosed as IgG4-RD because of respiratory symptoms.[39] Approximately 50% of patients with IgG4-RD with lung involvement note at least some respiratory symptoms, but the remainder are often asymptomatic.[2,38,40,41] Thoracic symptoms are nonspecific and can include cough (~65%), shortness of breath (~30%), and chest pain (~20%).[38,39,42] Hemoptysis is uncommon but has been reported[38]; like fever, it should raise concern for an alternative cause. Of note, cases of coronary involvement resulting in acute coronary syndrome (eg, chest pain) have been reported.[43–46] Patients with large vessel disease (eg, aorta) are often asymptomatic except in cases in which their disease has been complicated by dissection or flow-limiting vessel narrowing. Allergy and/or asthma are common comorbidities in patients with IgG4-RD and may lead to symptoms that are not related to IgG4-RD lesions.[2,40,47] The diagnosis of asthma in patients with IgG4-related lung disease may be related to airway inflammation resulting from IgG4-RD. The relationship between allergic conditions and IgG4-RD requires further study.

Chest manifestations

Chest computed tomography (CT) is frequently used for the detection and characterization of intrathoracic IgG4-RD, which can affect any structure in the chest, including the lungs, airways, mediastinum, and/or pleura.[2,38,48–50] Radiographs are less sensitive than CT for excluding IgG4-RD involvement in the chest. This article reviews the manifestations of IgG4-RD in the chest by framing the discussion around imaging findings.

Multiple simultaneous locations can be found to be affected by IgG4-RD with cross-sectional imaging and the constellation of features is often more specific for IgG4-RD than any single abnormality in isolation. Note that the thoracic radiological findings of IgG4-RD can resemble those associated with other conditions, most notably lymphoma, infection, and other inflammatory disorders, including sarcoidosis and ANCA-associated vasculitis.

Lymphadenopathy

The most common chest CT finding is lymphadenopathy (**Fig. 1**). This finding is usually symmetric and tends to involve multiple stations in the neck, axillae, hila, and mediastinum. Nodes are mildly enlarged, well defined, and often show enhancement following intravenous contrast administration. The nodes are often fluorodeoxyglucose (FDG) avid on PET scans (**Fig. 2**).

Paravertebral Mass

A striking mediastinal manifestation that occurs in a minority of patients with IgG4-RD is a paravertebral mass. It is most often right sided, spans multiple thoracic vertebral bodies, and does not typically encase the aorta, extend into the spine, or cause bony destruction (**Fig. 3**). Few disease entities other than IgG4-RD lead to this thoracic disease manifestation.

Airway Involvement

Airway involvement is seen in up to half of the patients with IgG4-RD with abnormalities on chest

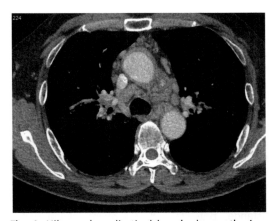

Fig. 1. Hilar and mediastinal lymphadenopathy in a 61-year-old man with IgG4-RD. Chest CT axial scan at the level of the aortopulmonary window on soft tissue windows. There is bilateral, mild mediastinal and hilar lymphadenopathy (*arrow*). In addition, soft tissue surrounds the ascending aorta, consistent with periaortitis (*arrowhead*).

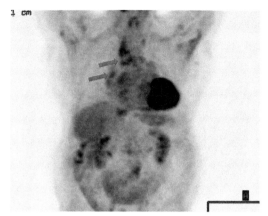

Fig. 2. FDG-avid lymphadenopathy in a 77-year-old man with IgG4-RD. Coronal PET CT shows FDG avidity in the hilar and mediastinal nodes (*arrows*).

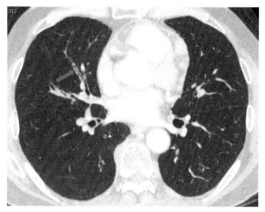

Fig. 4. Bronchial wall thickening in 61-year-old man with cough and IgG4-RD. Axial chest CT scan on lung windows shows diffuse, multifocal nodular thickening of the bronchial walls, best seen in the right middle lobe (*arrow*).

CT and is associated with pulmonary symptoms including cough and dyspnea.[51] Airway changes are characterized most frequently by smooth or nodular thickening of the airway wall (**Fig. 4**). Small airway obstruction and subsequent air trapping related to IgG4-RD can cause mosaic attenuation of the lung parenchyma on expiratory images. Saber sheath trachea, an abnormality in which the intrathoracic trachea becomes elongated in the sagittal dimension, can also be present in IgG4-RD (**Fig. 5**). This remodeling has been described in patients with other forms of chronic airflow obstruction and may be caused by chronically increased intrathoracic pressure from airway wall thickening.

Pleuropulmonary Manifestations

A variety of pulmonary parenchymal findings can be observed in IgG4-RD. These abnormalities are typically peripheral in location, often involving the subpleural lung. Consolidation, ground-glass opacities, pulmonary nodules, and/or septal thickening are the most frequent intrapulmonary manifestations (**Figs. 6 and 7**). Fibrosis has been observed but is less common; when present, it may rarely be associated with honeycombing and traction bronchiolectasis.

Pleural thickening and effusions may also be seen in IgG4-RD (see **Fig. 7**). The combination of pulmonary and pleural findings differentiates the disease from sarcoidosis or organizing pneumonia, both of which also cause subpleural,

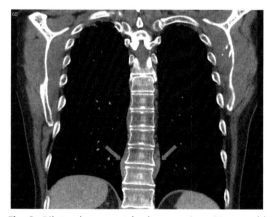

Fig. 3. Bilateral paravertebral masses in a 61-year-old man with IgG4-RD. Coronal reformatted image from a chest CT scan at the level of the thoracic spine on soft tissue windows. There are bilateral paravertebral masses, seen on the right at T8 and T10/11 and on the left at T10/11 (*arrows*). Biopsy confirmed IgG4-RD.

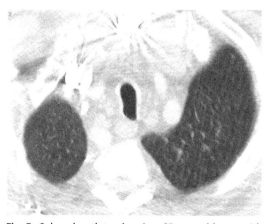

Fig. 5. Saber sheath trachea in a 65-year-old man with IgG4-RD. There is elongation in the sagittal plane of the trachea relative to the coronal plane.

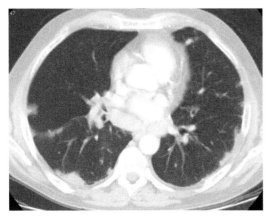

Fig. 6. Peripheral nodules and consolidation in 69-year-old man with IgG4-RD. Chest CT axial scan at the level of the aortic root on lung windows. There are multiple, bilateral peripheral lung nodules and consolidative opacities that also extend along the right major and minor fissures, in a perilymphatic distribution that is characteristic of IgG4-RD. The patient denied pulmonary symptoms.

peripheral, and peribronchiolar nodules and opacities but rarely involve the pleura.

Heart and Great Vessel Involvement

Chest CT also allows assessment of the heart and great vessels in IgG4-RD.[52] Cardiac features include coronary artery pseudotumors and aneurysms as well as pericardial thickening (**Fig. 8**). Periaortitis caused by IgG4-RD typically manifests as a soft tissue formation around the vessel with or

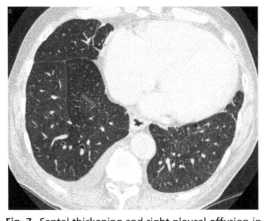

Fig. 7. Septal thickening and right pleural effusion in a 65-year-old man with IgG4-RD. Chest CT axial scan at the level of interventricular septum on lung windows shows smooth interlobular septal thickening (*arrow*) and a small right pleural effusion. The appearances mimic pulmonary edema. Echocardiogram showed normal cardiac function.

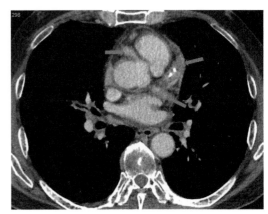

Fig. 8. Pseudotumors of the coronary arteries in a 61-year-old man with IgG4-RD. Chest CT axial scan at the level of the coronary arteries on mediastinal windows. There is soft tissue surrounding the right coronary artery and left anterior descending and circumflex arteries (*arrows*).

without vessel wall thickening and enhancement[53]; this can be found affecting the aorta, pulmonary artery, and/or great vessels (see **Fig. 1**).

Features Suggestive of Alternative Diagnoses

Certain manifestations of disease in the chest are uncommon in IgG4-RD. These manifestations include diffuse alveolar hemorrhage, large pleural or pericardial effusions, pulmonary hypertension, and airway stenosis or collapse. When present, clinicians should consider other explanations more commonly associated with these findings, such as vasculitis, systemic lupus erythematosus, systemic sclerosis, or relapsing polychondritis.

DIAGNOSING IMMUNOGLOBULIN G4–RELATED DISEASE
Overview

There is no single diagnostic test for IgG4-RD. The diagnosis of IgG4-RD requires a careful consideration of all available data, including the history, physical examination, laboratory results, imaging findings, and pathology.

Serum IgG4 concentration increases are neither sensitive nor specific for the diagnosis,[54–56] although they can support the diagnosis in the proper clinical setting. Moreover, although IgG4+ plasma cell infiltrates in the tissue are the sine qua non of the condition, these too are not specific for IgG4-RD and may be encountered in other conditions, including ANCA-associated vasculitis and malignancy.[57–59] Diagnostic criteria have previously been proposed by different groups around the world, some for specific organ manifestations and others for any manifestation of IgG4-RD.[60–62] These criteria often place excessive weight on histopathologic findings and serum IgG4 concentration increases, approaches that likely maximize specificity at the expense of sensitivity. Although they can help inform the approach to diagnosis, the authors do not strictly use these criteria in the day-to-day clinical care of patients with suspected IgG4-RD.

Considering Other Organ Involvement

The first step in diagnosing IgG4-RD is considering the full extent of potential organ involvement. For instance, when referred a patient because of abnormal findings in the lung, it is important to consider whether there is involvement of organs that may reveal key physical examination findings. The eyes and major salivary glands must be examined carefully. Lacrimal gland enlargement, readily detected on examination (**Fig. 9**A, B), may heighten the diagnostic suspicion for IgG4-RD but can also be found in IgG4-RD mimickers (eg, sarcoidosis, granulomatosis with polyangiitis, and Sjögren syndrome). Proptosis may be caused by IgG4-RD infiltrating and enlarging extraocular muscles.

Isolated submandibular gland enlargement (**Fig. 9**C) can be a major clue to IgG4-RD, but the parotid (**Fig. 9**D) and sublingual glands may also be strikingly enlarged.

Moreover, a careful history taking might reveal symptoms suggestive of organ involvement elsewhere. For instance, new-onset diabetes or loose and pale colored stool may suggest pancreatic disease. New lower back and/or groin pain may be suggestive of retroperitoneal fibrosis. The patient's medical history can also be useful when it suggests previous complications (eg, autoimmune pancreatitis, tubulointerstitial nephritis) likely related to what was unrecognized IgG4-RD at the time.

Cross-sectional imaging of the chest and the abdomen/pelvis can reveal asymptomatic disease in a distribution that supports a diagnosis of IgG4-RD. In the case of suspected pancreatohepatobiliary disease, magnetic resonance cholangiopancreatography may be useful for diagnosing IgG4-RD and ruling out alternative causes. Patients with significantly increased serum IgG4 concentrations (eg, >3× the upper limit of normal) are more likely to have multiorgan disease, and cross-sectional imaging may be higher yield in these patients.[3,39]

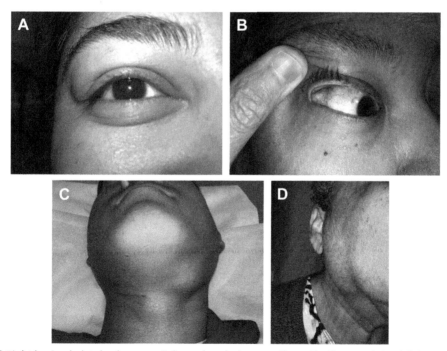

Fig. 9. (A) Right lacrimal gland enlargement shown by a bulge over the patient's upper lateral right eye. (B) Right lacrimal gland enlargement revealed by simple retraction of the eyelid. (C) Left submandibular gland enlargement in a 16-year-old boy with IgG4-related disease affecting the major salivary glands, lungs, kidneys, pancreas, and biliary tree. Note that the right submandibular gland has been resected (removed for diagnostic purposes). (D) Right parotid enlargement in a 75-year-old woman with IgG4-related disease affecting the major salivary glands, kidneys (interstitial nephritis), and pleura.

Considering Alternative Diagnoses

The second step is to consider the common mimickers of IgG4-RD and whether any of those conditions might better explain the patient's presentation or whether additional work-up is indicated to exonerate those conditions (**Table 1**). In the chest, the differential includes sarcoidosis, ANCA-associated vasculitis, Sjögren syndrome,[63] lymphoma and primary/metastatic lung cancer, Erdheim-Chester disease,[64] infections (including bacterial infections as well as atypical mycobacterial or fungal infections), and myofibroblastic tumors.[65] To exonerate these conditions, a new biopsy, a review of pathologic tissue available from earlier procedures, or additional laboratory testing can be helpful (see **Table 1**).

Biopsy Specimens to Diagnose Immunoglobulin G4–related Disease

In many cases, a biopsy of an affected lesion can help support a diagnosis of IgG4-RD and/or rule out alternative causes. Histopathologic confirmation was considered essential to diagnosing IgG4-RD in the years following its initial recognition. However, the full panoply of histopathologic findings associated with IgG4-RD may be difficult to detect in the more limited biopsy specimens that are often preferred now because they are less invasive and can help exonerate infection and malignancy. Review of an archived pathology sample from a biopsy of another affected site can be diagnostic, even if the sample is many years old. Fresh recuts of paraffin-embedded specimens can be stained for IgG4+ plasma cells

---

Table 1
Common mimickers of immunoglobulin G4–related disease in the chest

Disease	Differentiating Factors
Sjögren syndrome	• Parotid gland involvement more common • Positive anti-SSA (Ro) and/or anti-SSB generally (La) exclude IgG4-RD
Sarcoidosis	• Cutaneous disease more common than in IgG4-RD • ACE may be increased, not expected in IgG4-RD • Splenomegaly can be seen but would be atypical in IgG4-RD • Granulomas exclude IgG4-RD
AAV (eg, granulomatosis with polyangiitis, microscopic polyangiitis, EGPA)	• Fever and very high CRP may be present and atypical for IgG4-RD • A positive MPO-ANCA or PR3-ANCA generally excludes IgG4-RD; only present in ∼50% of EGPA cases • High-grade eosinophilia >3000/mm^3, as seen in EGPA, generally excludes IgG4-RD • Necrotizing vasculitis and/or granulomas exclude IgG4-RD
Giant cell arteritis	• Fever and very high CRP level may be present and atypical in IgG4-RD • Cranial symptoms (headache, scalp tenderness, jaw claudication, vision change) not typical in IgG4-RD
Lymphoma	• Fever may be present • Malignant pathology excludes IgG4-RD • Rapid progression across tissue planes not seen in IgG4-RD
Infection	• Fevers and very high CRP levels common, atypical in IgG4-RD • Rapid progression across tissue planes not seen in IgG4-RD
MCD	• Fever and very high CRP level often present and atypical in IgG4-RD • MCD pathology is distinct from IgG4-RD, although both may have IgG4+ plasma cells infiltrating tissue
Erdheim-Chester disease	• Classic long-bone abnormalities (eg, sclerosis) • Distinct pathology that includes foamy histiocytes excludes IgG4-RD • May have a *BRAF* mutation detectable in tissue and/or circulating blood
Inflammatory myofibroblastic tumor	• Much more common in pediatric patients than adult patients • Distinct pathology reveals spindle cells • *ALK, ROS-1,* and other gene rearrangements detectable in ∼50% of cases

Abbreviations: AAV, ANCA-associated vasculitis; ACE, angiotensin-converting enzyme; *ALK,* anaplastic lymphoma kinase; CRP, C-reactive protein; EGPA, eosinophilic granulomatosis with polyangiitis; MCD, multicentric Castleman disease; MPO, myeloperoxidase; PR3, proteinase-3; SSA, Sjögren syndrome A; SSB, Sjögren syndrome B.

even if immunostains were not performed originally. Lymphadenopathy is the most common manifestation of IgG4-RD in the chest, but note that histology of involved lymph nodes tends to show nonspecific hyperplastic or reactive histologic changes rather than the typical features of IgG4-RD[66–68]; fibrosis may be variably encountered in lymph node biopsies. Caution should be used when diagnosing IgG4-RD using only lymph node biopsies.

In 2012, an international group of experts published a consensus statement on the pathology of IgG4-RD.[69] Intended to act as diagnostic guidelines for practicing pathologists, this statement provides clear emphasis on 2 aspects of the pathology findings in IgG4-RD: a characteristic histologic appearance and a prominent infiltrate of IgG4-expressing plasma cells identified using immunostaining.

The characteristic histologic features include a dense lymphoplasmacytic infiltrate, fibrosis (often in a storiform pattern), and phlebitis (obliterative or nonobliterative) (**Fig. 10**). The collection of at least 2 of these features has classically formed the diagnostic foundation of IgG4-RD, but any single feature in isolation lacks specificity. Tumefactive pulmonary lesions often extend along the bronchovascular tree (see **Fig. 10**A) and can be subpleural (see **Fig. 10**B). The polyclonal lymphoplasmacytic infiltrate is diffusely distributed with lymphocytes, especially T lymphocytes, dominating plasma cells. CD20+ B cells are often present in extranodal germinal centers. A modest eosinophilic tissue infiltration can be seen but IgG4-RD is not considered to be a hypereosinophilic disorder. Consequently, a dominant eosinophilic infiltrate suggests an alternative cause. Macrophages may be a prominent feature, as in any inflammatory lesion, but discrete giant cells, granulomas, and predominant granulomatous inflammation should not be present in biopsies of IgG4-RD. Similarly, monoclonal cell populations, necrosis, and prominent histiocytic infiltrates are atypical of IgG4-RD.[69]

Fibrosis is a core feature of IgG4-RD lesions and, at least focally, should have a storiform or spiraling pattern (see **Fig. 10**A). In cases of limited tissue sampling, such as with retroperitoneal fibrosis, the fibrotic component may predominate. Phlebitis (obliterative or nonobliterative) represents destruction of the venous wall and filling of the lumen by infiltrating immune cells (see **Fig. 10**C). Pulmonary lesions related to IgG4-RD are unique in that pathology can reveal obliterative arteritis as well as obliterative phlebitis, neither of which should be confused with necrotizing

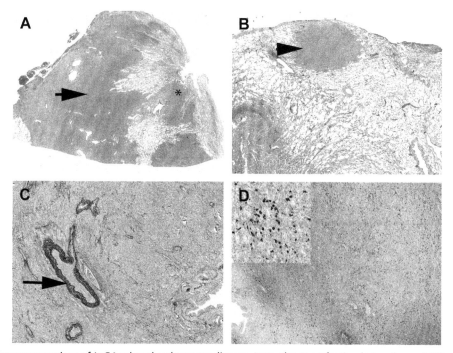

Fig. 10. Low-power view of IgG4-related pulmonary disease. Note the tumefactive lesion (*arrow*) (*A*), extension along the bronchovascular tree (*A*) (*asterisk*), and subpleural involvement (*B*) (*arrowhead*). An elastic stain highlights the focus of obliterative phlebitis (*C*) (*arrow*). An immunohistochemical stain shows a diffuse increase in IgG4+ plasma cells (*D* and *inset*). ([*A* and *B*]: H&E; [*C*]: elastin stain; [*D*]: IgG4 stain).

vasculitis. As in the vein, obliterative arteritis is characterized by a nonnecrotizing lymphoplasmacytic infiltrate with or without obliteration of the lumen. Elastin stains are often required to visualize obliterative phlebitis or arteritis because of the extensive vessel wall destruction.

Immunostaining for both IgG4+ and IgG+ plasma cells is essential to confirm a suspected histopathologic diagnosis (see **Fig. 10**D). Interpretation of IgG4 immunostaining relies on both the quantification of IgG4+ plasma cells per high-power field and the ratio of IgG4+/IgG+ plasma cells. The diagnostic cutoff for the former is organ specific, whereas a ratio greater than or equal to 40% is a general rule used to confirm the diagnosis. However, ratios of less than 40% are often encountered in cases of IgG4-RD, because much depends on adequate sampling and its converse: sampling error. Nevertheless, a true lack of IgG4+ plasma cells or a low proportion of IgG4+ plasma cells infiltrating tissue suggests that an alternative diagnosis should be considered. It is also critical to recognize that many important mimickers of IgG4-RD can be associated with a prominent IgG4+ plasma cell infiltrate.[57–59] Major examples include primary sclerosing cholangitis, ANCA-associated vasculitis, multicentric Castleman disease, B-cell lymphomas, and pancreatic cancer.

Although histopathology and immunostaining can be useful in suggesting or confirming an IgG4-RD diagnosis, clinicopathologic correlation remains critical in making this diagnosis. It is important to keep this in mind because the pathology of IgG4-RD in the lung may lack the typical storiform fibrosis and/or obliterative phlebitis often seen in biopsies from other organs affected by IgG4-RD.[40,69]

Laboratory Testing in Immunoglobulin G4–related Disease

Certain laboratory tests can be useful to screen for specific organ involvement by IgG4-RD (**Table 2**). Increases in the erythrocyte sedimentation rate (ESR) are common because of the hypergammaglobulinemia that typically accompanies untreated disease. However, ESR measurements greater than 100 mm/h are unusual. C-reactive protein (CRP) increases can be observed in IgG4-RD but these are less common than ESR increases. There is often an acute phase reactant discordance characterized by a high ESR and low CRP.

Other laboratory findings that make IgG4-RD less likely include pancytopenia (especially involving multiple lines) and the presence of disease-specific autoantibodies. Although

patients can be screened for many possible disease-specific autoantibodies (see **Table 1**), these are not meant to be checked in all patients in whom the diagnosis of IgG4-RD is being considered; they should be checked in patients with presentations that are suggestive of those specific diseases (eg, lupus, ANCA-associated vasculitis, Sjögren syndrome). Considering these diagnoses and interpreting laboratory results may require consultation with other specialists, such as a rheumatologist.

Perhaps the most commonly used laboratory test to evaluate for IgG4-RD is the serum IgG4 concentration. Although IgG4-RD was initially described in a cohort of patients with autoimmune

Table 2
Useful laboratory tests when evaluating patients for immunoglobulin G4–related disease

Laboratory Test	Reason for Test
General	
IgG subclasses	IgG4 level increased in ~70% of patients with IgG4-RD
IgE and peripheral eosinophilia	May be increased in patients with IgG4-RD; may predict risk of flare after treatment
Renal Disease	
CH50, C3, and C4	Often low in IgG4-related renal disease
Creatinine and glomerular filtration rate	To evaluate for potential IgG4-related renal disease
Urinalysis	Proteinuria may be present in IgG4-related renal disease
Pancreatic Disease	
Amylase and lipase	To evaluate for potential IgG4-related pancreatitis
Bilirubin	To evaluate for potential IgG4-related pancreatitis
A1c	To evaluate for potential IgG4-related pancreatitis causing endocrine insufficiency
Stool elastase	To evaluate for potential IgG4-related pancreatitis causing exocrine insufficiency

pancreatitis and uniform increases in serum IgG4 concentrations, it is now recognized that approximately 30% of patients with biopsy-proven IgG4-RD have normal serum IgG4 concentrations.[4] Moreover, increased serum IgG4 concentrations have been described in other conditions, including patients with interstitial lung disease, ANCA-associated vasculitis, and allergic conditions undergoing immunotherapy.[57–59] In sum, serum IgG4 concentrations have an approximate specificity for IgG4-RD of 83%.[70]

In the past, some patients with IgG4-RD and multiorgan disease were found to have surprisingly normal serum IgG4 concentrations that did not fit clinically. Ultimately, it was discovered that, in patients with very high serum IgG4 concentrations, a prozone effect caused falsely low measurements because of excess antigen that overwhelmed the assays.[71] To overcome this limitation, most commercial laboratories now use serial dilution of samples to avoid the prozone effect, but providers should be aware of this phenomenon when interpreting IgG4 concentrations.

Other laboratory anomalies commonly observed in IgG4 are increased levels of other IgG subclasses as well as increases of IgE levels.[20] Hypocomplementemia is often observed in patients with IgG4-related tubulointerstitial nephritis but is sometimes detected in patients without overt renal disease. The pattern of hypocomplementemia in IgG4-RD frequently calls to mind the hypocomplementemia observed in systemic lupus erythematosus or mixed cryoglobulinemia; namely, a reduced C3 level and an extremely low or even unmeasureable C4 level.

Pulmonary Function Tests

There is scant literature describing the frequencies of pulmonary function test (PFT) abnormalities in patients with IgG4-RD.[50,72] The authors suspect that findings on PFTs lack sensitivity and specificity to distinguish IgG4-RD from other conditions with thoracic involvement. PFTs may have a role in monitoring disease progression in certain patients but this requires further study.

INITIAL MANAGEMENT

Nearly all patients with IgG4-RD should be treated with immunosuppression to prevent accrual of additional organ involvement and damage in affected organs.[73,74] Exceptions to this include patients in whom lesions have been fully resected or those with asymptomatic and mild lymphadenopathy or salivary gland enlargement.[73,74] In those cases, watchful waiting may be considered. Glucocorticoids are the most frequently used first-

line treatment, but other strategies that incorporate glucocorticoid-sparing agents are often used. The goal of initial management is to achieve a complete remission. Note that in patients with increased pretreatment serum IgG4 concentrations, there is typically a decrease in the laboratory measurement following treatment, but levels may not normalize even in those achieving clinical remission.[18,20]

Glucocorticoids

Glucocorticoids have been the mainstay of treatment of IgG4-RD because of their efficacy as well as affordability. Failure to respond to glucocorticoid therapy suggests that the diagnosis is incorrect. In rare circumstances, a highly fibrotic lesion (eg, orbital lesion, retroperitoneal fibrosis) may not respond to glucocorticoid therapy, but this should be interpreted cautiously.

A single-arm clinical trial[75] found a response rate of greater than 93% to glucocorticoids and a complete remission rate of 66%, consistent with our general experience using glucocorticoids. However, patients in that study were maintained on significant doses of prednisone ($\geq$7.5 mg/d) throughout the 1-year follow-up period.

Glucocorticoids are typically used first line, with equivalent prednisone dosages ranging from 20 mg to 60 mg/d depending on the severity of the presentation. The general practice is to begin a slow taper of glucocorticoids after 2 to 4 weeks of therapy with the goal of discontinuation by 3 months, and sometimes sooner. During this time, the patient should be monitored for flares of disease, which are common, especially at lower doses and following discontinuation.[76,77] In the previously mentioned single-arm clinical trial, 15% of patients flared during follow-up.

The risks of glucocorticoid therapy must be weighed against these benefits, especially in light of the demographics of IgG4-RD. This group of patients is at increased risk for glucocorticoid-related toxicity (eg, diabetes mellitus, osteoporosis, infection) because of their age and comorbidities, especially those with pancreatic insufficiency. For instance, in the clinical trial of glucocorticoid therapy in IgG4-RD, more than 40% of patients experienced glucose intolerance and nearly half of these patients were newly diagnosed with diabetes mellitus. Because of the high incidence of glucocorticoid complications in this patient population, it is usually our practice to move quickly to treatment regimens that minimize glucocorticoids for long-term disease control.

Conventional Disease Modifying Antirheumatic Drugs

Much of our understanding of the efficacy of conventional disease modifying antirheumatic drugs (DMARDs; eg, methotrexate, azathioprine, mycophenolate mofetil) in IgG4-RD is extrapolated from the autoimmune pancreatitis literature.[21] Results from these uncontrolled observational studies have not suggested good efficacy of conventional DMARDs such as azathioprine for maintaining disease remission better than glucocorticoid monotherapy.[73] However, a recent open-label randomized clinical trial of patients with IgG4-RD with diverse manifestations suggests that mycophenolate mofetil added to glucocorticoids may be efficacious, especially for maintaining remission compared with maintenance therapy with glucocorticoid monotherapy.[78] Future studies are necessary to clarify the potential role of conventional DMARDs in IgG4-RD.

Rituximab

A small pilot clinical trial[18] as well as several cases series suggest that rituximab is effective for the treatment of IgG4-RD.[21–23] A unique benefit of rituximab in IgG4-RD is that it may be effective when used as monotherapy. When used, the dosing regimen is typically 1,000 mg administered twice over 2 weeks. A response may be observed over the first 8 weeks following treatment but the maximum benefit from rituximab may not be observed for approximately 12 weeks after treatment. If necessary, treatment may be repeated approximately 6 months after the initial doses, but many patients do not require retreatment at that time and can be monitored prospectively for evidence of a flare.[20,22] However, retreatment at 6 months may reduce the risk of subsequent flare.[23] One benefit of prospectively monitoring without preemptive retreatment at 6 month is a reduced risk of infection.[23]

General Approach

Most often, therapy is initiated with glucocorticoids and the decision of whether to combine glucocorticoids with an additional steroid-sparing immunosuppressant is guided by the severity of the presentation as well as the patient's comorbidities.[73] As discussed, some experts prefer to treat without glucocorticoids, which may be reasonable if the patient's presentation is not organ (eg, renal failure, aortitis, cholangitis) or life threatening. When organ-threatening or life-threatening disease is present, upfront glucocorticoids can be important for obtaining quick control of the disease. Regardless of the initial treatment strategy in patients with multiorgan disease, the various manifestations respond similarly to therapy, but some reports suggest that the response of thoracic IgG4-RD to treatment may not be synchronous with response elsewhere in the body.[2,40,79] Additional prospective studies are necessary to define optimal treatment strategies and to better characterize whether certain manifestations respond differently to treatment.

SUMMARY

IgG4-RD is an immune-mediated disease that causes fibroinflammatory lesions in nearly any organ, including structures in the chest. An accurate diagnosis requires careful clinicopathologic correlation. Neither increased serum IgG4 concentrations nor IgG4+ plasma cell infiltrates are diagnostic of IgG4-RD. Mimickers of IgG4-RD in the chest include malignancy, infection, and other immune-mediated diseases, such as vasculitis and sarcoidosis. Glucocorticoids and/or steroid-sparing agents are the cornerstone of treatment.

REFERENCES

1. Kamisawa T, Zen Y, Pillai S, et al. IgG4-related disease. Lancet 2015;385(9976):1460–71.
2. Fei Y, Shi J, Lin W, et al. Intrathoracic involvements of immunoglobulin G4-related sclerosing disease. Medicine (Baltimore) 2015;94(50):e2150.
3. Wallace ZS, Zhang Y, Perugino CA, et al. Clinical phenotypes of IgG4-related disease: an analysis of two international cross-sectional cohorts. Ann Rheum Dis 2019;78(3):406–12.
4. Wallace ZS, Deshpande V, Mattoo H, et al. IgG4-Related disease: clinical and laboratory features in one hundred twenty-five patients. Arthritis Rheumatol 2015;67(9):2466–75.
5. Inoue D, Yoshida K, Yoneda N, et al. IgG4-Related disease: dataset of 235 consecutive patients. Medicine (Baltimore) 2015;94(15):e680.
6. Huggett MT, Culver EL, Kumar M, et al. Type 1 autoimmune pancreatitis and IgG4-related sclerosing cholangitis is associated with extrapancreatic organ failure, malignancy, and mortality in a prospective UK cohort. Am J Gastroenterol 2014;109(10):1675–83.
7. Lin W, Lu S, Chen H, et al. Clinical characteristics of immunoglobulin G4-related disease: a prospective study of 118 Chinese patients. Rheumatology (Oxford) 2015;54(11):1982–90.
8. Goldoni M, Bonini S, Urban ML, et al. Asbestos and smoking as risk factors for idiopathic retroperitoneal

fibrosis: a case-control study. Ann Intern Med 2014; 161(3):181–8.

9. Uibu T, Oksa P, Auvinen A, et al. Asbestos exposure as a risk factor for retroperitoneal fibrosis. Lancet 2004;363(9419):1422–6.

10. Wallwork R, Choi HK, Perugino CA, et al. Cigarette smoking is a risk factor for IgG4-related disease [abstract]. Arthritis Rheumatol 2018;70(suppl 10).

11. Wallace ZS, Wallace CJ, Lu N, et al. Association of IgG4-related disease with history of malignancy. Arthritis Rheumatol 2016;68(9):2283–9.

12. de Buy Wenniger LJ, Culver EL, Beuers U. Exposure to occupational antigens might predispose to IgG4-related disease. Hepatology 2014;60(4):1453–4.

13. Kawa S, Ota M, Yoshizawa K, et al. HLA DRB10405-DQB10401 haplotype is associated with autoimmune pancreatitis in the Japanese population. Gastroenterology 2002;122(5):1264–9.

14. Brandt AS, Kamper L, Kukuk S, et al. Associated findings and complications of retroperitoneal fibrosis in 204 patients: results of a urological registry. J Urol 2011;185(2):526–31.

15. Mattoo H, Mahajan VS, Della-Torre E, et al. De novo oligoclonal expansions of circulating plasmablasts in active and relapsing IgG-related disease. J Allergy Clin Immunol 2014;134(3):679–87.

16. Wallace ZS, Mattoo H, Carruthers M, et al. Plasmablasts as a biomarker for IgG4-related disease, independent of serum IgG4 concentrations. Ann Rheum Dis 2015;74(1):190–5.

17. Lin W, Zhang P, Chen H, et al. Circulating plasmablasts/plasma cells: a potential biomarker for IgG4-related disease. Arthritis Res Ther 2017;19(1):25.

18. Carruthers MN, Topazian MD, Khosroshahi A, et al. Rituximab for IgG4-related disease: a prospective, open-label trial. Ann Rheum Dis 2015;74(6):1171–7.

19. Khosroshahi A, Carruthers MN, Deshpande V, et al. Rituximab for the treatment of IgG4-related disease: lessons from 10 consecutive patients. Medicine (Baltimore) 2012;91(1):57–66.

20. Wallace ZS, Mattoo H, Mahajan VS, et al. Predictors of disease relapse in IgG4-related disease following rituximab. Rheumatology (Oxford) 2016;55(6): 1000–8.

21. Hart PA, Topazian MD, Witzig TE, et al. Treatment of relapsing autoimmune pancreatitis with immunomodulators and rituximab: the Mayo Clinic experience. Gut 2013;62(11):1607–15.

22. Ebbo M, Grados A, Samson M, et al. Long-term efficacy and safety of rituximab in IgG4-related disease: data from a French nationwide study of thirty-three patients. PLoS One 2017;12(9):e0183844.

23. Majumder S, Mohapatra S, Lennon RJ, et al. Rituximab maintenance therapy reduces rate of relapse of pancreaticobiliary immunoglobulin G4-related disease. Clin Gastroenterol Hepatol 2018;16(12): 1947–53.

24. Du H, Shi L, Chen P, et al. Prohibitin is involved in patients with IgG4 related disease. PLoS One 2015; 10(5):e0125331.

25. Perugino CA, AlSalem SB, Mattoo H, et al. Identification of galectin-3 as an autoantigen in patients with IgG4-related disease. J Allergy Clin Immunol 2018; 143(2):736–45.e6.

26. Shiokawa M, Kodama Y, Sekiguchi H, et al. Laminin 511 is a target antigen in autoimmune pancreatitis. Sci Transl Med 2018;10(453) [pii:eaaq0997].

27. Akiyama M, Yasuoka H, Yamaoka K, et al. Enhanced IgG4 production by follicular helper 2 T cells and the involvement of follicular helper 1 T cells in the pathogenesis of IgG4-related disease. Arthritis Res Ther 2016;18:167.

28. Nirula A, Glaser SM, Kalled SL, et al. What is IgG4? A review of the biology of a unique immunoglobulin subtype. Curr Opin Rheumatol 2011; 23(1):119–24.

29. Vidarsson G, Dekkers G, Rispens T. IgG subclasses and allotypes: from structure to effector functions. Front Immunol 2014;5:520.

30. Sugimoto M, Watanabe H, Asano T, et al. Possible participation of IgG4 in the activation of complement in IgG4-related disease with hypocomplementemia. Mod Rheumatol 2016;26(2):251–8.

31. Culver EL, van de Bovenkamp FS, Derksen NI, et al. Unique patterns of glycosylation in immunoglobulin subclass G4-related disease and primary sclerosing cholangitis. J Gastroenterol Hepatol 2018. [Epub ahead of print].

32. Shiokawa M, Kodama Y, Kuriyama K, et al. Pathogenicity of IgG in patients with IgG4-related disease. Gut 2016;65(8):1322–32.

33. Shiokawa M, Kodama Y, Yoshimura K, et al. Risk of cancer in patients with autoimmune pancreatitis. Am J Gastroenterol 2013;108(4):610–7.

34. Mahajan VS, Mattoo H, Deshpande V, et al. IgG4-Related disease. Annu Rev Pathol 2014;9:315–47.

35. Mattoo H, Mahajan VS, Maehara T, et al. Clonal expansion of CD4(+) cytotoxic T lymphocytes in patients with IgG4-related disease. J Allergy Clin Immunol 2016;138(3):825–38.

36. Maehara T, Mattoo H, Ohta M, et al. Lesional CD4+ IFN-gamma+ cytotoxic T lymphocytes in IgG4-related dacryoadenitis and sialoadenitis. Ann Rheum Dis 2017;76(2):377–85.

37. Stone JH, Zen Y, Deshpande V. IgG4-related disease. N Engl J Med 2012;366(6):539–51.

38. Sun X, Liu H, Feng R, et al. Biopsy-proven IgG4-related lung disease. BMC Pulm Med 2016;16:20.

39. Corcoran JP, Culver EL, Anstey RM, et al. Thoracic involvement in IgG4-related disease in a UK-based patient cohort. Respir Med 2017;132:117–21.

40. Zen Y, Inoue D, Kitao A, et al. IgG4-related lung and pleural disease: a clinicopathologic study of 21 cases. Am J Surg Pathol 2009;33(12):1886–93.

41. Matsui S, Hebisawa A, Sakai F, et al. Immunoglobulin G4-related lung disease: clinicoradiological and pathological features. Respirology 2013;18(3): 480–7.

42. Hui P, Mattman A, Wilcox PG, et al. Immunoglobulin G4-related lung disease: a disease with many different faces. Can Respir J 2013;20(5):335–8.

43. Ruggio A, Iaconelli A, Panaioli E, et al. Coronary artery aneurysms presenting as acute coronary syndrome: an unusual case of IgG4-related disease vascular involvement. Can J Cardiol 2018;34(8). 1088.e1087–10.

44. Barbu M, Lindstrom U, Nordborg C, et al. Sclerosing aortic and coronary arteritis due to IgG4-related disease. Ann Thorac Surg 2017;103(6):e487–9.

45. Keraliya AR, Murphy DJ, Aghayev A, et al. IgG4-Related disease with coronary arteritis. Circ Cardiovasc Imaging 2016;9(3):e004583.

46. Bito Y, Sasaki Y, Hirai H, et al. A surgical case of expanding bilateral coronary aneurysms regarded as immunoglobulin G4-related disease. Circulation 2014;129(16):e453–6.

47. Della Torre E, Mattoo H, Mahajan VS, et al. Prevalence of atopy, eosinophilia, and IgE elevation in IgG4-related disease. Allergy 2014;69(2):269–72.

48. Inoue D, Zen Y, Abo H, et al. Immunoglobulin G4-related lung disease: CT findings with pathologic correlations. Radiology 2009;251(1):260–70.

49. Keenan JC, Miller E, Jessurun J, et al. IgG4-related lung disease: a case series of 6 patients and review of the literature. Sarcoidosis Vasc Diffuse Lung Dis 2016;32(4):360–7.

50. Saraya T, Ohkuma K, Fujiwara M, et al. Clinical characterization of 52 patients with immunoglobulin G4-related disease in a single tertiary center in Japan: special reference to lung disease in thoracic high-resolution computed tomography. Respir Med 2017;132:62–7.

51. Lim SY, McInnis M, Wallace Z, et al. Intrathoracic manifestations of IgG4-related disease: findings in a cohort study from North America [abstract]. Arthritis Rheumatol 2016;68(suppl 10).

52. Oyama-Manabe N, Yabusaki S, Manabe O, et al. IgG4-related cardiovascular disease from the aorta to the coronary arteries: multidetector CT and PET/CT. Radiographics 2018;38(7):1934–48.

53. Perugino CA, Wallace ZS, Meyersohn N, et al. Large vessel involvement by IgG4-related disease. Medicine (Baltimore) 2016;95(28):e3344.

54. Carruthers MN, Khosroshahi A, Augustin T, et al. The diagnostic utility of serum IgG4 concentrations in IgG4-related disease. Ann Rheum Dis 2015;74(1): 14–8.

55. Ryu JH, Horie R, Sekiguchi H, et al. Spectrum of disorders associated with elevated serum IgG4 levels encountered in clinical practice. Int J Rheumatol 2012;2012:232960.

56. Yamamoto M, Tabeya T, Naishiro Y, et al. Value of serum IgG4 in the diagnosis of IgG4-related disease and in differentiation from rheumatic diseases and other diseases. Mod Rheumatol 2012;22(3):419–25.

57. Chang SY, Keogh KA, Lewis JE, et al. IgG4-positive plasma cells in granulomatosis with polyangiitis (Wegener's): a clinicopathologic and immunohistochemical study on 43 granulomatosis with polyangiitis and 20 control cases. Hum Pathol 2013;44(11): 2432–7.

58. Bledsoe J, Wallace Z, Deshpande V, et al. Atypical IgG4+ plasmacytic proliferations and lymphomas: characterization of 11 cases. Am J Clin Pathol 2017;148(3):215–35.

59. Kiil K, Bein J, Schuhmacher B, et al. A high number of IgG4-positive plasma cells rules out nodular lymphocyte predominant Hodgkin lymphoma. Virchows Arch 2018;473(6):759–64.

60. Chari ST, Smyrk TC, Levy MJ, et al. Diagnosis of autoimmune pancreatitis: the Mayo Clinic experience. Clin Gastroenterol Hepatol 2006;4(8):1010–6 [quiz: 1934].

61. Otsuki M, Chung JB, Okazaki K, et al. Asian diagnostic criteria for autoimmune pancreatitis: consensus of the Japan-Korea Symposium on Autoimmune Pancreatitis. J Gastroenterol 2008;43(6): 403–8.

62. Shimosegawa T, Chari ST, Frulloni L, et al. International consensus diagnostic criteria for autoimmune pancreatitis: guidelines of the International Association of Pancreatology. Pancreas 2011;40(3):352–8.

63. Ahuja J, Arora D, Kanne JP, et al. Imaging of pulmonary manifestations of connective tissue diseases. Radiol Clin North Am 2016;54(6):1015–31.

64. Mirmomen SM, Sirajuddin A, Nikpanah M, et al. Thoracic involvement in Erdheim-Chester disease: computed tomography imaging findings and their association with the BRAFV600E mutation. Eur Radiol 2018;28(11):4635–42.

65. Surabhi VR, Chua S, Patel RP, et al. Inflammatory myofibroblastic tumors: current update. Radiol Clin North Am 2016;54(3):553–63.

66. Cheuk W, Chan JK. Lymphadenopathy of IgG4-related disease: an underdiagnosed and overdiagnosed entity. Semin Diagn Pathol 2012;29(4): 226–34.

67. Sato Y, Notohara K, Kojima M, et al. IgG4-related disease: historical overview and pathology of hematological disorders. Pathol Int 2010;60(4):247–58.

68. Cheuk W, Yuen HK, Chu SY, et al. Lymphadenopathy of IgG4-related sclerosing disease. Am J Surg Pathol 2008;32(5):671–81.

69. Deshpande V. The pathology of IgG4-related disease: critical issues and challenges. Semin Diagn Pathol 2012;29(4):191–6.

70. Hao M, Liu M, Fan G, et al. Diagnostic value of serum IgG4 for IgG4-related disease: a

PRISMA-compliant systematic review and meta-analysis. Medicine (Baltimore) 2016;95(21):e3785.

71. Khosroshahi A, Cheryk LA, Carruthers MN, et al. Brief Report: spuriously low serum IgG4 concentrations caused by the prozone phenomenon in patients with IgG4-related disease. Arthritis Rheumatol 2014;66(1):213–7.

72. Cao L, Chen YB, Zhao DH, et al. Pulmonary function tests findings and their diagnostic value in patients with IgG4-related disease. J Thorac Dis 2017;9(3):547–54.

73. Khosroshahi A, Wallace ZS, Crowe JL, et al. International consensus guidance statement on the management and treatment of IgG4-related disease. Arthritis Rheumatol 2015;67(7):1688–99.

74. Shimizu Y, Yamamoto M, Naishiro Y, et al. Necessity of early intervention for IgG4-related disease–delayed treatment induces fibrosis progression. Rheumatology (Oxford) 2013;52(4):679–83.

75. Masaki Y, Matsui S, Saeki T, et al. A multicenter phase II prospective clinical trial of glucocorticoid for patients with untreated IgG4-related disease. Mod Rheumatol 2017;27(5):849–54.

76. Hart PA, Kamisawa T, Brugge WR, et al. Long-term outcomes of autoimmune pancreatitis: a multicentre, international analysis. Gut 2013;62(12):1771–6.

77. Masamune A, Nishimori I, Kikuta K, et al. Randomised controlled trial of long-term maintenance corticosteroid therapy in patients with autoimmune pancreatitis. Gut 2017;66(3):487–94.

78. Yunyun F, Yu P, Panpan Z, et al. Efficacy and safety of low dose Mycophenolate mofetil treatment for immunoglobulin G4-related disease: a randomized clinical trial. Rheumatology (Oxford) 2019;58(1):52–60.

79. Wang L, Zhang P, Wang M, et al. Failure of remission induction by glucocorticoids alone or in combination with immunosuppressive agents in IgG4-related disease: a prospective study of 215 patients. Arthritis Res Ther 2018;20(1):65.

Thoracic Manifestations of Ankylosing Spondylitis, Inflammatory Bowel Disease, and Relapsing Polychondritis

Abhijeet Danve, MD

KEYWORDS

- Thoracic • Pulmonary • Respiratory • Ankylosing spondylitis • Inflammatory bowel disease
- Relapsing polychondritis • Axial spondyloarthritis

KEY POINTS

- Ankylosing spondylitis, inflammatory bowel disease, and relapsing polychondritis are multisystem immune-mediated inflammatory diseases associated with variable involvement of airways, lungs, and thoracic wall.
- Obstructive sleep apnea, restrictive physiology, apical fibrosis, and spontaneous pneumothorax are well known but less frequent pulmonary manifestations in ankylosing spondylitis.
- Inflammatory bowel diseases can be associated with tracheobronchitis, bronchiectasis, and necrobiotic lung nodules.
- Airway involvement is seen in half of the patients with relapsing polychondritis and contributes significantly to morbidity and mortality. Early recognition is important to prevent long-term complications.

INTRODUCTION

The term spondyloarthropathy or spondyloarthritis (SpA) refers to a group of immune-medicated rheumatic diseases that are characterized by inflammation of axial and peripheral skeleton, entheses as well as involvement of skin, eyes, and intestines (**Fig. 1**). This group includes axial SpA, psoriatic arthritis, arthritis associated with inflammatory bowel disease (IBD), and reactive arthritis.[1] The term "axial spondyloarthritis (axSpA)" is a combined term used for ankylosing spondylitis (AS) (also called radiographic axSpA), and Its earlier stage is called nonradiographic axSpA (nr-axSpA). These diseases are also referred to as "seronegative spondyloarthropathy" because rheumatoid factor and antinuclear antibody are usually negative. Relapsing polychondritis (RP) is a systemic disease that primarily affects cartilaginous portion of several different organs mainly including upper and lower airways, ears, and eyes but can also involve joints, skin, and cardiovascular system.[2] Patients with SpA and RP can have variable cardiopulmonary involvement. This review focuses on the pulmonary manifestations of axSpA, RP, and IBD.

AXIAL SPONDYLOARTHRITIS

Chronic inflammation in sacroiliac (SI) joints and joints of the spine, leading to chronic inflammatory low back pain is the most characteristic feature of axSpA. These patients can also have enthesitis (inflammation of the insertion site of tendons or

Disclosure Statement: The author has served on advisory board or has received research grants from Janssen and Novartis.

Section of Rheumatology, Department of Medicine, Yale School of Medicine, 300 Cedar Street, TACS-525, New Haven, CT 06520-8031, USA

E-mail address: abhijeet.danve@yale.edu

chestmed.theclinics.com

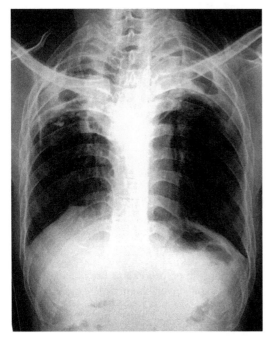

Fig. 1. Chest radiograph showing bilateral upper zone fibrocavitary/bullous changes with volume loss. The trachea is deviated to the right side and both the hila are pulled up. (*From* Madan K, Guleria R. Bamboo spine and the lungs. *BMJ Case Rep.* 2013 Oct 8;2013. pii: bcr2013201006. https://doi.org/10.1136/bcr-2013-201006; with permission.)

ligaments into the bones) and peripheral inflammatory arthritis commonly affecting the joints of lower extremities. Chronic inflammation may result in structural damage and new bone formation in SI joints and spine, causing fusion of the SI joint and spine in late stages (called bamboo spine). Preradiographic stage is called "nonradiographic axial spondyloarthritis", whereas the term "ankylosing spondylitis" is used when there is obvious sacroiliitis on radiograph. Common extraarticular manifestations of axSpA include anterior uveitis (25%–35%), asymptomatic (up to 60%) or symptomatic (7%) colitis, and psoriasis (10%), but this disease is also associated with various other extra-articular manifestations, which include osteoporosis, respiratory abnormalities, cardiac conduction abnormalities, valvular insufficiency, immunoglobulin A nephropathy, and secondary amyloidosis. This disease tends to affect young adults in their third decade of life with male to female ratio of 2:1. There is strong genetic association between HLA-B27 and axSpA. About 85% to 95% patients with AS have positive HLA B27 and about 50% patients with nr-axSpA have positive HLA B27. Most of the data in literature about the thoracic manifestations pertain to AS. The thoracic manifestations of AS can be divided into those

affecting chest wall, airways, lung parenchyma, heart, and great vessels (**Table 1**).

Abnormalities of Chest Wall and Ventilatory Apparatus

Anterior chest wall pain

Anterior chest wall (ACW) pain is a classic symptom of patients with SpA. Pain can be diffuse or localized to sternocostal, sternoclavicular, and manubriosternal areas. Usually the ACW pain is acute, sharp, and worse with respiratory movements and movements of the arm. It tends to present in flares lasting few weeks and frequent recurrences. It is relieved by nonsteroidal antiinflammatory drugs and tumor necrosis factor (TNF) inhibitors.[3] ACW pain arises from enthesitis of rib cage and inflammation of sternoclavicular or manubriosternal joints. It can occur in earlier as well as later stages of the disease.[4,5] Overall 30% to 60% patients with axSpA develop ACW pain during the course of the disease. About 4% to 6% patients can have ACW pain as the first manifestation of SpA,[3,5] but most of the patients experience ACW pain after the onset of back pain. ACW is associated with longer disease duration, severe disease, radiographic sacroiliitis, and higher enthesitis scores.[5] Involvement of sternoclavicular joints has been reported in 17% to 50% patients[4,6] and manubriosternal joints in 51% of patients.[6]

Restrictive lung disease

Prevalence of restrictive lung disease in AS has been variably reported between 20% and 57%.[7] Patients with late stages of AS tend to have

Table 1 Thoracic manifestations of ankylosing spondylitis	
Chest wall and ventilatory apparatus	Anterior chest wall pain Restrictive lung disease Obstructive sleep apnea
Pleuroparenchymal disease	Apical fibrosis Spontaneous pneumothorax Asymptomatic HRCT abnormalities
Airway disease	Cricoarytenoid arthritis COPD
Cardiac and great vessels	Valvular heart disease, Conduction abnormalities, Aortitis, Periaortitis

Abbreviations: COPD, chronic obstructive pulmonary disease; HRCT, high-resolution computed tomography.

restrictive lung physiology due to involvement of thoracic cage as well as parenchymal disease (apical fibrosis). Chest expansion is reduced in advanced AS due to pain and stiffness in thoracic spine and costovertebral joints as well as fusion in the vertebral joints.[8] Inflammation in the thoracic vertebrae and costovertebral joints can lead to fusion, kyphosis, rigidity, and immobility of chest wall causing reduced chest expansion.[9] Thus, restrictive physiology in AS can be from a fixed component of structural damage to thoracic cage and lung parenchyma as well as a dynamic component of inflammation causing pain, stiffness, and resultant reduced mobility. In a cross-sectional study of 147 patients, reduced pulmonary function was associated with decreased spinal mobility and chest wall mobility.[10]

Obstructive sleep apnea

The prevalence of obstructive sleep apnea (OSA) in AS is reported to be higher than that in general population. Kang and colleagues found a prevalence of 0.85% among 1411 patients with AS compared with 0.50% in control population.[11] In an observational study using 6679 patients with AS and 19,951 matched controls from national claims database, OSA was found to be more prevalent (8.8%) as compared with controls (5.1%). Risk was increased in older patients with AS (>45 years).[12] In a small prospective study of 31 patients, 22% patients were found to have OSA.[13] OSA was found to be common in older patients with AS (>35 years), with longer disease duration. Mean body mass index (BMI) was higher in patients with AS with OSA but not statistically significant as compared with patients without OSA.[13] Several mechanisms have been suggested which include restriction of the oropharyngeal airway from cervical spine disease, compression of the respiratory center in the medulla from cervical spine involvement resulting in central depression of respiration or restrictive pulmonary physiology.[14] Patients with OSA suffer from worse fatigue and increased risk of hypertension and cardiovascular disease, which are also known comorbidities of AS. Therefore, it is important to have low threshold to evaluate patients with AS for OSA in the appropriate clinical setting. Treatment with TNF inhibitors was associated with improved sleep quality but not the polysomnography parameters in 34 patients with AS.[15] Also, OSA seems to be a chronic proinflammatory state by virtue of hypoxia-induced release of cytokines. Interestingly, patients with OSA are found to be at elevated risk of developing autoimmune inflammatory conditions, mainly rheumatoid arthritis (RA) but also AS and systemic lupus erythematosus.[11]

Pleuroparenchymal Diseases

Prevalence of pleuroparenchymal involvement in AS varies with the methods used for detection and the disease duration. Studies using high-resolution computed tomography (HRCT) of the chest find that 40% to 90% patients with AS have abnormalities detected in lung parenchyma,[8,16–18] 20% to 57% using spirometry[8,19,20] and 1% to 8% using radiograph of the chest.[21,22] In routine clinical practice, symptomatic pleuroparenchymal disease is encountered less frequently than that reported in previous studies.

Apical fibrosis

Apical fibrosis is a known complication of late stages of AS and also the most common lung parenchymal abnormality reported. Apical fibrosis in AS can be unilateral, bilateral, and can be associated with cystic changes (**Fig. 1**). It was the first pulmonary manifestation of AS described in literature by Dunham and Kautz.[7] Histologic sections of the apices have shown chronic inflammatory infiltrates within the alveolus and accompanied by areas of interstitial fibrosis with foci of dense collagen deposits. Apical fibrosis is not unique to AS and may be seen in other inflammatory rheumatic disorders such as RA.[23] In a systematic review by Maghraoui and colleagues, 6.9% of 303 patients with AS had apical fibrosis.[24] Prevalence of apical fibrosis increases with the disease duration. Recurrent aspiration pneumonitis was the suggested mechanism for apical fibrosis, but exact cause is not known.[25] Apical fibrosis can be complicated by bullous or cavitary changes and misdiagnosed as pulmonary tuberculosis given the similar radiological appearance.[26,27] Also, apical fibrosis is a risk factor for superinfection with tuberculosis (TB) and aspergillus. It is important to differentiate pulmonary fibro bullous disease from TB in patients with AS, especially because the TNF inhibitors used for the treatment of AS themselves increase the risk of TB. Apical fibrosis is an independent risk factor for colonization by aspergillus and formation of aspergilloma.[28] It is not clear if TNF inhibitors prevent initiation or progression of apical fibrosis.

Spontaneous pneumothorax

Presence of apical bullae increases the likelihood of spontaneous pneumothorax. The estimated incidence of spontaneous pneumothorax in patients with AS was 0.29%, which is higher than that in the general population.[29] Unilateral as well as bilateral spontaneous pneumothoraces have been reported.[30] Smoking and thin body habitus haven been reported as risk factors for spontaneous pneumothorax in AS.[7]

Imaging abnormalities

Studies using chest HRCT in patients with AS show several nonspecific findings. Various studies have reported abnormal HRCT findings in 40% to 98% patients. Whether these abnormalities are clinically relevant is not entirely clear. In a systematic review of 10 studies (303 patients), the prevalence of pulmonary abnormalities on chest HRCT of patients with AS was 61%. A total of 185 patients (61%) had an abnormal thoracic HRCT: upper lobe fibrosis in 21 (6.9%), emphysema in 55 (18.1%), bronchiectasis in 33 (10.8%), and ground glass attenuation in 34 (11.2%). Nonspecific interstitial abnormalities were observed in 101 (33%) patients.[17] In a more recent study involving 41 patients with AS, nodules, peribronchial thickening, pleural thickening, bronchiectasis, apical fibrosis, and emphysema were the most frequent abnormalities.[31]

Other

There are few reports of cricoarytenoid joint arthritis associated with AS.[32] Cricoarytenoid arthritis causing dysphonia is more common in RA than in AS. Also, there are case reports of alveolar hemorrhage in patients with AS and association between chronic obstructive pulmonary disease and AS.[33,34]

Cardiac and Great Vessel Abnormalities

Valvular heart disease and conduction abnormalities

Both asymptomatic as well as symptomatic valvular heart disease and cardiac conduction abnormalities have been associated with AS. Valvular disease and conduction blocks have been linked to aortitis and positive HLA B27.[35] Previous studies have reported that up to 82% patients with AS may have subclinical echocardiographic abnormalities.[36] Different case series report prevalence of aortic insufficiency to be 0% to 34%, whereas mitral regurgitation was reported in 5% to 74% patients. Valvular insufficiency is typically mild and associated with long-standing AS. Clinically significant valvular disease occurs in 2% to 12% patients with AS.[37–39] The thickening of the valvular cusps, dilatation of the aortic root, and abnormal cusp displacement via the thickened subaortic tissue that lead to aortic regurgitation are observed on echocardiography.[40] It is not clear whether patients with AS should be routinely screened for valvular disease and conduction abnormalities. A recent study suggested that the lifetime prevalence of valvular heart disease and pacemaker use in elderly patients with ankylosing spondylitis was only slightly higher than in controls, and this slight increase does not support

screening for subclinical heart disease in patients with AS.[41] Asymptomatic conduction abnormalities can be found in 10% to 33% patients with AS and they mainly include first-degree atrioventricular block and QRS prolongation.[42,43] Complete heart block has been reported in 0% to 9% patients with AS.[36]

Aortitis

Clinically silent aortitis is found in 10% to 20% patients with AS in autopsy studies.[44] Typically, the ascending aorta is affected late in the course of disease. Aortitis is only rarely seen in routine clinical practice. Chronic periaortitis has also been described in patients with AS.[45]

INFLAMMATORY BOWEL DISEASE

IBD is a combined term used for 2 conditions, Crohn's disease (CD) and ulcerative colitis (UC), which are characterized by chronic inflammation in the digestive tract. UC mainly affects mucosal layer of continuous sections of colon, whereas CD causes transmural inflammation and skip lesions throughout the entire gastrointestinal tract, ileocolitis being the most common feature. Extraintestinal manifestations (EIMs) occur commonly in UC as well as CD and involve joints (axial and peripheral inflammatory arthritis), eyes (uveitis and episcleritis), skin (erythema nodosum and pyoderma gangrenosum), and liver (primary sclerosing cholangitis, fatty liver). Although less frequent, pulmonary disease has been reported as a distinct extraintestinal manifestation in both UC and CD. Lung involvement is characterized by airway disease, serositis, parenchymal disease, pulmonary thromboembolism, and asymptomatic abnormalities found on pulmonary function tests (PFTs) and imaging (**Table 2**).

Prevalence of pulmonary disease in IBD is variably reported in the literature (see **Table 2**).[46,47] Airway complications are more frequent in women, whereas serositis occurs among men and women in equal frequency. Airways and parenchymal lung disease does not correlate with severity of IBD; rather airway disease developing after colectomy is known.[46] Serositis on the other hand affects patients who have active IBD symptoms. In most of the patients, lung involvement follows gastrointestinal disease; however, rarely lung disease can be the initial symptom of IBD.

Airway Disease

IBD can be associated with inflammation of trachea, bronchi, and bronchioles.[46,48,49] Upper airway disease can manifest as subglottic stenosis, tracheitis, and tracheal stenosis.[50–52] Patients

Table 2
Pulmonary manifestations of inflammatory bowel diseases

Airways	Bronchiectasis
	Chronic bronchitis
	Bronchiolitis
	Subglottic stenosis
	Fistulae
Serositis	Pericarditis
	Pleuritis
	Myopericarditis
Parenchymal disease	COOP
	ILD
	Necrobiotic nodules
	Sarcoidosis
Thromboembolic disease	Pulmonary thromboembolism
Medication-induced lung injury	Methotrexate
	Mesalamine, Sulfasalazine
	Infliximab,
	Vedolizumab
Asymptomatic abnormalities	Reduced DLCO
	Bronchial wall thickening

Abbreviations: COOP, cryptogenic organizing pneumonia; DLCO, diffusing capacity of the lung for carbon monoxide; ILD, interstitial lung disease.

may present with cough, dyspnea, dysphonia, and stridor.

Chronic bronchitis and more commonly bronchiectasis occur in variable frequency in patients with UC more than CD.[53,54] IBD-related bronchiectasis differs from usual bronchiectasis in that the symptoms are more steroid responsive. Bronchiectasis is more common in UC than CD. Patients typically have copious secretions and chronic cough. Granulomatous airway inflammation can be seen in CD. Patients can develop symptoms of airway disease even after colectomy.[52]

Bronchiolitis also can occur with IBD-related lung disease. With the use of HRCT, it is being more frequently observed than before. The airway disease in IBD responds well to inhaled and systemic steroids.[55]

Fistulae between intestines and airways and lungs have been reported in patients with CD. They include colobronchial, ileobronchial, and enteric-pulmonary fistulae.[56,57] Rarely colopleural fistula and fecopneumothorax have been reported as complications and these need urgent surgical intervention.[58,59]

Serositis

Pleurisy, pericarditis, and myopericarditis are uncommon complications of IBD.[60,61] Usually these

occur in young men with quiescent UC.[55] Sometimes serositis can can be an adverse effect of medications, especially TNF inhibitors or mesalamine.

Parenchymal Disease

About one-fourth of the patients with IBD-related lung disease have involvement of lung parenchyma.[46] Most common presentations include cryptogenic organizing pneumonia (COOP) and interstitial lung disease (ILD).[51,62] Acute or subacute onset cough and shortness of breath are most common symptoms. COOP is usually treated with systemic steroids but sometimes can remit spontaneously. COOP can be also seen in other autoimmune diseases such as RA, myositis, and vasculitis and can also occur as adverse reaction to medications.

ILD in IBD can present as COOP, nonspecific interstitial pneumonia, usual interstitial pneumonia, and eosinophilic pneumonia.[51] Bronchioalveolar lavage fluid in IBD-associated ILD is commonly lymphocytic with elevated CD4:CD8 ratio similar to sarcoidosis.[51,63]

Necrobiotic pulmonary nodules have been frequently reported in CD.[64-66] Radiologically these cavitating nodules can mimic septic emboli or granulomatosis with polyangiitis. Several features of lung disease in CD share similarities with granulomatosis with polyangiitis, including COOP, granulomatous inflammation, and necrobiotic nodules.[64] Histologically these nodules demonstrate sterile aggregates of neutrophils with necrosis.[67]

There are numerous reports of coexisting sarcoidosis and UC or CD in the literature.[68,69] Sarcoidosis and CD both being granulomatous diseases may share pathologic and genetic aspects,[56,70] although they run independent course in same patient.[71] Men with IBD are at higher risk of developing sarcoidosis.[72]

Thromboembolic Disease

IBD is now a known risk factor for venous thromboembolism.[73,74] Patients with IBD have 3- to 4-fold higher risk of venous thromboembolism (VTE) than in age-matched control subjects.[75,76] VTE is an important cause of mortality in IBD and tends to occur when IBD is clinically active.[74]

Medication-Induced Lung Injury

There are several reports of pneumonitis from sulfasalazine, mesalamine, and methotrexate in patients with IBD.[77-79] Infliximab can cause serositis and a lupus-like syndrome. Infliximab-induced interstitial pneumonitis also has been reported.[80,81] There is one case report of development of symptomatic necrobiotic nodules in a patient with IBD, 4 months after starting vedolizumab. Symptoms and radiological findings resolved after treatment with steroids and stopping vedolizumab.[82]

Asymptomatic Abnormalities

Asymptomatic abnormalities on PFTs are observed in up to 50% patients with IBD and these include restrictive physiology and reduced diffusion capacity.[47,83] In an observational study of 601 patients, 167 patients with UC and 93 patients with CD had abnormal chest HRCT, most common findings being centrilobular nodules (49% and 45%, respectively) and bronchial wall thickening (31% and 54%, respectively). There was no correlation between disease activity and HRCT findings.[84]

RELAPSING POLYCHONDRITIS

RP is an inflammatory immune-mediated disease mainly involving cartilaginous structures in the body but can also involve other organs. RP predominantly affects the cartilaginous portions of ear, nose, respiratory tract, and joints. Exact pathogenesis is unknown, but it seems to be autoimmune response to type II collagen, which is abundant in cartilage and sclera.[85] RP tends to affect both sexes equally. It has been reported in all age groups and ethnicities with predilection toward adults in their 50s. Patients with RP have diverse manifestations with episodic or smoldering diseases that evolve and recur over time; there is no specific laboratory or imaging test, and the diagnosis is made on clinical grounds. Antineutrophil cytoplasmic antibodies (ANCA) can be present in patients with RP.[86] McAdam and colleagues suggested diagnostic criterion for RP where a patient needs to have the presence of any 3 out of the following 6 clinical features: (1) bilateral auricular chondritis, (2) nonerosive seronegative inflammatory arthritis, (3) nasal chondritis, (4) ocular inflammation, (5) respiratory tract chondritis, or (6) audiovestibular damage.[87]

Auricular chondritis is most common and usually the presenting feature of RP.[88,89] Ocular disease is characterized by scleritis, episcleritis, peripheral ulcerative keratitis, and uveitis.[90,91] Nasal chondritis can lead to saddle nose deformity. Other associations of RP include arthralgia and arthritis, cutaneous involvement, valvular heart diseases, and hematological abnormalities, mainly myelodysplastic syndrome.

Respiratory tract is involved in 30% to 50% of the patients with RP and is associated with poor prognosis.[92,93] RP mainly affects the cartilaginous portions of the large airways; pulmonary parenchymal or vascular involvement is rare.[88] Involvement of larynx, trachea, and bronchi can occur slowly over years and can lead to life-threatening complications.[88] Laryngotracheal disease can lead to tracheal stenosis and stricture formation in about 25% of patients with air way involvement.[88] Tracheomalacia, bronchomalacia, or tracheobronchomalacia is caused by recurrent airway chondritis and is associated with poor prognosis.[94] Sometimes, large air way disease can be the isolated manifestation of RP.[95] Destruction of cartilaginous portion of trachea can cause dynamic airway collapse during the forced expiration and sleep apnea. The clinical features from the airway involvement in RP are variable depending on the extent and severity of the inflammation and damage. Lower respiratory tract infection is an important cause of death in RP. Patients can present with cough, shortness of breath, dysphonia, stridor, or hoarseness of voice. Tenderness of thyroid cartilage, laryngeal, and tracheal rings is a feature of active RP. Patients with severe tracheal stenosis may need tracheal stenting.[96] Many patients with RP are initially misdiagnosed to have asthma and remain undiagnosed until late phases because frequent treatment with steroid tapers for presumed asthma, thus masking the underlying polychondritis.[97] Contrary to asthma, the airway inflammation in RP does not respond to inhaled steroids and bronchodilators. The spirometry can reveal upper airway obstruction, and CT scan demonstrates thickening and stenosis of the large airways with dynamic collapse during forced expiration. *Bronchoscopy* can show inflammation, narrowing, or collapse of the airways. If detected early, airway disease in RP can be treated with steroids and TNF inhibitors.[88,98] In late stages, however, patients may need tracheostomy, stenting, or reconstructive procedures.[93,99]

ACKNOWLEDGMENTS

The author would like to thank Ms Melissa Funaro MLS, MS (Yale Medical Library) for her assistance with literature search.

REFERENCES

1. Raychaudhuri SP, Deodhar A. The classification and diagnostic criteria of ankylosing spondylitis. J Autoimmun 2014;48-49:128–33.
2. Lahmer T, Treiber M, von Werder A, et al. Relapsing polychondritis: an autoimmune disease with many faces. Autoimmun Rev 2010;9(8):540–6.
3. Elhai M, Paternotte S, Burki V, et al. Clinical characteristics of anterior chest wall pain in

spondyloarthritis: an analysis of 275 patients. Joint Bone Spine 2012;79(5):476–81.

4. Fournie B, Boutes A, Dromer C, et al. Prospective study of anterior chest wall involvement in ankylosing spondylitis and psoriatic arthritis. Rev Rhum Engl Ed 1997;64(1):22–5.

5. Wendling D, Prati C, Demattei C, et al. Anterior chest wall pain in recent inflammatory back pain suggestive of spondyloarthritis. data from the DESIR cohort. J Rheumatol 2013;40(7): 1148–52.

6. Jurik AG. Anterior chest wall involvement in seronegative arthritides. A study of the frequency of changes at radiography. Rheumatol Int 1992;12(1): 7–11.

7. Kanathur N, Lee-Chiong T. Pulmonary manifestations of ankylosing spondylitis. Clin Chest Med 2010;31(3):547–54.

8. Dincer U, Cakar E, Kiralp MZ, et al. The pulmonary involvement in rheumatic diseases: pulmonary effects of ankylosing spondylitis and its impact on functionality and quality of life. Tohoku J Exp Med 2007;212(4):423–30.

9. Fisher LR, Cawley MI, Holgate ST. Relation between chest expansion, pulmonary function, and exercise tolerance in patients with ankylosing spondylitis. Ann Rheum Dis 1990;49(11):921–5.

10. Berdal G, Halvorsen S, van der Heijde D, et al. Restrictive pulmonary function is more prevalent in patients with ankylosing spondylitis than in matched population controls and is associated with impaired spinal mobility: a comparative study. Arthritis Res Ther 2012;14(1):R19.

11. Kang JH, Lin HC. Obstructive sleep apnea and the risk of autoimmune diseases: a longitudinal population-based study. Sleep Med 2012;13(6): 583–8.

12. Walsh JA, Song X, Kim G, et al. Evaluation of the comorbidity burden in patients with ankylosing spondylitis using a large US administrative claims data set. Clin Rheumatol 2018;37(7):1869–78.

13. Solak O, Fidan F, Dundar U, et al. The prevalence of obstructive sleep apnoea syndrome in ankylosing spondylitis patients. Rheumatology (Oxford) 2009; 48(4):433–5.

14. Erb N, Karokis D, Delamere JP, et al. Obstructive sleep apnoea as a cause of fatigue in ankylosing spondylitis. Ann Rheum Dis 2003;62(2):183–4.

15. Karatas G, Bal A, Yuceege M, et al. Evaluation of sleep quality in patients with ankylosing spondylitis and efficacy of anti-TNF-alpha therapy on sleep problems: a polisomnographic study. Int J Rheum Dis 2018;21(6):1263–9.

16. Turetschek K, Ebner W, Fleischmann D, et al. Early pulmonary involvement in ankylosing spondylitis: assessment with thin-section CT. Clin Radiol 2000; 55(8):632–6.

17. El-Maghraoui A, Chaouir S, Bezza A, et al. Thoracic high resolution computed tomography in patients with ankylosing spondylitis and without respiratory symptoms. Ann Rheum Dis 2003; 62(2):185–6.

18. Altin R, Ozdolap S, Savranlar A, et al. Comparison of early and late pleuropulmonary findings of ankylosing spondylitis by high-resolution computed tomography and effects on patients' daily life. Clin Rheumatol 2005;24(1):22–8.

19. Ayhan-Ardic FF, Oken O, Yorgancioglu ZR, et al. Pulmonary involvement in lifelong non-smoking patients with rheumatoid arthritis and ankylosing spondylitis without respiratory symptoms. Clin Rheumatol 2006;25(2):213–8.

20. Baser S, Cubukcu S, Ozkurt S, et al. Pulmonary involvement starts in early stage ankylosing spondylitis. Scand J Rheumatol 2006;35(4):325–7.

21. Rosenow E, Strimlan CV, Muhm JR, et al. Pleuropulmonary manifestations of ankylosing spondylitis. Mayo Clin Proc 1977;52(10):641–9.

22. Sampaio-Barros PD, Cerqueira EM, Rezende SM, et al. Pulmonary involvement in ankylosing spondylitis. Clin Rheumatol 2007;26(2):225–30.

23. Cohen AA, Natelson EA, Fechner RE. Fibrosing interstitial pneumonitis in ankylosing spondylitis. Chest 1971;59(4):369–71.

24. El Maghraoui A, Dehhaoui M. Prevalence and characteristics of lung involvement on high resolution computed tomography in patients with ankylosing spondylitis: a systematic review. Pulm Med 2012; 2012:965956.

25. Davies D. Lung fibrosis in ankylosing spondylitis. Thorax 1972;27(2):262.

26. Pamuk ON, Harmandar O, Tosun B, et al. A patient with ankylosing spondylitis who presented with chronic necrotising aspergillosis: report on one case and review of the literature. Clin Rheumatol 2005;24(4):415–9.

27. Kim DY, Lee SJ, Ryu YJ, et al. Progressive pulmonary fibrocystic changes of both upper lungs in a patient with ankylosing spondylitis. Tuberc Respir Dis (Seoul) 2015;78(4):459–62.

28. Thai D, Ratani RS, Salama S, et al. Upper lobe fibrocavitary disease in a patient with back pain and stiffness. Chest 2000;118(6):1814–6.

29. Lee CC, Lee SH, Chang IJ, et al. Spontaneous pneumothorax associated with ankylosing spondylitis. Rheumatology (Oxford) 2005;44(12):1538–41.

30. Ersoy E, Akgol G, Ozgocmen S. Bilateral spontaneous pneumothorax in a patient with longstanding ankylosing spondylitis. Acta Reumatol Port 2014; 39(4):353–4.

31. Yuksekkaya R, Almus F, Celikyay F, et al. Pulmonary involvement in ankylosing spondylitis assessed by multidetector computed tomography. Pol J Radiol 2014;79:156–63.

32. Desuter G, Duprez T, Huart C, et al. The use of adalimumab for cricoarytenoid arthritis in ankylosing spondylitis–an effective therapy. Laryngoscope 2011;121(2):335–8.

33. Hara S, Sakamoto N, Ishimatsu Y, et al. Diffuse alveolar hemorrhage in a patient with ankylosing spondylitis. Intern Med 2013;52(17):1963–6.

34. Lai SW, Lin CL. Association between ankylosing spondylitis and chronic obstructive pulmonary disease in Taiwan. Eur J Intern Med 2018;57:e28–9.

35. O'Neill TW, Bresnihan B. The heart in ankylosing spondylitis. Ann Rheum Dis 1992;51(6):705–6.

36. Roldan CA, Chavez J, Wiest PW, et al. Aortic root disease and valve disease associated with ankylosing spondylitis. J Am Coll Cardiol 1998;32(5):1397–404.

37. Graham DC, Smythe HA. The carditis and aortitis of ankylosing spondylitis. Bull Rheum Dis 1958;9(3):171–4.

38. Gran JT, Skomsvoll JF. The outcome of ankylosing spondylitis: a study of 100 patients. Br J Rheumatol 1997;36(7):766–71.

39. Szabo SM, Levy AR, Rao SR, et al. Increased risk of cardiovascular and cerebrovascular diseases in individuals with ankylosing spondylitis: a population-based study. Arthritis Rheum 2011;63(11):3294–304.

40. Moyssakis I, Gialafos E, Vassiliou VA, et al. Myocardial performance and aortic elasticity are impaired in patients with ankylosing spondylitis. Scand J Rheumatol 2009;38(3):216–21.

41. Ward MM. Lifetime risks of valvular heart disease and pacemaker use in patients with ankylosing spondylitis. J Am Heart Assoc 2018;7(20):e010016.

42. Forsblad-d'Elia H, Wallberg H, Klingberg E, et al. Cardiac conduction system abnormalities in ankylosing spondylitis: a cross-sectional study. BMC Musculoskelet Disord 2013;14:237.

43. Dik VK, Peters MJ, Dijkmans PA, et al. The relationship between disease-related characteristics and conduction disturbances in ankylosing spondylitis. Scand J Rheumatol 2010;39(1):38–41.

44. Davidson P, Baggenstoss AH, Slocumb CH, et al. Cardiac and aortic lesions in rheumatoid spondylitis. Proc Staff Meet Mayo Clin 1963;38:427–35.

45. Palazzi C, Salvarani C, D'Angelo S, et al. Aortitis and periaortitis in ankylosing spondylitis. Joint Bone Spine 2011;78(5):451–5.

46. Camus P, Piard F, Ashcroft T, et al. The lung in inflammatory bowel disease. Medicine (Baltimore) 1993;72(3):151–83.

47. Tunc B, Filik L, Bilgic F, et al. Pulmonary function tests, high-resolution computed tomography findings and inflammatory bowel disease. Acta Gastroenterol Belg 2006;69(3):255–60.

48. Bayraktaroglu S, Basoglu O, Ceylan N, et al. A rare extraintestinal manifestation of ulcerative colitis: tracheobronchitis associated with ulcerative colitis. J Crohns Colitis 2010;4(6):679–82.

49. Kuzniar T, Sleiman C, Brugiere O, et al. Severe tracheobronchial stenosis in a patient with Crohn's disease. Eur Respir J 2000;15(1):209–12.

50. Rickli H, Fretz C, Hoffman M, et al. Severe inflammatory upper airway stenosis in ulcerative colitis. Eur Respir J 1994;7(10):1899–902.

51. Black H, Mendoza M, Murin S. Thoracic manifestations of inflammatory bowel disease. Chest 2007;131(2):524–32.

52. Vasishta S, Wood JB, McGinty F. Ulcerative tracheobronchitis years after colectomy for ulcerative colitis. Chest 1994;106(4):1279–81.

53. Spira A, Grossman R, Balter M. Large airway disease associated with inflammatory bowel disease. Chest 1998;113(6):1723–6.

54. Eaton TE, Lambie N, Wells AU. Bronchiectasis following colectomy for Crohn's disease. Thorax 1998;53(6):529–31.

55. Ji XQ, Wang LX, Lu DG. Pulmonary manifestations of inflammatory bowel disease. World J Gastroenterol 2014;20(37):13501–11.

56. Storch I, Sachar D, Katz S. Pulmonary manifestations of inflammatory bowel disease. Inflamm Bowel Dis 2003;9(2):104–15.

57. Casella G, Villanacci V, Di Bella C, et al. Pulmonary diseases associated with inflammatory bowel diseases. J Crohns Colitis 2010;4(4):384–9.

58. Alameel T, Maclean DA, Macdougall R. Colobronchial fistula presenting with persistent pneumonia in a patient with Crohn's disease: a case report. Cases J 2009;2:9114.

59. Barisiae G, Krivokapiae Z, Adziae T, et al. Fecopneumothorax and colopleural fistula - uncommon complications of Crohn's disease. BMC Gastroenterol 2006;6:17.

60. Faller M, Gasser B, Massard G, et al. Pulmonary migratory infiltrates and pachypleuritis in a patient with Crohn's disease. Respiration 2000;67(4):459–63.

61. Patwardhan RV, Heilpern RJ, Brewster AC, et al. Pleuropericarditis: an extraintestinal complication of inflammatory bowel disease. Report of three cases and review of literature. Arch Intern Med 1983;143(1):94–6.

62. Casey MB, Tazelaar HD, Myers JL, et al. Noninfectious lung pathology in patients with Crohn's disease. Am J Surg Pathol 2003;27(2):213–9.

63. Bewig B, Manske I, Bottcher H, et al. Crohn's disease mimicking sarcoidosis in bronchoalveolar lavage. Respiration 1999;66(5):467–9.

64. Nelson BA, Kaplan JL, El Saleeby CM, et al. Case records of the Massachusetts General Hospital. Case 39-2014. A 9-year-old girl with Crohn's disease and pulmonary nodules. N Engl J Med 2014;371(25):2418–27.

65. Freeman HJ, Davis JE, Prest ME, et al. Granulomatous bronchiolitis with necrobiotic pulmonary nodules in Crohn's disease. Can J Gastroenterol 2004; 18(11):687–90.

66. El-Kersh K, Fraig M, Cavallazzi R, et al. Pulmonary necrobiotic nodules in Crohn's disease: a rare extra-intestinal manifestation. Respir Care 2014; 59(12):e190–2.

67. Kasuga I, Yanagisawa N, Takeo C, et al. Multiple pulmonary nodules in association with pyoderma gangrenosum. Respir Med 1997;91(8):493–5.

68. Smiejan JM, Cosnes J, Chollet-Martin S, et al. Sarcoid-like lymphocytosis of the lower respiratory tract in patients with active Crohn's disease. Ann Intern Med 1986;104(1):17–21.

69. Theodoropoulos G, Archimandritis A, Davaris P, et al. Ulcerative colitis and sarcoidosis: a curious association-report of a case. Dis Colon Rectum 1981;24(4):308–10.

70. Fellermann K, Stahl M, Dahlhoff K, et al. Crohn's disease and sarcoidosis: systemic granulomatosis? Eur J Gastroenterol Hepatol 1997;9(11):1121–4.

71. Fries W, Grassi SA, Leone L, et al. Association between inflammatory bowel disease and sarcoidosis. Report of two cases and review of the literature. Scand J Gastroenterol 1995;30(12): 1221–3.

72. Halling ML, Kjeldsen J, Knudsen T, et al. Patients with inflammatory bowel disease have increased risk of autoimmune and inflammatory diseases. World J Gastroenterol 2017;23(33):6137–46.

73. Yuhara H, Steinmaus C, Corley D, et al. Meta-analysis: the risk of venous thromboembolism in patients with inflammatory bowel disease. Aliment Pharmacol Ther 2013;37(10):953–62.

74. Solem CA, Loftus EV, Tremaine WJ, et al. Venous thromboembolism in inflammatory bowel disease. Am J Gastroenterol 2004;99(1):97–101.

75. Miehsler W, Reinisch W, Valic E, et al. Is inflammatory bowel disease an independent and disease specific risk factor for thromboembolism? Gut 2004;53(4):542–8.

76. Bernstein CN, Blanchard JF, Houston DS, et al. The incidence of deep venous thrombosis and pulmonary embolism among patients with inflammatory bowel disease: a population-based cohort study. Thromb Haemost 2001;85(3):430–4.

77. Parry SD, Barbatzas C, Peel ET, et al. Sulphasalazine and lung toxicity. Eur Respir J 2002;19(4): 756–64.

78. Jain N, Petruff C, Bandyopadhyay T. Mesalamine lung toxicity. Conn Med 2010;74(5):265–7.

79. Margagnoni G, Papi V, Aratari A, et al. Methotrexate-induced pneumonitis in a patient with Crohn's disease. J Crohns Colitis 2010;4(2):211–4.

80. Perez-Alvarez R, Perez-de-Lis M, Diaz-Lagares C, et al. Interstitial lung disease induced or exacerbated by TNF-targeted therapies: analysis of 122 cases. Semin Arthritis Rheum 2011;41(2): 256–64.

81. Heraganahally SS, Au V, Kondru S, et al. Pulmonary toxicity associated with infliximab therapy for ulcerative colitis. Intern Med J 2009;39(9):629–30.

82. Myc LA, Girton MR, Stoler MH, et al. Necrobiotic pulmonary nodules of Crohn's disease in a patient receiving vedolizumab. Am J Respir Crit Care Med 2019;199(1):e1–2.

83. Marvisi M, Borrello PD, Brianti M, et al. Changes in the carbon monoxide diffusing capacity of the lung in ulcerative colitis. Eur Respir J 2000;16(5):965–8.

84. Sato H, Okada F, Matsumoto S, et al. Chest high-resolution computed tomography findings in 601 patients with inflammatory bowel diseases. Acad Radiol 2018;25(4):407–14.

85. Letko E, Zafirakis P, Baltatzis S, et al. Relapsing polychondritis: a clinical review. Semin Arthritis Rheum 2002;31(6):384–95.

86. Papo T, Piette JC, Le Thi Huong D, et al. Antineutrophil cytoplasmic antibodies in polychondritis. Ann Rheum Dis 1993;52(5):384–5.

87. McAdam LP, O'Hanlan MA, Bluestone R, et al. Relapsing polychondritis: prospective study of 23 patients and a review of the literature. Medicine (Baltimore) 1976;55(3):193–215.

88. Kent PD, Michet CJ Jr, Luthra HS. Relapsing polychondritis. Curr Opin Rheumatol 2004;16(1):56–61.

89. Chuah TY, Lui NL. Relapsing polychondritis in Singapore: a case series and review of literature. Singapore Med J 2017;58(4):201–5.

90. Sainz-de-la-Maza M, Molina N, Gonzalez-Gonzalez LA, et al. Scleritis associated with relapsing polychondritis. Br J Ophthalmol 2016;100(9): 1290–4.

91. Isaak BL, Liesegang TJ, Michet CJ Jr. Ocular and systemic findings in relapsing polychondritis. Ophthalmology 1986;93(5):681–9.

92. Hazra N, Dregan A, Charlton J, et al. Incidence and mortality of relapsing polychondritis in the UK: a population-based cohort study. Rheumatology (Oxford) 2015;54(12):2181–7.

93. Ernst A, Rafeq S, Boiselle P, et al. Relapsing polychondritis and airway involvement. Chest 2009; 135(4):1024–30.

94. Sarodia BD, Dasgupta A, Mehta AC. Management of airway manifestations of relapsing polychondritis: case reports and review of literature. Chest 1999; 116(6):1669–75.

95. Suzuki S, Ikegami A, Hirota Y, et al. Fever and cough without pulmonary abnormalities on CT: relapsing polychondritis restricted to the airways. Lancet 2015;385(9962):88.

96. Gorard C, Kadri S. Critical airway involvement in relapsing polychondritis. BMJ Case Rep 2014;2014 [pii:bcr2014205036].

97. Sato R, Ohshima N, Masuda K, et al. A patient with relapsing polychondritis who had been diagnosed as intractable bronchial asthma. Intern Med 2012; 51(13):1773–8.

98. Mpofu S, Estrach C, Curtis J, et al. Treatment of respiratory complications in recalcitrant relapsing polychondritis with infliximab. Rheumatology (Oxford) 2003;42(9):1117–8.

99. Xie C, Shah N, Shah PL, et al. Laryngotracheal reconstruction for relapsing polychondritis: case report and review of the literature. J Laryngol Otol 2013;127(9):932–5.

Interstitial Pneumonia with Autoimmune Features

Aryeh Fischer, MD

KEYWORDS

- Idiopathic interstitial pneumonias • Connective tissue diseases • Interstitial lung disease
- Pulmonary fibrosis

KEY POINTS

- Interstitial pneumonia with autoimmune features (IPAF) is a classification or diagnosis of the subset of patients that reside at the intersection between idiopathic interstitial pneumonia and connective tissue disease (CTD)-associated interstitial lung disease.
- Patients with IPAF require longitudinal surveillance for potential evolution to a characterizable CTD.
- The IPAF designation represents an important first step toward studying and furthering our understanding of the natural history of this cohort of patients with interstitial lung disease using uniform nomenclature and a standardized set of criteria.
- Prospective evaluations and, ideally, interdisciplinary and multicenter collaborations will inform best practices for treatment and management and will guide future refinement to the IPAF criteria.

INTRODUCTION

Interstitial lung disease (ILD) is characterized by inflammation or fibrosis of the lung parenchyma, classified based on the integration of clinical, radiographic, and histopathologic features and broadly grouped into those considered idiopathic versus those with an identifiable cause. Comprehensive assessment of ILD includes detailed history and physical examination, pulmonary function testing, high-resolution computed tomography (HRCT) scanning, and often surgical lung biopsy. The integration of the clinical, radiologic, and histopathologic data via multidisciplinary engagement among clinicians, radiologists, and pathologists is useful to provide the most accurate diagnosis and distinguish an idiopathic interstitial pneumonia (IIP) from ILD with an identifiable etiology.[1]

Systemic autoimmune disease—often referred to as connective tissue disease (CTD)—is a common cause of ILD and may be identified in up to 30% of new ILD diagnoses.[2] Distinguishing CTD-associated ILD (CTD-ILD) from an IIP, particularly IPF, is important because CTD-ILD has a more favorable prognosis and the available therapeutic options differ significantly.[3–5] There is no standardized approach to assess for CTD, and the extent of evaluation varies by center, is often practitioner dependent, and is impacted by the composition of the multidisciplinary team, particularly with regard to rheumatologic engagement.

Moreover, despite extensive efforts to identify occult CTD in patients with IIP, in many instances, features suggesting background autoimmunity are identified yet the patient may not have a characterizable CTD.[6] The terms undifferentiated CTD, lung-dominant CTD, or autoimmune-featured ILD have all been used to describe these patients and each term has been associated with different sets of criteria,[7–9] leading to concerns that diverse cohorts are being identified with the application of each unique set of criteria. Indeed, a recent study

Funding: None.
Divisions of Rheumatology, Pulmonary Sciences and Critical Care Medicine, University of Colorado Anschutz Medical Campus, University of Colorado School of Medicine, 12631 East 17th Avenue, Academic Office Building One, Aurora, CO 80045, USA
E-mail address: aryeh.fischer@ucdenver.edu

Clin Chest Med 40 (2019) 609–616
https://doi.org/10.1016/j.ccm.2019.05.007

Table 1
Classification criteria for IPAF

1. Presence of an interstitial pneumonia by HRCT or SLB *and*
2. Exclusion of alternative etiologies *and*
3. Does not meet criteria for a defined CTD *and*
4. At least 1 feature from at least 2 of the following domains:

A. Clinical domain	B. Serologic domain	C. Morphologic domain

1. Distal digital fissuring (ie, "mechanic hands")
2. Distal digital tip ulceration
3. Inflammatory arthritis *or* polyarticular morning joint stiffness ≥60 min
4. Palmar telangiectasia
5. Raynaud's phenomenon
6. Unexplained digital edema
7. Unexplained fixed rash on the digital extensor surfaces (Gottron's sign)
	1. ANA ≥1:320 titer, diffuse, speckled, homogeneous patterns *or*
	  a. ANA nucleolar pattern (any titer) *or*
	  b. ANA centromere pattern (any titer)
	2. Rheumatoid factor ≥2 × the upper limit of normal
	3. Anti-CCP
	4. Anti-dsDNA
	5. Anti-Ro (SS-A)
	6. Anti-La (SS-B)
	7. Anti-ribonucleoprotein
	8. Anti-Smith
	9. Anti-topoisomerase (Scl-70)
	10. Anti-tRNA synthetase (eg, Jo-1, PL-7, PL-12; others are: EJ, OJ, KS, Zo, tRS)
	11. Anti–PM-Scl
	12. Anti–MDA-5
		1. Suggestive radiology patterns by HRCT:
		  a. NSIP
		  b. OP
		  c. NSIP with OP overlap
		  d. LIP
		2. Histopathology patterns or features by surgical lung biopsy:
		  a. NSIP
		  b. OP
		  c. NSIP with OP overlap
		  d. LIP
		  e. Interstitial lymphoid aggregates with germinal centers
		  f. Diffuse lymphoplasmacytic infiltration (with or without lymphoid follicles)
		3. Multicompartment involvement (in addition to interstitial pneumonia):
		  a. Unexplained pleural effusion or thickening
		  b. Unexplained pericardial effusion or thickening
		  c. Unexplained intrinsic airways disease[a] (by PFT, imaging or pathology)
		  d. Unexplained pulmonary vasculopathy

Abbreviations: ANA, antinuclear antibody; LIP, lymphocytic interstitial pneumonia; NSIP, nonspecific interstitial pneumonia; OP, organizing pneumonia; PFT, pulmonary function testing; SLB, surgical lung biopsy.

[a] Includes airflow obstruction, bronchiolitis or bronchiectasis.

Reproduced with permission of the © ERS 2019. European Respiratory Journal 2015;46(4):976–87; DOI: 10.1183/13993003.00150.

that applied these sets of criteria to a cohort of 119 patients with IIP demonstrated that 56% of patients fulfilled criteria for at least one of these sets, but only 18% fulfilled all sets.[10] Application of the broadest, least specific criteria[8] captured 41% of the cohort, but the narrowest, most specific[3] of the 4 criteria, only encompassed 21%.[10]

The European Respiratory Society/American Thoracic Society Task Force on Undifferentiated Forms of Connective Tissue Disease-associated Interstitial Lung Disease put forth the research classification interstitial pneumonia with autoimmune features (IPAF)—and a set of criteria—as an initial step to more uniformly describe patients with ILD that have features of autoimmunity without a characterizable CTD.[11]

CRITERIA FOR INTERSTITIAL PNEUMONIA WITH AUTOIMMUNE FEATURES

Several a priori requirements must be fulfilled for the classification of IPAF (**Table 1**): individuals must have evidence of interstitial pneumonia by HRCT imaging and/or by surgical lung biopsy, known causes for interstitial pneumonia must have been excluded after comprehensive evaluation, and patients do not meet criteria for a characterizable CTD. The classification criteria are then organized around 3 domains: a clinical domain consisting of specific extrathoracic features, a serologic domain consisting of specific circulating autoantibodies, and a morphologic domain consisting of specific chest imaging features,

Table 2
Comparison of retrospectively identified IPAF cohorts

	Oldham et al,[12] 2016	Chartrand et al,[15] 2016	Ahmad et al,[17] 2017	Ito et al,[19] 2017	Dai et al,[20] 2018	Yoshimura et al,[21] 2018	Kelly & Moua,[22] 2018
Patients	n = 144	n = 56	n = 57	n = 98	n = 177	n = 32	n = 101
Age, y (mean ± SD)	63.2 ± 11	54.6 ± 10.3	64.4 ± 14	67.5 ± 9	67.6 ± 8.6	63.4 ± 12.6	56.9 ± 14.2
Female	52.1	71.4	49.1	58.2	55.9	40.6	39
Ever smoker	54.9	32.1	34	38.8	19.2	56.2	31
Clinical	49.3	62.5	47.3	NR	20.3	53.1	NR
Serologic	91.7	91.1	93	100[a]	92.1	71.9	NR
Morphologic	85.4	98.2	78.9	100[b]	95.5	96.9	NR
Clinical and serologic	14.6	2	NR	NR	NR	3.1	4
Clinical and morphologic	8.3	9	NR	NR	NR	28.1	14
Serologic and morphologic	50.7	37.5	NR	100	NR	46.9	26
All 3 domains	26.4	52	28	NR	NR	21.9	56
UIP by HRCT	54.6	8.9	28	0	4.5	NR	NR
Underwent SLB, n (%)	83 (57.6)	36 (64.3)	16 (28.1)	17 (17.3)	0[c]	22 (68.8)	51 (50.5)
UIP on SLB, n (%)	61 (73.5)	8 (22.2)	3 (18.8)	3 (17.6)	—	—	12 (23.5)
Treatment							
Corticosteroids	32.2	81.8	67.9	17.3	72.3	59.4	NR
Antifibrotic	NR	NR	5.4	2	NR	25	NR
Outcome							
Death	39.6	0	12.3	27.6	19.8	NR	28
Lung transplant	10.8	NR	NR	NR	NR	NR	NR

Data presented as % unless otherwise stated.

Abbreviations: NR, not reported; UIP, usual interstitial pneumonia pattern.

[a] Based on study design, inclusion criteria was positive serologic evaluation.
[b] Based on reported HRCT findings of nonspecific interstitial pneumonia (NSIP), organizing pneumonia (OP) or NSIP + OP in 98 of 98 subjects.
[c] All histopathology from transbronchial biopsies.

Reprinted with permission of the American Thoracic Society. Copyright © 2019 American Thoracic Society. Graney BA, Fischer A. Interstitial pneumonia with autoimmune features. Ann Am Thorac Soc 2019;16(5):525–33. Annals of the American Thoracic Society is an official journal of the American Thoracic Society.

histopathologic features, or pulmonary physiologic features. To be classified as IPAF, the individual must meet all of the a priori requirements and have at least 1 feature from at least 2 of the 3 domains (see **Table 1**).[11]

RETROSPECTIVE RESEARCH STUDIES OF INTERSTITIAL PNEUMONIA WITH AUTOIMMUNE FEATURES

A number of studies have retrospectively described cohorts of patients with ILD that fulfill IPAF criteria (**Table 2**). Each study is impacted by the retrospective—and differing—application of the criteria. Oldham and colleagues[12] identified 422 patients with either IIP or undifferentiated CTD from their ILD database and 144 (34%) met the criteria for IPAF. The mean age of the IPAF group was 63.2 years, with a majority being female (52%) and former smokers (55%). The most common clinical feature was Raynaud's phenomenon (27.8%) and the most common serologic feature was antinuclear antibody (ANA) positivity (77.6%). The majority of the cohort demonstrated an usual interstitial pneumonia pattern (UIP) pattern on HRCT (54.6%) and on surgical lung biopsy (61 of 83 patients biopsied [73.5%]). Twenty-six percent of patients met criteria in all 3 domains. Those meeting IPAF criteria had slightly better outcomes than IPF, but worse than those with CTD-ILD.[12] After stratifying for the presence of UIP pattern on HRCT or surgical lung biopsy, non–UIP-IPAF had a similar survival to CTD-ILD (P = .45), whereas UIP-IPAF demonstrated similar survival to IPF (P = .51). Predictors of increased mortality after multivariate analysis included age and diffusing capacity for carbon monoxide, suggesting that the gender, age, physiology scoring system,[13] validated for mortality prediction in IPF, may be useful in IPAF as well. In a follow-up study, Chung and colleagues[14] identified that the imaging findings of honeycombing or pulmonary artery enlargement were associated with worse survival experience.

Chartrand and colleagues[15] characterized a cohort of 56 patients from a tertiary ILD referral center who met IPAF criteria. The mean age was 55 years, was female predominant (71%), and most were never smokers (68%). Raynaud's phenomenon (39%) and ANA positivity (48%) were the most common clinical and serologic domain features, respectively. Fifty-five of the 56 patients (98%) fulfilled IPAF morphologic criteria. By HRCT, the predominant pattern was nonspecific interstitial pneumonia (NSIP [57%]) followed by the combination of NSIP and organizing pneumonia (OP [18%]). Of the 36 patients who underwent surgical lung biopsy, 12 (33%) had NSIP and 8 (22%) had UIP. A majority of patients (52%) met criteria in all 3 domains. Thirty-six percent of the cohort had a positive transfer RNA (tRNA) synthetase antibody, suggesting that these individuals could be considered to have a partial presentation of the antisynthetase syndrome.[16]

Ahmad and colleagues[17] identified patients over a 3-year period via a hospital discharge database searching for those with IIP or CTD-ILD. Of 778 patients screened, 156 (20.1%) had IPF, 167 (21.5%) had CTD-ILD, and 57 (7.3%) met the criteria for IPAF. Patients had a mean age of 64 years and gender distribution was equal. Raynaud's phenomenon (74%) and ANA positivity (82%) were the most common clinical and serologic features, respectfully. Clinical features were identified in 47% of patients. Morphologically, 53% had a NSIP pattern and 28% had a UIP pattern on HRCT. Sixteen patients with IPAF underwent surgical lung biopsy; a NSIP pattern was identified in 5 patients (31%) and UIP pattern in 3 patients (19%). Survival at 1 year was not different between those with IPAF (83.6%) and IPF (94.8%; P = .05). Among those with IPAF, a UIP pattern on HRCT was not associated with worse survival. Twenty-three percent had abnormal nailfold capillaroscopy, suggesting that such individuals may have partial presentation of systemic sclerosis.[18]

Ito and colleagues[19] sought to identify prognostic factors of the serologic and morphologic IPAF domains from a cohort of 98 patients retrospectively determined as having IPAF. The cohort had a mean age of 67.5 years, was predominantly female (58.2%) and never smokers (61.2%). Sixty-four percent of patients had a NSIP pattern on HRCT. Advancing age as well as a NSIP pattern on HRCT as compared with NSIP with OP overlap or OP alone were associated with shortened survival.

Dai and colleagues[20] retrospectively identified a cohort of 177 patients from an ILD database who fulfilled the criteria for IPAF and compared them with a group of 1252 patients with ILD who did not fulfill the IPAF criteria. The IPAF cohort had a mean age of 60.2 years, was 55.9% female, and 80.8% never smokers. Raynaud's phenomenon (12.9%), ANA positivity (49.2%), and NSIP on HRCT (61.6%) were the most common features from the 3 domains. Twenty percent of the cohort had an identified clinical feature of IPAF. Eight (4.5%) had a UIP pattern on HRCT. None of the patients underwent surgical lung biopsy. Multivariate analysis demonstrated age, smoking history, anti-RNP positivity, and OP pattern as predictors for worsened survival.

Yoshimura and colleagues[21] retrospectively applied the IPAF criteria to a cohort of 194 patients from their center, of whom 163 (84%) had a clinical diagnosis of IPF. Thirty-two patients (16.5%) met the criteria for IPAF. Patients with IPAF were significantly younger and included a higher proportion of women, never smokers, and patients with NSIP compared with those without IPAF. Fulfillment of the IPAF criteria was an independent predictor of overall survival (95% confidence interval, 0.017–0.952; $P = .045$) and incidence of acute exacerbations (95% confidence interval, 0.054–0.937; $P = .040$).[21]

Kelly and Moua[22] reviewed the charts of 101 patients from their tertial ILD referral center who they had defined as having undifferentiated CTD-ILD and noted that the vast majority (91%) also met the criteria for IPAF. They too highlighted frequent clinical findings of Raynaud's phenomenon, a positive ANA, and HRCT features suggestive of NSIP. Nineteen percent had features of UIP either on histopathology or computed tomography imaging. As compared with IPF, patients with IPAF had an overall better survival, except in those with a UIP pattern.[22]

The cohort studies described reflect the retrospective application of IPAF criteria from individual centers around the world. Each study is limited by referral bias, methodologic limitations of cohort identification, and how the specifics of the IPAF criteria were applied. Despite these limitations, these cohort studies provide important insights about IPAF. For example, these studies demonstrate that there is significant heterogeneity within the IPAF phenotype—similar to what is encountered in CTD-ILD—which may have prognostic implications, because fibrotic patterns may portend a worse prognosis.[23] Further, similar to IIP,[24] an underlying pattern of UIP in patients with IPAF seems to be associated with worse survival. These studies also point to a need for revisions to the IPAF criteria, particularly with respect to the morphologic domain. Because the IPAF criteria do not rigorously define how to characterize aspects of the morphology domain, individual providers, investigators, and studies define them differently.

PROPOSED FUTURE DIRECTIONS

IPAF represents an initial consensus classification scheme put forth by a relatively small panel of experts in the field. The designation has spurred healthy interdisciplinary dialogue, generated widespread interest, and it has become clear that modifications are needed to refine the original classification criteria. As acknowledged in a recent expert commentary, the IPAF criteria have an intrinsically changing structure and perhaps "the most important effect of these criteria is the identification of a gray zone of not well-defined rheumatology conditions."[25] Numerous questions exist about the individual items within each domain. With the next iteration, other than expanding and diversifying the panel, a more systematic approach (eg, Delphi exercise) and global input should be considered.

One major advantage of IPAF is that a uniform nomenclature has been adopted, prospective research studies from diverse programs are using similar classification criteria, data are being gathered to allow for the anticipated refinement of the criteria in an evidence-based manner, and there is far more interdisciplinary engagement within this arena.

There has been controversy around the exclusion of antineutrophil cytoplasmic antibody and the inclusion of anti-tRNA synthetase antibodies.[26,27] Should the serologic domain include antineutrophil cytoplasmic antibody, PR-3, and myeloperoxidase antibodies? Indeed, antineutrophil cytoplasmic antibody positivity in various forms of fibrotic interstitial pneumonia has been described in patients with or without features of systemic vasculitis.[28,29] Controversy exists regarding the inclusion of anti-tRNA synthetase antibodies, because this ultimately raises the question of the definition of the antisynthetase syndrome and whether the presence of ILD with a tRNA synthetase antibody is sufficient for this classification. According to the current idiopathic inflammatory myositis scheme,[30] these 2 features alone would not meet the criteria. Fortunately, in part owing to interdisciplinary interests in IPAF and the relationship to antisynthetase syndrome, there is now an international effort to develop consensus classification criteria for antisynthetase syndrome.[25] And as novel autoantibodies associated with ILD continue to be identified, changes to the serologic domain will be needed.

The morphologic domain may remain the most important and yet also the most challenging. One common critique is that the UIP pattern—unlike the other IIP patterns—is not included in the morphologic domain.[31] It is worth emphasizing that the presence of a UIP pattern does not exclude a designation of IPAF; indeed, many of the published cohorts have substantial proportions of patients with IPAF with UIP. Outcomes for patients with UIP-IPAF have been variable in the retrospective cohorts and this may be due to how cohorts were identified. Prospective studies should provide valuable insights regarding the prevalence and outcomes of patients with IPAF that have the UIP pattern.

Studies comparing CTD-ILD with a UIP pattern on HRCT or surgical lung biopsy have consistently demonstrated improved survival as compared with idiopathic UIP (IPF),[24,32–34] with the exception of rheumatoid arthritis UIP, for which the data are conflicting.[33,35] These studies suggest that patients with an autoimmune-mediated basis to their lung disease have improved survival even with similar radiographic or histologic pattern of fibrosis—highlighting the importance of etiology in ILD natural history. As such, identifying and distinguishing between patients with truly idiopathic disease and UIP (ie, the clinical diagnosis of IPF) from those with clinical, serologic, and/or morphologic features of autoimmune disease and UIP (ie, UIP-IPAF) may have significant prognostic implications. Furthermore, it is likely to alter management decisions. In the current era, the use of antifibrotic therapy is limited to those with IPF because clinical trials have shown a benefit in this patient population.[36,37] Data from prospective clinical trials are needed to determine whether antifibrotic therapy has a similar role in the management of other cohorts with UIP pattern of lung injury, including those with IPAF or fibrotic ILD in general.

We have learned from the divergent application of the morphologic domain features in retrospective cohorts that there needs to be more uniform specifications regarding how to define multicompartment involvement in patients beyond unexplained airways disease or unexplained pulmonary vasculopathy. How best to define the presence of pulmonary vasculopathy is a particularly interesting question, given that studies that defined it by PFT,[12] imaging,[14] or histopathology[38] all suggest that its presence is associated with worse outcomes.

Clarity is also needed with regard to the extent of germinal centers or lymphoplasmacytic infiltration on histopathology required to fulfill these morphologic domain features. As an example, a recent study[38] designated at least 3 germinal centers in any 1 low-power field and the presence of lymphocytes and 40 or more plasma cells in a high-power field as meeting criteria, but to date there has been no consensus on this definition.

Although initially considered a research classification, there is a growing appreciation that IPAF reflects a clinical diagnosis residing between the intersection of IIP and CTD-ILD. Fundamental questions about the natural history of IPAF and how these patients should be managed remain unanswered. Is IPAF a distinct disease entity or do these patients evolve to CTD? Is it merely the underlying lung injury pattern (eg, UIP vs NSIP) that predicts prognosis or treatment responsiveness, or are there specific autoimmune clinical, serologic, or other morphologic features of importance? Should patients with IPAF be treated similar to those with CTD-ILD by using immunosuppressive therapies, or should they be treated with an antifibrotic similar to IPF? We eagerly await subset analysis from the phase II clinical trial with pirfenidone for unclassifiable ILD, because a subset of the enrolled subjects fulfill IPAF criteria (clinicaltrials.gov identifier: NCT03099187).[39] Undoubtedly, prospective, randomized controlled clinical trials will augment our understanding of how to manage patients with IPAF.

SUMMARY

IPAF describes patients with ILD who have features of autoimmunity without a characterizable CTD. Before IPAF, diverse nomenclature and classification schemes had been proposed to characterize such patients. IPAF has provided uniform nomenclature and criteria that has fostered interdisciplinary engagement and research into this previously amorphous subset of ILD. Retrospective studies of cohorts with IPAF have demonstrated the substantial heterogeneity within the IPAF phenotype, that the underlying lung histopathology of these patients likely impacts prognosis, and a recognition that modifications to the criteria are needed. Although initially considered a research classification, there is a growing appreciation that IPAF reflects a clinical diagnosis residing between the intersection of IIP and CTD-ILD. Longitudinal surveillance of patients with IPAF is needed, because some patients evolve to a defined CTD and prospective research studies are needed to inform how to best manage patients with IPAF.

REFERENCES

1. Raghu G, Remy-Jardin M, Myers JL, et al, American Thoracic Society, European Respiratory Society, Japanese Respiratory Society, and Latin American Thoracic Society. Diagnosis of idiopathic pulmonary fibrosis. An official ATS/ERS/JRS/ALAT clinical practice guideline. Am J Respir Crit Care Med 2018;198: e44–68.

2. Lee CT, Oldham JM. Interstitial pneumonia with autoimmune features: overview of proposed criteria and recent cohort characterization. Clin Pulm Med 2017;24:191–6.

3. Corte TJ, Copley SJ, Desai SR, et al. Significance of connective tissue disease features in idiopathic interstitial pneumonia. Eur Respir J 2012;39:661–8.

4. Fischer A, du Bois R. Interstitial lung disease in connective tissue disorders. Lancet 2012;380:689–98.

5. Cottin V. Significance of connective tissue diseases features in pulmonary fibrosis. Eur Respir Rev 2013;22:273–80.

6. Collins BF, Spiekerman CF, Shaw MA, et al. Idiopathic interstitial pneumonia associated with autoantibodies: a large case series followed over 1 year. Chest 2017;152:103–12.

7. Fischer A, West SG, Swigris JJ, et al. Connective tissue disease-associated interstitial lung disease: a call for clarification. Chest 2010;138:251–6.

8. Kinder BW, Collard HR, Koth L, et al. Idiopathic nonspecific interstitial pneumonia: lung manifestation of undifferentiated connective tissue disease? Am J Respir Crit Care Med 2007;176: 691–7.

9. Vij R, Noth I, Strek ME. Autoimmune-featured interstitial lung disease: a distinct entity. Chest 2011; 140:1292–9.

10. Assayag D, Kim EJ, Elicker BM, et al. Survival in interstitial pneumonia with features of autoimmune disease: a comparison of proposed criteria. Respir Med 2015;109:1326–31.

11. Fischer A, Antoniou KM, Brown KK, et al, ERS/ATS Task Force on Undifferentiated Forms of CTD-ILD. An official European Respiratory Society/American Thoracic Society research statement: interstitial pneumonia with autoimmune features. Eur Respir J 2015;46:976–87.

12. Oldham JM, Adegunsoye A, Valenzi E, et al. Characterisation of patients with interstitial pneumonia with autoimmune features. Eur Respir J 2016;47: 1767–75.

13. Ley B, Ryerson CJ, Vittinghoff E, et al. A multidimensional index and staging system for idiopathic pulmonary fibrosis. Ann Intern Med 2012;156:684–91.

14. Chung JH, Montner SM, Adegunsoye A, et al. CT findings, radiologic-pathologic correlation, and imaging predictors of survival for patients with interstitial pneumonia with autoimmune features. AJR Am J Roentgenol 2017;208:1229–36.

15. Chartrand S, Swigris JJ, Stanchev L, et al. Clinical features and natural history of interstitial pneumonia with autoimmune features: a single center experience. Respir Med 2016;119:150–4.

16. Chartrand S, Lee JS, Fischer A. Longitudinal assessment of interstitial pneumonia with autoimmune features is encouraged. Respir Med 2017; 132:267.

17. Ahmad K, Barba T, Gamondes D, et al. Interstitial pneumonia with autoimmune features: clinical, radiologic, and histological characteristics and outcome in a series of 57 patients. Respir Med 2017;123:56–62.

18. Cutolo M, Pizzorni C, Sulli A, et al. Early diagnostic and predictive value of capillaroscopy in systemic sclerosis. Curr Rheumatol Rev 2013;9:249–53.

19. Ito Y, Arita M, Kumagai S, et al. Serological and morphological prognostic factors in patients with interstitial pneumonia with autoimmune features. BMC Pulm Med 2017;17:111.

20. Dai J, Wang L, Yan X, et al. Clinical features, risk factors, and outcomes of patients with interstitial pneumonia with autoimmune features: a population-based study. Clin Rheumatol 2018;37: 2125–32.

21. Yoshimura K, Kono M, Enomoto Y, et al. Distinctive characteristics and prognostic significance of interstitial pneumonia with autoimmune features in patients with chronic fibrosing interstitial pneumonia. Respir Med 2018;137:167–75.

22. Kelly BT, Moua T. Overlap of interstitial pneumonia with autoimmune features with undifferentiated connective tissue disease and contribution of UIP to mortality. Respirology 2018;23:600–5.

23. Solomon JJ, Chung JH, Cosgrove GP, et al. Predictors of mortality in rheumatoid arthritis-associated interstitial lung disease. Eur Respir J 2016;47: 588–96.

24. Park JH, Kim DS, Park IN, et al. Prognosis of fibrotic interstitial pneumonia: idiopathic versus collagen vascular disease-related subtypes. Am J Respir Crit Care Med 2007;175:705–11.

25. Cavagna L, Gonzalez Gay MA, Allanore Y, et al. Interstitial pneumonia with autoimmune features: a new classification still on the move. Eur Respir Rev 2018;27:30.

26. Jee AS, Bleasel JF, Adelstein S, et al. A call for uniformity in implementing the IPAF (interstitial pneumonia with autoimmune features) criteria. Eur Respir J 2016;48:1811–3.

27. Jee AS, Adelstein S, Bleasel J, et al. Role of autoantibodies in the diagnosis of connective-tissue disease ILD (CTD-ILD) and interstitial pneumonia with autoimmune features (IPAF). J Clin Med 2017;6 [pii:E51].

28. Hozumi H, Enomoto N, Oyama Y, et al. Clinical implication of proteinase-3-antineutrophil cytoplasmic antibody in patients with idiopathic interstitial pneumonias. Lung 2016;194:235–42.

29. Hozumi H, Oyama Y, Yasui H, et al. Clinical significance of myeloperoxidase-anti-neutrophil cytoplasmic antibody in idiopathic interstitial pneumonias. PLoS One 2018;13:e0199659.

30. Lundberg IE, Tjarnlund A, Bottai M, et al, International Myositis Classification Criteria Project Consortium, the Euromyositis Register, and the Juvenile Dermatomyositis Cohort Biomarker Study and Repository (UK and Ireland). 2017 European league against rheumatism/American college of rheumatology classification criteria for adult and Juvenile idiopathic inflammatory myopathies and their major subgroups. Arthritis Rheumatol 2017;69: 2271–82.

31. Collins B, Raghu G. Interstitial pneumonia with autoimmune features: the new consensus-based definition for this cohort of patients should be broadened. Eur Respir J 2016;47:1293–5.

32. Aggarwal R, McBurney C, Schneider F, et al. Myositis-associated usual interstitial pneumonia has a better survival than idiopathic pulmonary fibrosis. Rheumatology (Oxford) 2017;56:384–9.

33. Moua T, Zamora Martinez AC, Baqir M, et al. Predictors of diagnosis and survival in idiopathic pulmonary fibrosis and connective tissue disease-related usual interstitial pneumonia. Respir Res 2014;15:154.

34. Strand MJ, Sprunger D, Cosgrove GP, et al. Pulmonary function and survival in idiopathic vs secondary usual interstitial pneumonia. Chest 2014;146:775–85.

35. Song JW, Lee HK, Lee CK, et al. Clinical course and outcome of rheumatoid arthritis-related usual interstitial pneumonia. Sarcoidosis Vasc Diffuse Lung Dis 2013;30:103–12.

36. Richeldi L, du Bois RM, Raghu G, et al, INPULSIS Trial Investigators. Efficacy and safety of nintedanib in idiopathic pulmonary fibrosis. N Engl J Med 2014;370:2071–82.

37. King TE Jr, Bradford WZ, Castro-Bernardini S, et al. A phase 3 trial of pirfenidone in patients with idiopathic pulmonary fibrosis. N Engl J Med 2014;370:2083–92.

38. Adegunsoye A, Oldham JM, Valenzi E, et al. Interstitial pneumonia with autoimmune features: value of histopathology. Arch Pathol Lab Med 2017;141:960–9.

39. Maher TM, Corte TJ, Fischer A, et al. Pirfenidone in patients with unclassifiable progressive fibrosing interstitial lung disease: design of a double-blind, randomised, placebo-controlled phase II trial. BMJ Open Respir Res 2018;5:e000289.

Connective Tissue Disease–Associated Interstitial Lung Disease
Evaluation and Management

Danielle Antin-Ozerkis, MD[a],*, Monique Hinchcliff, MD, MS[b]

KEYWORDS

- Interstitial lung disease • Connective tissue disease • Pulmonary fibrosis • Immunosuppression
- Scleroderma • Rheumatoid arthritis • Supportive care

KEY POINTS

- Interstitial lung disease is common among patients with connective tissue disease and contributes to morbidity and mortality in this population.
- Comprehensive assessment is required for appropriate diagnosis and includes consideration of infection and drug-induced pneumonitis.
- A multidisciplinary team approach should focus on indications for treatment, relevant comorbidities, assessment of response, and prevention of therapeutic complications.
- Controlled trials of therapeutic agents for connective tissue disease–associated interstitial lung disease are needed.

INTRODUCTION

Thoracic involvement, particularly interstitial lung disease (ILD), is common and is an important contributor to morbidity and mortality in the connective tissue diseases (CTDs). When CTD-associated ILD (CTD-ILD) is clinically apparent, presentations may range from mild, nonspecific symptoms to fulminant respiratory failure. In addition, ILD may be the first manifestation of systemic rheumatologic tissue disease. The radiographic findings and histopathologic appearance of CTD-ILD mirror those of the idiopathic interstitial pneumonias. However, specific findings may offer clues to a diagnosis of underlying CTD. When evaluating patients with parenchymal abnormalities, other causes, such as drug toxicity or opportunistic infection, must be considered in the diagnostic pathway.

The general diagnostic approach to such patients depends on the presenting scenario. Some patients do not carry a preexisting CTD diagnosis and therefore require a full evaluation of the ILD, including a careful search for CTD. Such a diagnosis changes the prognosis and specific therapies. For other patients, ILD presents in the setting of known CTD. For these patients it is important to remember the basic tenets of ILD diagnosis. In either case, multidisciplinary discussion is often beneficial.

When considering therapy, initial considerations include an assessment of disease severity through

Disclosures: Dr D. Antin-Ozerkis has received grants and contracts to her institution from Biogen, Boehringer Ingelheim, FibroGen, Genentech, and Promedior. Dr M. Hinchcliff has received grants and research support from Gilead Sciences and Actelion Pharmaceuticals.
[a] Section of Pulmonary and Critical Care Medicine, Yale School of Medicine, PO Box 208057, New Haven, CT 06520-8057, USA; [b] Section of Rheumatology, Allergy and Immunology, Yale School of Medicine, PO Box 208031, New Haven, CT 06520-8031, USA
* Corresponding author.
E-mail address: danielle.antin-ozerkis@yale.edu

Clin Chest Med 40 (2019) 617–636
https://doi.org/10.1016/j.ccm.2019.05.008
0272-5231/19/© 2019 Elsevier Inc. All rights reserved.

both objective and subjective means as well as a determination of the rate of progression. Extrathoracic disease activity is also a strong consideration when deciding whether to initiate therapy and which among the many immunosuppressive and immunomodulatory agents to choose. Many decisions are based on reports of case series and clinical experience because there are few large randomized controlled trials in CTD-ILD. With therapy, determinations of response and toxicity help guide clinicians in tailoring the regimen. Supportive care and management of comorbidities are vital considerations in the comprehensive care of patients with CTD-ILD.

EPIDEMIOLOGY

ILD refers to a group of lung disorders that share many characteristics, including clinical manifestations, radiographic appearance, and pathologic findings. Clinical course and treatment approach differ between types of ILD. In particular, idiopathic pulmonary fibrosis (IPF) is a distinct clinical entity that must be differentiated from other forms, particularly CTD-ILD.[1,2] ILD has long been recognized to affect patients with CTD (**Table 1**). Most commonly, patients with rheumatoid arthritis (RA) and systemic sclerosis (SSc) are affected.[3,4] However, ILD is frequently seen polymyositis/dermatomyositis (PM/DM) spectrum disorders; Sjögren syndrome; mixed CTD (MCTD); and, less commonly, in systemic lupus erythematosus (SLE).[5]

The recognition of ILD depends on the methods used to detect disease as well as the definition of clinically significant disease. When using chest radiographs alone, an early series of patients with

RA at presentation found fewer than 5% of patients to have rheumatoid lung.[6] When pulmonary function was tested, prevalence ranged from 33% to 45%,[7,8] and findings on high-resolution chest computed tomography (HRCT) suggest a prevalence as high as 61%.[8–10] A review of patients with RA at autopsy showed that more than one-third of patients had pathologic findings of ILD.[11] Strikingly high numbers are found in the SSc population, in which the presence of ILD at autopsy is reported to be 74% and by HRCT between 64% and 91%.[12] Although some patients remain asymptomatic and do not experience progression of disease, ILD remains an important contributor to morbidity and mortality in CTD.[13–15]

Clinically, the presence of ILD is most frequently confirmed by HRCT. The radiographic patterns are described using the terminology developed for diagnosing the idiopathic interstitial pneumonias, which is based on a histopathologic correlate.[16] When idiopathic, the usual interstitial pneumonia (UIP) pattern is the most common of these and is the hallmark characteristic of IPF, a progressive fatal disease. The UIP pattern is characterized by basilar and subpleural reticulation with or without traction bronchiectasis, as well as subpleural honeycomb cysts without features of another disease (**Fig. 1**).[1] In idiopathic disease, the radiographic UIP pattern is highly predictive of the histologic UIP pattern.[17,18] At least in RA, this seems to also hold true.[19,20] The nonspecific interstitial pneumonia (NSIP) pattern, which can be subcategorized into cellular and fibrotic NSIP, generally carries a more favorable prognosis, particularly the cellular form.[21,22] NSIP is radiographically characterized by ground-glass opacities in combination with reticulation and traction bronchiectasis (**Fig. 2**).[23,24] UIP is the most common pattern in

Table 1
Frequency of interstitial lung disease in connective tissue diseases

Disease	ILD	CT Pattern
Systemic sclerosis	++++	NSIP, UIP
Myositis	++++	NSIP, OP, DAD, UIP
RA	+++	UIP, NSIP, OP
Sjögren syndrome	++	NSIP, LIP
Systemic lupus erythematosus	+	NSIP, DAH
Ankylosing spondylitis	+	Upper lobe fibrosis

Abbreviations: CT, computed tomography; DAD, diffuse alveolar damage; DAH, diffuse alveolar hemorrhage; LIP, lymphocytic interstitial pneumonitis; NSIP, nonspecific interstitial pneumonitis; OP, organizing pneumonia; RA, Rheumatoid arthritis; UIP, usual interstitial pneumonia.

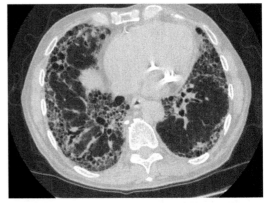

Fig. 1. The UIP pattern, characterized by lower lobe and peripheral predominant fibrosis, traction bronchiectasis, and honeycombing.

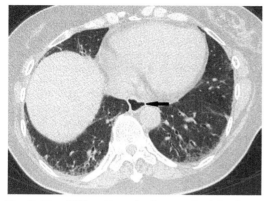

Fig. 2. The NSIP pattern is characterized by lower lobe–predominant traction bronchiectasis with ground glass. Note the dilated esophagus (*arrow*) in this patient with systemic sclerosis.

patients with RA-ILD and seems to carry a worse prognosis than other patterns of lung disease.[19,25] NSIP is more common in SSc and is frequently seen in other CTDs, such as PM/DM, Sjögren syndrome, and SLE.[26,27] Other characteristic patterns in CTD-ILD include that of organizing pneumonia (OP), often seen in PM/DM (**Fig. 3**), and lymphocytic interstitial pneumonia, frequently associated with Sjögren syndrome.

GENERAL APPROACH TO DIAGNOSIS AND TREATMENT
Diagnosis

In the approach to diagnosis of CTD-ILD, the underlying scenario is of key importance. There are 2 categories of patients: those with a preexisting diagnosis of underlying CTD and those presenting with new-onset ILD who are given a new diagnosis of CTD as an explanation for the ILD. For those patients presenting with ILD but without known CTD, updated clinical practice guidelines and

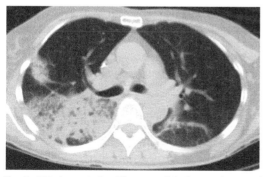

Fig. 3. OP, characterized by consolidation and ground glass, often peripheral and peribronchovascular in distribution, and frequently nodular in appearance.

consensus statements offer important management recommendations for diagnostic evaluation.[1,2]

Patients with no prior connective tissue disease diagnosis
For this group of patients, detailed clinical history can lead to a specific ILD diagnosis. This history includes a thorough evaluation of environmental and occupational exposures (including organic exposures such as mold and bird feathers/droppings), a review of prior medications to assess for drug toxicity, and a thorough assessment for signs and symptoms of CTD.[28–30] For example, the presence of muscle weakness, heliotrope rash, Gottron papules, or so-called mechanic's hands may suggest DM.[31] A history of skin thickening, telangiectasias, Raynaud, or digital nail pitting may lead to a diagnosis of SSc.[32] The presence of acid reflux, regurgitation of food, or dysphagia may indicate esophageal dysmotility, suggesting SSc or MCTD.[31,32] Joint pain, swelling, inflammation, and morning stiffness may all be seen in RA.[33] Specialized testing, such as nailfold capillaroscopy and esophageal manometry, may assist in the diagnosis.[34,35]

The most recent American Thoracic Society (ATS)/European Respiratory Society (ERS) guidelines recommend serologic testing to exclude CTD as a potential cause of the ILD.[1] Many ILD centers commonly use extensive panels (**Table 2**); however, no consensus exists on which tests to use or whether particular patients benefit more than others. With careful identification of clinical CTD features, it is estimated that at least 15% of patients presenting with ILD have evidence of underlying CTD.[36]

Radiographic features in CTD-ILD include ground-glass opacities (hazy areas of increased parenchymal density that do not obscure the underlying lung markings), reticulation (a series of crisscrossing lines resulting in a weblike pattern), and centrilobular nodules, in addition to more advanced fibrotic features such as architectural distortion, traction bronchiectasis, and honeycombing.[37–40] In addition to parenchymal abnormalities, air trapping from obstructive small airways disease, as seen with bronchiolitis obliterans, may be observed. UIP and NSIP patterns are common. However, although specific patterns, such as that of UIP, may be prognostically useful, mixed or unclassifiable patterns are frequent in CTD.[21,41]

Surgical lung biopsy is infrequently obtained when a new diagnosis of CTD is confirmed, because pathologic findings often do not change clinical management.[42] Atypical features, such as

Table 2
Commonly used laboratory tests and autoantibodies in connective tissue disease–associated interstitial lung disease diagnosis

Disease	Autoantibodies
Reumatoid arthritis	Anti-CCP RF
Sjögren syndrome	Anti-Ro (SSA) Anti-La (SSB)
Polymyositis/ dermatomyositis/ antisynthetase syndrome	CPK/CK Aldolase Anti-ARS antibodies: • Anti–Jo-1 • Anti–PL-7 • Anti–PL-12 • Anti–EJ • Anti–OJ • Anti–KS • Anti–Zo • Anti–Ha Specific autoantibodies: • Anti- MDA5 • Mi-2 (helicase) • SRP
Systemic sclerosis	Anti–Scl-70 RNA polymerase-III
Systemic lupus erythematosus	ANA dsDNA Sm
ANCA-associated vasculitis	ANCA MPO Pr-3
General markers of inflammation	CRP ESR

Abbreviations: ANA, antinuclear antibody; ANCA, antineutrophil cytoplasmic antibodies; ARS, aminoacyl transfer RNA synthetase; CCP, cyclic citrullinated peptide; CPK/CK, creatine phosphokinase; CRP, C-reactive protein; dsDNA, double-stranded DNA; ESR, erythrocyte sedimentation rate; MDA5, melanoma differentiation-associated gene 5; MPO, myeloperoxidase; Pr-3, proteinase-3; RF, rheumatoid factor; Sm, Smith antigen; SRP, Signal recognition particle; SSA, Sjögren syndrome–related antigen A; SSB, Sjögren syndrome–related antigen B; TRNA, transfer RNA.

unilateral or upper lobe predominance, parenchymal nodules, or any other features suggestive of infection or malignancy, may be indications to consider invasive testing. Bronchoscopy with bronchoalveolar lavage (BAL) is most useful in ruling out alternative diagnoses such as eosinophilic pneumonia, diffuse alveolar hemorrhage, or opportunistic infection.[43–46] Transbronchial biopsy may be helpful when infection, malignancy, OP, or granulomatous disease (including drug toxicity) is suspected, but is still controversial in the evaluation of undifferentiated fibrotic lung disease.[47] In the past, BAL was used prognostically in SSc but is no longer routine.[48] Ultimately, the decision to pursue a lung biopsy of any type should include an individualized assessment of risk and benefit and multidisciplinary discussion.[49]

Patients with a prior connective tissue disease diagnosis

In patients with known CTD and a new diagnosis of ILD, a similar process to the described earlier must be pursued before attributing a finding of ILD to the CTD itself. This process includes a careful search for suspect environmental and occupational exposures and a thorough review of prior medications. Of note, many of the disease-modifying antirheumatic drugs (DMARDs) used in the management of CTD have been reported to cause pulmonary toxicity. The most commonly implicated drugs include methotrexate and leflunomide.[30] Anti–tumor necrosis factor (TNF) agents have also been reported to cause drug-induced ILD, although evidence is controversial.[50] Reports of pneumonitis from tocilizumab and rituximab are more commonly seen in the oncology population.[30] A challenge in this body of literature is the difficulty in establishing definitive proof of a causal relationship between these DMARDs and CTD-ILD. It is possible that disease severity, immunologic background, or genetic predisposition may be confounders.[50] Nonetheless, for any individual patient, the possibility of drug-induced lung disease must be assessed by examining the timing of ILD onset relative to the initiation of the drug. Clinical improvement with drug discontinuation can be diagnostic.

Infections, both community acquired and opportunistic, are another major consideration in the differential diagnosis of abnormal HRCT findings in patients with underlying CTD.[51] These patients may experience immune dysregulation related to their underlying disease and may also be receiving immunosuppressive medications.[52] HRCT findings (such as tree-in-bud opacities) sometimes suggest infection but may also be nonspecific (ground glass and consolidation). The use of prophylactic antibiotics before diagnosis may reduce suspicion for certain types of infection, such as pneumocystis pneumonia; however, suspicion must remain high, particularly in patients receiving corticosteroids.[53] Bronchoscopy is often considered in cases in which uncertainty remains.

Assessment of Disease Severity

Symptoms

Often patients are asymptomatic early in the course of CTD-ILD. When present, symptoms are typically nonspecific, including dyspnea on exertion or cough. Progressive lung disease typically leads to increasing breathlessness, related to both lung stiffness and hypoxemia.[54] In addition to the ILD, other reasons for dyspnea include deconditioning, muscle weakness, pulmonary hypertension (PH), pleural involvement, and thoracic cage restriction caused by skin involvement (in SSc). Symptoms alone are generally not the sole consideration in the decision to treat CTD-ILD, but patient-centered outcomes are an important factor. Some centers recommend the routine use of standardized dyspnea indices such as the Multidimensional Health Assessment Questionnaire, University of California San Diego Dyspnea Questionnaire, or Dyspnea 12 Questionnaire in order to longitudinally follow the degree of subjective dyspnea.[42]

Pulmonary function tests and walking oximetry

Often the earliest physiologic finding in CTD-ILD is a decrement in the diffusing capacity of the lungs for carbon monoxide (DLCO). This diffusion defect may manifest as exertional hypoxemia as assessed by the 6-minute walk distance (6MWD). Longitudinal changes in DLCO and 6MWD have been shown to be prognostically important in IPF[55,56] but in CTD-ILD it is less clear whether these variables carry the same specificity, because they may be affected by the presence of other cardiopulmonary disease such as PH as well as by musculoskeletal weakness or pain.[57] Nonetheless, both are measures typically considered in treatment decisions, particularly in the setting of progressive decline. The forced vital capacity (FVC) is frequently used as a primary outcome measure in clinical trials.[58] This value too may be affected by other factors, such as muscle weakness or thoracic cage restriction, but is nevertheless used longitudinally in combination with other factors. Several studies in SSc have identified FVC and DLCO as predictors of progression and mortality.[59,60] Similarly, among patients with RA, a lower baseline FVC as well as a 10% decline in FVC from baseline to any time during follow-up were associated with increased risk of death.[61] The ILD-GAP model, a composite mortality prediction model initially developed in IPF, found that incorporating ILD subtype, gender, age, and physiology (FVC and DLCO) may be useful in predicting mortality in CTD-ILD.[62] Note that a normal FVC cannot rule out the presence of ILD, particularly in patients at high risk for developing lung disease, because this value may still reflect significant loss of lung function from a patient's premorbid status.[63]

Radiographic extent of fibrosis

Among patients with SSc, visual assessment of lung involvement greater than 20% on HRCT is a predictor for mortality, particularly as part of a staging system in combination with an FVC threshold of 70%.[64] Regardless of whether this visual method or computer-assisted fibrosis scoring is used, increased extent of fibrosis on HRCT is associated with greater FVC decline.[65] Similarly, in RA-ILD, radiographic assessment performed using the SSc scoring system, IPF guidelines, or computer-assisted scoring all led to strong predictions of outcome.[66] There are few studies in other forms of CTD-ILD and it is unknown whether similar assessment is similarly applicable.

General Strategies in Treatment of Connective Tissue Disease–Associated Interstitial Lung Disease

Therapeutic decision making must be tailored to the individual patient. Considerations include severity and tempo of disease course, extrathoracic disease activity, and presence of comorbid conditions. For some patients with stable chronic, fibrotic disease or with early and mild subclinical disease, it is appropriate to monitor closely without treatment, whereas for those with acute-onset inflammatory disease or progressive disease an aggressive strategy may be undertaken. If an expectant strategy is undertaken, it is our practice to monitor with pulmonary function tests (PFTs) every 3 to 6 months. In those patients requiring treatment of lung disease who also have extrathoracic manifestations requiring therapy, close collaboration between pulmonologists and rheumatologists is required for appropriate decision making. Because patients with preexisting ILD may be more at risk for lung toxicity from methotrexate,[67] the authors typically avoid this drug in patients with preexisting ILD both for this reason and because it may be difficult to distinguish progressive CTD-ILD from drug toxicity. Although anti-TNF agents have also been reported to cause pneumonitis, our approach is to assess time course and activity of the underlying CTD in making these decisions, often using them for management of joint symptoms with caution and close observation. Frequently, DMARDs with activity against synovitis and myositis, such as the anti-TNF drugs or rituximab, are used in combination with agents directed at the lung disease, such as mycophenolate mofetil (MMF) and azathioprine. Other investigators have reported similar practices.[68]

Assessment of comorbidities is crucial in the therapeutic decision pathway. Some affect drug choice, whereas others confound assessment of disease severity or response to treatment. For example, in patients with diabetes, obesity, and severe osteoporosis, there must be significant hesitation in the choice to use corticosteroids, with a goal to taper to the lowest possible dose as quickly as able. Adjunctive therapy designed to prevent further complications (aggressive glucose control, osteoporosis treatment) should be undertaken. Some comorbidities may make assessment of disease severity and response to treatment more difficult. In particular, PH may lead to additional breathlessness and can affect diffusing capacity measurements. Any muscle weakness can lead to worsened dyspnea and can affect FVC measurements. Obstructive airways disease affects subjective sensation of breathlessness and, when severe, can lead to pseudorestriction from air trapping.

With the choice to initiate therapy for CTD-ILD, clinicians must establish a plan for assessment of response, length of therapy, and safety. It is our practice to consider a patient's subjective assessment but also establish baseline values for objective evaluation of response, including PFTs, walking oximetry, and frequently HRCT. In some cases, although improvement is not obtained, stabilization of previous progression may be considered a success. In others, it is the ability to reduce or even eliminate corticosteroids. Baseline and regular laboratory monitoring, tailored to the therapy chosen, should be considered. Preventive measures, including *Pneumocystis jirovecii* (PJP) prophylaxis and bone health monitoring (as outlined later), should be considered. For patients with SSc-ILD, longer term maintenance of immunosuppression may be warranted.[69] In others, is our practice to consider taper of medications after a period of 6 to 12 months of stability, but length of therapy must be individualized.

MEDICAL THERAPIES
Corticosteroids

Corticosteroids are the mainstay for many patients with CTD-ILD, although few data support their use.[70–72] SSc-ILD is one important exception to this rule because the benefits of glucocorticoid therapy are less well established.[73] Daily prednisone greater than or equal to 15 mg has been associated with the onset of SSc renal crisis.[74] High-dose corticosteroid treatment is indicated in patients with SSc-associated inflammatory myositis; however, daily blood pressure monitoring should be advised, and patients cautioned about the need for emergent evaluation of persistently increased blood pressure readings.

Normotensive SSc renal crisis can also occur, and patients with SSc taking prednisone should undergo regular kidney function tests. Inflammation, often indicated by ground-glass or consolidative opacity on HRCT, tends to be more responsive to steroid therapy, whereas patients with high fibrotic burden are less likely to experience improvement.[75]

Azathioprine

Azathioprine is a prodrug that is metabolized in the liver and gastrointestinal tract to its active metabolites.[76] Individuals with genetic variants in thiopurine methyltransferase (TPMT) or nucleoside diphosphate–linked motif 15 (NUDT15), liver disease, or who are taking allopurinol or febuxostat are at increased risk for azathioprine-induced bone marrow toxicity.[77] Genetic testing or assessment of TPMT enzymatic activity should be considered before use, and complete blood counts and liver function tests should be monitored during therapy.[77]

Azathioprine has been primarily studied in CTD-ILD as maintenance treatment following induction with cyclophosphamide, particularly in the SSc population.[71,78–82] It is difficult to determine the benefit of azathioprine because of the lack of prospective placebo-controlled trials and the potential for confounding by indication.[83] Retrospective studies of patients with SSc-ILD who were treated with azathioprine are inconsistent.[84,85] When assessed in patients with fibrotic CTD-ILD (all types), azathioprine was less well tolerated than mycophenolate mofetil but led to equal rates of stability.[86]

Mycophenolate Mofetil

Mycophenolate mofetil (MMF) is a potent inhibitor of lymphocyte proliferation.[87] In our experience, titration to 2 to 3 g/d is usually well tolerated and avoids the need for enteric-coated mycophenolate sodium, which has fewer gastrointestinal side effects but is much costlier. MMF use in patients with SSc has not been associated with progressive multifocal leukoencephalopathy, as has been reported in SLE, but there is concern for lymphocyte suppression and liver and kidney toxicity warranting regular complete blood counts and comprehensive chemistry monitoring. Serologic testing for hepatitis B virus and hepatitis C virus infection as well as screening for latent tuberculosis is recommended before treatment.

A retrospective study of 125 patients with CTD-ILD showed that MMF was well tolerated and resulted in FVC and DLCO stabilization (in patients with UIP) or improvement (patients without UIP).[88]

In addition, there are limited data in SLE-ILD, myositis-ILD, and RA-ILD, comprising uncontrolled case series or retrospective studies that show a potential benefit.[71,89,90] MMF has been best studied in SSc. The prospective, multicenter, randomized Scleroderma Lung Study II examined lung function in 73 patients with SSc treated with oral cyclophosphamide for 12 months plus placebo for 12 months versus 69 patients treated with MMF (1500 mg twice a day) for 24 months.[91] Both drugs led to improvement in prespecified outcome (percentage predicted FVC change 2.19 for MMF and 2.88 for cyclophosphamide), but fewer adverse events were seen in the MMF group. MMF has become the new gold-standard initial treatment of SSc-ILD.

Cyclophosphamide

Cyclophosphamide is an alkylating agent originally used for cancer chemotherapy. It has historically been the standard treatment of rapidly progressive CTD-ILD,[71,90,92,93] but there are few prospective, randomized studies.[71,72,91,94–98] Because of its toxicity profile, including ovarian failure, cyclophosphamide is best reserved for these high-risk patients rather than for chronic lung disease. Of note, it is possible that early institution of cyclophosphamide in SSc-ILD, before FVC decline, may offer better outcomes. Analysis of 111 out of 148 patients with SSc randomized to the cyclophosphamide arms of Scleroderma Lung Studies I and II showed that patients with higher baseline FVC fared better.[69]

Cyclosporine/tacrolimus

Cyclosporine A and tacrolimus and are calcineurin inhibitors that primarily affect T lymphocytes, decreasing production of IL-2 and other proinflammatory cytokines.[99] They are used in CTD-ILD refractory to other immunosuppressive treatment but must be used with care because of significant drug interactions and the potential for renal toxicity.[100–103] They may be useful in the treatment of inflammatory myositis-associated ILD, especially in patients with rapidly progressive ILD who also carry the antimelanoma differentiation-associated gene 5 (MDA-5) antibody.[93,104,105] A meta-analysis of 553 patients with myositis-associated chronic ILD revealed functional improvement in objective outcomes in 80.7% (95% confidence interval [CI] 49.6–94; 6 studies, n = 38) for patients treated with cyclosporine A and 86.2% (95% CI, 61.5–96; 2 studies, n = 23) for patients treated with tacrolimus.[72] Small studies in severe SSc-ILD showed no improvement in FVC or DLCO with significant renal toxicity.[106–109]

Rituximab

Rituximab is an anti-CD20 monoclonal antibody that results in plasma cell depletion typically lasting 6 to 9 months. Based on the mechanism of action, rituximab seems to be helpful in CTD-ILD cases in which the production of serum autoantibodies is associated with the presence and/or severity of ILD (ie, rheumatoid factor and anti–cyclic citrullinated peptide antibodies in RA and anti–transfer RNA synthetase antibodies in myositis).[90,110] Results from a retrospective study of 700 patients with RA-ILD showed improvement or stabilization in ILD as assessed by HRCT or PFT after treatment with rituximab.[70] Several studies have described the use of rituximab for the treatment of myositis-associated ILD.[93,111] Small studies suggest that rituximab is a reasonable therapy to consider for other CTD-ILDs, especially in patients who have failed conventional treatments.[112–118] Note that there are increasing numbers of case reports of rituximab-associated lung injury. This pneumonitis may be asymptomatic and often responds to steroids.[119] The protocol for a multicenter, prospective, randomized, double-blind, controlled trial of rituximab versus cyclophosphamide over the course of 24 weeks in CTD-ILD (RECITAL [Rituximab versus cyclophosphamide for the treatment of connective tissue disease-associated interstitial lung disease]) has been published.[120] Results from this study will add to the understanding of the role of rituximab in these patients.

Tocilizumab

Interleukin (IL)-6 has been shown to be expressed in the synovium of patients with RA and in SSc skin biopsies; it also has pleiotropic inflammatory effects, making it an attractive therapeutic target for CTD-ILD.[121,122] Tocilizumab is an IL-6 receptor α antibody, approved for use in RA. Despite concerns regarding an association with RA-ILD,[123–125] large postmarketing studies have not supported this.[126] Tocilizumab can be administered as a monotherapy without methotrexate in patients in whom methotrexate-associated lung toxicity is a concern; however, results of a recent retrospective study found no benefit in ILD HRCT changes in 7 patients who received tocilizumab for the treatment of RA-ILD.[127] Results of the phase II FaSScinate (Safety and efficacy of subcutaneous tocilizumab in adults with systemic sclerosis) Trial were published in 2016 showing that weekly tocilizumab for 48 weeks in patients with

SSc-ILD resulted in a favorable change in FVC percentage predicted between weeks 24 and 48, although skin disease was the primary outcome.[128] A phase III study of tocilizumab in SSc-ILD is now underway. The role of tocilizumab in other CTD-ILDs is currently limited to case reports.[129]

Abatacept

Abatacept is a fully humanized monoclonal antibody against CD80/86, a receptor present on antigen presenting cells that binds with CD28 on the surface of T cells. Abatacept CD80/86 binding prevents the second signal required for T-cell activation. In one single-center small retrospective study of 49 patients with RA who received biologics, abatacept use and prevalent airway disease were negative risk factors for incident or progressive airway disease or ILD.[127] One case report describes a patient with Sjögren syndrome and ILD who improved during treatment with tacrolimus and abatacept.[100] There have been no studies that have specifically assessed the utility of abatacept for CTD-ILD, but a rationale for use in SSc-ILD exists based on its mechanism.[130]

Intravenous Immunoglobulin

Intravenous immunoglobulin (IVIG) may be useful in PM/DM-ILD specifically, MDA-5–associated ILD.[131,132] Its use in SSc-ILD is of unclear benefit.[133] In spite of its high cost, IVIG is increasingly being used as adjunctive therapy for refractory CTD-ILD.[134] Care must be taken to administer IVIG slowly to avoid side effects, including aseptic meningitis.

Stem Cell Transplant

Results of 3 randomized studies have been published that suggest that autologous stem cell transplant (ASCT) may be advantageous in carefully selected patients with SSc with associated ILD. Note that hospital stays after ASCT can be long and complicated, and mortalities related to the transplant (ie, infection) ranged from 5% to 10% in these studies. Moreover, ASCT does not cure SSc and patients need to remain on immune suppression following ASCT to prevent disease recurrence. To reduce transplant-related mortality, pretransplant protocols were redesigned to include cardiac MRI and/or PET scans to assess for subclinical myocardial disease. Patients with extensive cardiac disease who may be unable to increase cardiac output in response to infection are often excluded. ASCT regimens are either lymphoablative or myeloablative and there is controversy about which approach is best. Proponents of lymphoablative regimens hail the potential for improved safety, including less risk of treatment-related serious infections and death, whereas proponents of myeloablative regimens cite better response duration. The results of 3 studies in patients with SSc that underwent ASCT have been published (**Table 3**). Referral to specialty centers with experience in ASCT can be considered for patients with severe disease.

Antifibrotic Therapies

A host of antifibrotic therapies have been studied, mainly in SSc-ILD, not all successful. CAT192 is a human IgG4 monoclonal antibody developed as a transforming growth factor (TGF)-β1 receptor–specific antagonist. In a randomized study of 32 patients with SSc, there was no added benefit in skin scoring, and there were more deaths (4 deaths vs 0 in the placebo group), more adverse events, and more serious adverse events in the active treatment group.[135]

Tyrosine kinase inhibitors (imatinib mesylate, dasatinib, and nilotinib) alter signaling cascades for TGF-β and platelet-derived growth factor, important profibrotic cytokines. These agents have been studied in patients with SSc,[136–138] but concern for drug-induced toxicity exists.[139–142] One open-label study of 31 patients with SSc-ILD treated with dasatinib showed no lung fibrosis progression in 65% and no progression of total ILD in 39%.[138] The phase III SENSCIS (Safety and Efficacy of Nintedanib in Systemic SClerosIS) clinical trial in patients with SSc-ILD treated with nintedanib, a newer tyrosine kinase inhibitor approved for treatment of IPF, has completed enrollment, and the US Food and Drug Administration has granted the drug fast-track designation that will enable more rapid approval evaluation. Limited data on the use of nintedanib in other CTD-ILDs are available.[143] Information from the PF-ILD (progressive fibrosing interstitial lung disease) trial of nintedanib for non-IPF ILD, which includes patients with various fibrotic CTD-ILDs, is anticipated.[144]

Pirfenidone is another antifibrotic drug approved for use in IPF. It has several mechanisms of action, including downregulation of TGF-β and TNF-α, as well as reduction of collagen synthesis and fibroblast proliferation.[145] Data from 2 case reports and an open-label phase II trial of pirfenidone for SSc-ILD treatment have been published that showed acceptable tolerability and possible efficacy, but large prospective trials are needed.[146–148] The results of a study of 30 patients with early amyopathic dermatomyositis-associated rapidly progressive ILD who received

Table 3
Autologous stem cell transplant in systemic sclerosis

Study (Year Results Published)	SCOT[94] (2018)	ASTIS[96] (2014)	ASSIST[95] (2013)
Study Design	Multicenter Prospective ITT	Multicenter Prospective ITT	Single center Retrospective
Sponsor	NIH NIAID	Investigator initiated	Investigator initiated
SSc Characteristics	Severe SSc duration <5 y and lung or renal	dcSSc duration <4 y; mRSS>15; and cardiac, lung, or renal dcSSc <2 y without organ involvement	dcSSc and mRSS >14 and lung, cardiac, or gastrointestinal
Control Group Treatment	Induction: CYC 500 mg/m^2 Maintenance: CYC 750 mg/m^2	CYC 750 mg/m^2	CYC 1 g/m^2 monthly
Patient Number	75 (226 targeted)	156	90
Total Body Irradiation	Yes (800 cGy)	No	No
Approach	Myeloablative	Lymphoablative	Lymphoablative
Mobilization	CYC 120 mg/kg G-CSF	CYC 4 g/m^2 ~100 mg/kg G-CSF	CYC 2 g/m^2 ~50 mg/kg G-CSF
Conditioning Regimen	ATG 90 mg/kg	CYC 200 mg/kg over 4 d ATG 7.5 mg/kg over 3 d GC 1 mg/kg	CYC 200 mg/kg ATG 0.5 mg/kg day −5 GC 250–1000 mg
Posttransplant Care	G-CSF GC Lisinopril Acyclovir	ACEI EBV load monitoring	G-CSF ACEI/ARB and CCB Cef/pip-tazo,val/acyclovir Fluconazole Bactrim/pentamidine
Transplant-related Mortality	3%	10.7% (CI, 4.5–19) during year 1	6% (4 deaths caused by cardiac complications)
Follow-up (y), median	4.5–6	5.8–7y	2.6 y, mean
Primary End Point	Global rank composite score at 54 mo	Event-free (heart, lung, kidney) survival	Decrease in mRSS >25% or increase in FVC >10%
Public Availability of Data	Yes	No	No

Abbreviations: ACEI, angiotensin-converting enzyme inhibitor; ARB, angiotensin receptor blocker; ASSIST, autologous stem cell systemic sclerosis immune suppression trial; ASTIS, autologous hematopoietic stem cell transplantation versus intravenous pulse cyclophosphamide in diffuse cutaneous systemic sclerosis; ATG, antithymocyte globulin; CCB, calcium channel blocker; Cef/pip-taza, cefepime/piperacillin-tazobactam; CYC, cyclophosphamide; dcSSc, diffuse cutaneous SSc; EBV, Epstein-Barr virus; GC, glucocorticoids; G-CSF, granulocyte colony–stimulating factor; ITT, intention to treat; mRSS, modified Rodnan skin score; NIH NIAID, National Institutes of Health National Institute of Allergy and Infectious Diseases; SCOT, scleroderma: cyclophosphamide or transplant.

pirfenidone plus conventional treatment versus 27 historical controls that received conventional treatment only revealed no survival benefit with pirfenidone.[149]

Lung Transplant

Despite advances in therapy for both ILD and PH, a considerable number of patients with CTD progress to end-stage respiratory failure, prompting consideration for lung transplant.[150] It has been recognized that extrapulmonary disease manifestations affect posttransplant outcomes, leading many centers in the recent past to consider CTD and particularly SSc as a relative, if not absolute, contraindication to lung transplant in part because of the concern that esophageal dysmotility will cause recurrent microaspiration and have negative early effects on allograft function and lead to chronic rejection.[151,152] In all CTDs, musculoskeletal limitations may impair mobility and the ability to participate in rehabilitation programs before and following transplant. Patients with CTD may have increased risk for thromboembolism, allosensitization, and renal failure. However, more recent evidence has shown that posttransplant outcomes can be similar to those of patients without CTD in carefully selected populations, suggesting that the diagnosis of CTD alone should not prevent consideration for transplant.[153–156] Despite these data, there remains wide variability between centers in the approach to patient selection and methods of testing. It is recommended that a multidisciplinary evaluation of these patients occur as early as feasible to improve optimization of relevant comorbidities.[152,157]

ADDITIONAL SUPPORTIVE TREATMENT STRATEGIES
Oxygen

Exertional hypoxemia in patients with CTD-ILD is typically caused by both diffusion impairment and ventilation-perfusion mismatch; the development of pulmonary vascular abnormalities may also contribute.[158] This desaturation may be profound and can contribute significantly to dyspnea, which is itself linked with depression and poor functional status.[159] Chronic hypoxemia may also lead to worsening PH.[160] Multiple small studies suggest that exercise capacity and quality of life are improved by the use of oxygen therapy.[161–165] However, the use of long-term oxygen in ILD remains poorly studied and recommendations for its use rely on data from the mortality benefit seen in its use in patients with chronic obstructive lung disease.[166,167] No such data exist in ILD, and questions regarding the potential harm caused by oxidative stress have not been fully answered.[168] Results from ongoing studies may better address these questions.[169]

Despite these uncertainties, the authors and many physicians continue to recommend oxygen supplementation for resting and exertional hypoxemia, as do most national guidelines in ILD.[170] Additional study is needed in this population, because some patients are negatively affected by the weight of the device, personal expectations, and stigma associated with oxygen use.[171–173] Our practice is to work individually with patients and caregivers to assess specific lifestyle considerations and allow the dispensing of units tailored to these needs wherever possible. Despite a lack of data, the authors generally titrate

oxygen flow to achieve a saturation greater than 90%, which is similar to other ILD centers.[171] We encourage oxygen use in the setting of pulmonary rehabilitation and other exercise because oxygen supplementation does augment endurance and the utility of such programs.[174] However, in patients with severe disease, high flow rates and use of pendant devices may limit portability.[175] Particularly in patients with CTD, musculoskeletal limitations may lead to challenges with managing devices. Multidisciplinary services are greatly needed in this population to assist patients and their caregivers.

Pulmonary Rehabilitation

Pulmonary rehabilitation (PR) is a structured and comprehensive program designed for patients with pulmonary disease. A multidisciplinary team develops an individualized therapy program, which may include exercise training, education, and behavioral interventions.[176] Recent studies lend support to the benefit of PR in patients with ILD, showing significantly increased 6MWD, dyspnea, muscle strength, and health-related quality of life.[177–179] It is unclear whether patients with CTD-ILD benefit as much as those with IPF or other forms of ILD, because of comorbid conditions and therapy (such as corticosteroids), musculoskeletal pain and weakness, or other factors. However, benefits are nonetheless observed in this group.[177] PR seems to benefit patients with both mild and severe diffusion impairment.[180] Although most PR participants in a large survey of European and American patients reported improvements in symptoms, activities of daily living, mood or sense of emotional wellbeing, understanding of their lung condition, and social functioning, many potentially eligible patients had never heard of such a program or had difficulty with accessing one.[181]

Pneumocystis Jirovecii Pneumonia Prophylaxis

P jirovecii, formerly known as Pneumocystis carinii, is associated with a potentially life-threatening pneumonia in patients with CTD-ILD receiving immune suppression.[182] Pneumocystis colonization is common (present in 30% of patients with systemic autoimmune diseases), but infections are rare, in part because of effective prophylaxis strategies.[182] Although formal guidelines are lacking for patients with CTD, Pneumocystis prophylaxis is recommended in patients treated with prednisone greater than 15 to 20 mg daily for greater than 4 weeks or with immunosuppressive therapy (**Table 4**).[183]

Table 4
Pneumocystis jirovecii pneumonia prophylaxis

Agent	Dosage	Notes
Trimethoprim-sulfamethoxazole	80 mg/400 PO QD 160 mg/800 mg PO TIW	If normal renal function Avoid in sulfa allergy
Dapsone	50–100 mg PO QD	Avoid if G6PD deficient Avoid in sulfa allergy
Atovaquone	1500 mg PO QD	Often expensive
Pentamidine	300 mg aerosolized Q 3–4 wk	Can cause cough and bronchospasm
Clindamycin + primaquine	300 mg + 15 mg PO QD or TIW	GI side effects common

Abbreviations: G6PD, glucose-6-phosphate dehydrogenase; GI, gastrointestinal; PO, by mouth; Q, every; QD, every day; TIW, 3 times a week.

  Data extracted from Martin SI, Fishman JA, AST Infectious Diseases Community of Practice. Pneumocystis pneumonia in solid organ transplantation. Am J Transplant 2013;13 Suppl 4:272–9.

Bone Health Management

The American College of Rheumatology 2017 clinical practice guidelines recommend that consideration be given to instituting prophylaxis for glucocorticoid-induced osteoporosis (GIOP) based on patient and disease factors.[184,185] At a minimum, calcium and vitamin D should be prescribed, a fall assessment should be conducted, and patients should be advised to participate in weight-bearing exercise (walking, running, or weight lifting as opposed to cycling or swimming).[184,185] Patient factors to consider when making the decision to start prophylaxis for GIOP include age, menopausal status, sex, race, prior osteoporotic fracture, a parent with a prior osteoporotic fracture, alcohol and tobacco consumption, fall risk, and body mass.[186] Disease factors include the presence of RA and intended glucocorticoid dose, route, and duration. The Fracture Risk Assessment Tool (FRAX) calculator (https://www.sheffield.ac.uk/FRAX/) with and without bone mineral density provides the 10-year probability of fracture and can help inform the decision regarding antiresorptive (bisphosphonates) or bone anabolic (teriparatide) treatment.[186] Prophylaxis should be considered for patients at low or medium risk for fracture who will be receiving in excess of 7.5 mg daily prednisone or patients with high fracture risk who will be receiving in excess of 5 mg daily prednisone for greater than 3 months. Oral bisphosphonates should be avoided in patients with esophageal dysmotility because they are a leading cause of pill esophagitis.[187]

Vaccinations

All patients with CTD-ILD in whom glucocorticoids and immune suppression are indicated should be vaccinated, if possible, with influenza vaccine and 1 or both pneumonia vaccines before therapy is commenced.[188] For patients more than 50 years of age, consider administering a shingles (zoster) vaccine. Intervals of 2 weeks for inactivated vaccines (recombinant zoster vaccine/Shingrix) and 4 weeks for live vaccines (zoster vaccine live/Zostavax) before the start of immune suppression are deemed optimal.[188] If the patient is pneumococcal vaccine naive, the 13-valent vaccine (PCV13) should be given first and the 23-valent vaccine (PPSV23) given greater than or equal to 8 weeks later. If the patient has received PPSV23 at least 8 weeks prior, PCV13 can be given. Zostavax should not be given at the same time as PCV13 or PPSV23. Separate Zostavax and PCV13 or PPSV23 injections by 4 weeks to maximize immunity. It is permissible to administer Shingrix or Zostavax and the influenza vaccine concurrently.

Assessment and Management of Comorbidities

PH is common in patients with CTD-ILD and may be in 1 or more of several categories based on classification by the Sixth World Symposium on Pulmonary Hypertension.[189] Often, patients with ILD are in group 3 (caused by chronic lung disease and/or hypoxia). However, it is important to consider group 1 (pulmonary arterial hypertension caused by CTD) as well as group 2 (caused by left heart disease), particularly in the setting of SSc, in which diastolic dysfunction may be present.[190] Many of the screening guidelines for PH are focused on pulmonary arterial hypertension in the SSc population and may not be applicable to other forms of CTD.[191] Current screening guidelines recommend annual transthoracic echocardiography. Composite measures such as the DETECT (Early, Simple and Reliable Detection of

Pulmonary Arterial Hypertension in Systemic Sclerosis) and ASIG (Australian Scleroderma Interest Group) algorithms, which include biomarkers such as brain natriuretic peptide and PFTs, have increased sensitivity.[192] Disproportionate decline in DLCO compared with FVC should increase suspicion for coexistent PH.[193] Right heart catheterization remains the gold standard for diagnosis. Evaluation by a specialized PH center is recommended to address individualized therapeutic decisions in the setting of combined PH and ILD.[193]

Gastroesophageal reflux disease is common in the CTD population, particularly in patients with SSc and MCTD because of motility disorders. Decline in esophageal peristalsis and loss of lower esophageal sphincter function may lead to recurrent microaspiration. Esophageal abnormalities are associated with increased pulmonary fibrosis, although the exact mechanism of this association is still unproved.[194] Consultation with a gastroenterologist familiar with motility testing and the use of promotility drugs may be useful, but the utility of such an approach requires further study.[195]

Patients with CTD-ILD are at risk for premature atherosclerosis and this should be considered in the assessment of patients with dyspnea and may be a factor in therapeutic decisions.[196–198] In addition, patients with ILD have increased risk for lung cancer beyond smoking history alone.[199] Lesions of concern should be addressed with this in mind and tobacco cessation should be encouraged. Obstructive sleep apnea seems to be particularly prevalent among patients with ILD, even in the absence of excessive sleepiness or obesity, and may portend a worse prognosis because of the effects of nocturnal hypoxemia.[200] Patients with all forms of ILD, and particularly patients with CTD, seem to be at increased risk for development of thromboembolic disease and should have new complaints of leg swelling, shortness of breath, or otherwise unexplained decline in diffusing capacity evaluated with this in mind.[201–203]

Palliative Care

Patients with ILD often experience dyspnea, cough, fatigue, anxiety, and depression.[204] Palliative care in this population is a significant unmet need, often leaving patients and their caregivers without effective pharmacologic and psychosocial interventions to improve symptoms, quality of life, and family distress at the end of life.[205,206] However, this is a growing area of research, with improved focus on validated outcome measures, longitudinal symptom measures, and improved evaluation of interventions. Whether early palliative

care intervention is helpful will be examined in the IPF population.[207] Given the different patient population and prognosis in many cases, patients with CTD-ILD require individualized study.

Benzodiazepines and opioids can reduce the sensation of breathlessness. Many physicians limit prescriptions of these drugs because of fear of increased mortality and respiratory suppression. In a recent population-based longitudinal cohort study of patients with progressive fibrotic ILD, higher-dose benzodiazepines were associated with higher mortality, whereas lower doses were not.[208] The higher doses may also reflect the setting of end-of-life care. Small studies suggest that morphine may also be used safely in patients with ILD.[209] Care must be taken if lung transplant is still a viable option, because chronic narcotic use may be a relative contraindication to listing in some centers. Multiple nonpharmacologic interventions, including relaxation and breathing exercises, cool air fans, positioning, and cognitive therapy, may be helpful.[205]

Cough can be a deeply troubling symptom; opiates, gabapentin, low-dose prednisolone, and thalidomide may all be considered.[205,210] A search for contributory features, such as postnasal drip and gastroesophageal reflux, should be undertaken. Similarly, for systemic symptoms such as fatigue, a search for alternative underlying causes, such as obstructive sleep apnea, endocrine disorders, and anemia, should be sought. Psychosocial interventions for depression and anxiety are a useful component of a multidisciplinary approach to care.[211,212]

SUMMARY

ILD is common among patients with CTD and remains a challenging area for diagnosis and treatment. The approach should always include an assessment for alternative causes for lung findings, including infection and drug toxicity. Immunosuppression remains a mainstay of therapy despite few controlled trials supporting its use. Additional information regarding novel agents is anticipated. A multidisciplinary approach is crucial and should include supportive and nonpharmacologic management strategies.

REFERENCES

1. Raghu G, Remy-Jardin M, Myers JL, et al. Diagnosis of idiopathic pulmonary fibrosis. An official ATS/ERS/JRS/ALAT clinical practice guideline. Am J Respir Crit Care Med 2018;198(5):e44–68.
2. Lynch DA, Sverzellati N, Travis WD, et al. Diagnostic criteria for idiopathic pulmonary fibrosis: a

Fleischner Society white paper. Lancet Respir Med 2018;6(2):138–53.

3. Price TM, Skelton MO. Rheumatoid arthritis with lung lesions. Thorax 1956;11(3):234–40.

4. Weaver AL, Divertie MB, Titus JL. The lung scleroderma. Mayo Clin Proc 1967;42(11):754–66.

5. Castelino FV, Varga J. Interstitial lung disease in connective tissue diseases: evolving concepts of pathogenesis and management. Arthritis Res Ther 2010;12(4):213.

6. Stack BH, Grant IW. Rheumatoid interstitial lung disease. Br J Dis Chest 1965;59(4):202–11.

7. Frank ST, Weg JG, Harkleroad LE, et al. Pulmonary dysfunction in rheumatoid disease. Chest 1973; 63(1):27–34.

8. Robles-Perez A, Luburich P, Rodriguez-Sanchon B, et al. Preclinical lung disease in early rheumatoid arthritis. Chron Respir Dis 2016;13(1):75–81.

9. Dawson JK, Fewins HE, Desmond J, et al. Fibrosing alveolitis in patients with rheumatoid arthritis as assessed by high resolution computed tomography, chest radiography, and pulmonary function tests. Thorax 2001;56(8):622–7.

10. Gochuico BR, Avila NA, Chow CK, et al. Progressive preclinical interstitial lung disease in rheumatoid arthritis. Arch Intern Med 2008;168(2):159–66.

11. Suzuki A, Ohosone Y, Obana M, et al. Cause of death in 81 autopsied patients with rheumatoid arthritis. J Rheumatol 1994;21(1):33–6.

12. Lee JS, Fischer A. Current and emerging treatment options for interstitial lung disease in patients with rheumatic disease. Expert Rev Clin Immunol 2016;12(5):509–20.

13. Bongartz T, Nannini C, Medina-Velasquez YF, et al. Incidence and mortality of interstitial lung disease in rheumatoid arthritis: a population-based study. Arthritis Rheum 2010;62(6):1583–91.

14. Olson AL, Swigris JJ, Sprunger DB, et al. Rheumatoid arthritis-interstitial lung disease-associated mortality. Am J Respir Crit Care Med 2011;183(3): 372–8.

15. Morisset J, Vittinghoff E, Elicker BM, et al. Mortality risk prediction in scleroderma-related interstitial lung disease: the SADL model. Chest 2017; 152(5):999–1007.

16. Travis WD, Costabel U, Hansell DM, et al. An official American Thoracic Society/European Respiratory Society statement: update of the international multidisciplinary classification of the idiopathic interstitial pneumonias. Am J Respir Crit Care Med 2013;188(6):733–48.

17. Hunninghake GW, Lynch DA, Galvin JR, et al. Radiologic findings are strongly associated with a pathologic diagnosis of usual interstitial pneumonia. Chest 2003;124(4):1215–23.

18. Lynch DA, Godwin JD, Safrin S, et al. High-resolution computed tomography in idiopathic pulmonary fibrosis: diagnosis and prognosis. Am J Respir Crit Care Med 2005;172(4):488–93.

19. Assayag D, Elicker BM, Urbania TH, et al. Rheumatoid arthritis-associated interstitial lung disease: radiologic identification of usual interstitial pneumonia pattern. Radiology 2014;270(2): 583–8.

20. Kim EJ, Collard HR, King TE Jr. Rheumatoid arthritis-associated interstitial lung disease: the relevance of histopathologic and radiographic pattern. Chest 2009;136(5):1397–405.

21. Travis WD, Hunninghake G, King TE Jr, et al. Idiopathic nonspecific interstitial pneumonia: report of an American Thoracic Society project. Am J Respir Crit Care Med 2008;177(12):1338–47.

22. Bjoraker JA, Ryu JH, Edwin MK, et al. Prognostic significance of histopathologic subsets in idiopathic pulmonary fibrosis. Am J Respir Crit Care Med 1998;157(1):199–203.

23. Batra K, Butt Y, Gokaslan T, et al. Pathology and radiology correlation of idiopathic interstitial pneumonias. Hum Pathol 2018;72:1–17.

24. MacDonald SL, Rubens MB, Hansell DM, et al. Nonspecific interstitial pneumonia and usual interstitial pneumonia: comparative appearances at and diagnostic accuracy of thin-section CT. Radiology 2001;221(3):600–5.

25. Yunt ZX, Chung JH, Hobbs S, et al. High resolution computed tomography pattern of usual interstitial pneumonia in rheumatoid arthritis-associated interstitial lung disease: relationship to survival. Respir Med 2017;126:100–4.

26. Fischer A, Swigris JJ, Groshong SD, et al. Clinically significant interstitial lung disease in limited scleroderma: histopathology, clinical features, and survival. Chest 2008;134(3):601–5.

27. Urisman A, Jones KD. Pulmonary pathology in connective tissue disease. Semin Respir Crit Care Med 2014;35(2):201–12.

28. Salisbury ML, Gross BH, Chughtai A, et al. Development and validation of a radiological diagnosis model for hypersensitivity pneumonitis. Eur Respir J 2018;52(2) [pii:1800443].

29. Vasakova M, Morell F, Walsh S, et al. Hypersensitivity pneumonitis: perspectives in diagnosis and management. Am J Respir Crit Care Med 2017; 196(6):680–9.

30. Skeoch S, Weatherley N, Swift AJ, et al. Drug-induced interstitial lung disease: a systematic review. J Clin Med 2018;7(10) [pii:E356].

31. Khan S, Christopher-Stine L. Polymyositis, dermatomyositis, and autoimmune necrotizing myopathy: clinical features. Rheum Dis Clin North Am 2011; 37(2):143–58, v.

32. Hachulla E, Launay D. Diagnosis and classification of systemic sclerosis. Clin Rev Allergy Immunol 2010;40(2):78–83.

33. Arnett FC, Edworthy SM, Bloch DA, et al. The American Rheumatism Association 1987 revised criteria for the classification of rheumatoid arthritis. Arthritis Rheum 1988;31(3):315–24.

34. Minier T, Guiducci S, Bellando-Randone S, et al. Preliminary analysis of the very early diagnosis of systemic sclerosis (VEDOSS) EUSTAR multicentre study: evidence for puffy fingers as a pivotal sign for suspicion of systemic sclerosis. Ann Rheum Dis 2014;73(12):2087–93.

35. Carlson DA, Hinchcliff M, Pandolfino JE. Advances in the evaluation and management of esophageal disease of systemic sclerosis. Curr Rheumatol Rep 2015;17(1):475.

36. Strange C, Highland KB. Interstitial lung disease in the patient who has connective tissue disease. Clin Chest Med 2004;25(3):549–59, vii.

37. Tanaka N, Kim JS, Newell JD, et al. Rheumatoid arthritis-related lung diseases: CT findings. Radiology 2004;232(1):81–91.

38. Miller W. Diagnostic thoracic imaging. McGraw-Hill; 2006.

39. Mori S, Cho I, Koga Y, et al. Comparison of pulmonary abnormalities on high-resolution computed tomography in patients with early versus longstanding rheumatoid arthritis. J Rheumatol 2008;35(8):1513–21.

40. Kocheril SV, Appleton BE, Somers EC, et al. Comparison of disease progression and mortality of connective tissue disease-related interstitial lung disease and idiopathic interstitial pneumonia. Arthritis Rheum 2005;53(4):549–57.

41. Walsh SL, Hansell DM. Diffuse interstitial lung disease: overlaps and uncertainties. Eur Radiol 2010;20(8):1859–67.

42. Fischer A, Chartrand S. Assessment and management of connective tissue disease-associated interstitial lung disease. Sarcoidosis Vasc Diffuse Lung Dis 2015;32(1):2–21.

43. Costabel U, Guzman J, Bonella F, et al. Bronchoalveolar lavage in other interstitial lung diseases. Semin Respir Crit Care Med 2007;28(5):514–24.

44. Schnabel A, Richter C, Bauerfeind S, et al. Bronchoalveolar lavage cell profile in methotrexate induced pneumonitis. Thorax 1997;52(4):377–9.

45. Ramirez P, Valencia M, Torres A. Bronchoalveolar lavage to diagnose respiratory infections. Semin Respir Crit Care Med 2007;28(5):525–33.

46. Meyer KC, Raghu G, Baughman RP, et al. An official American Thoracic Society clinical practice guideline: the clinical utility of bronchoalveolar lavage cellular analysis in interstitial lung disease. Am J Respir Crit Care Med 2012;185(9):1004–14.

47. Lentz RJ, Argento AC, Colby TV, et al. Transbronchial cryobiopsy for diffuse parenchymal lung disease: a state-of-the-art review of procedural techniques, current evidence, and future challenges. J Thorac Dis 2017;9(7):2186–203.

48. Kowal-Bielecka O, Kowal K, Highland KB, et al. Bronchoalveolar lavage fluid in scleroderma interstitial lung disease: technical aspects and clinical correlations: review of the literature. Semin Arthritis Rheum 2010;40(1):73–88.

49. Mathai SC, Danoff SK. Management of interstitial lung disease associated with connective tissue disease. BMJ 2016;352:h6819.

50. Hallowell RW, Horton MR. Interstitial lung disease in patients with rheumatoid arthritis: spontaneous and drug induced. Drugs 2014;74(4):443–50.

51. Rutherford AI, Subesinghe S, Hyrich KL, et al. Serious infection across biologic-treated patients with rheumatoid arthritis: results from the British Society for Rheumatology biologics register for rheumatoid arthritis. Ann Rheum Dis 2018;77(6):905–10.

52. Falagas ME, Manta KG, Betsi GI, et al. Infection-related morbidity and mortality in patients with connective tissue diseases: a systematic review. Clin Rheumatol 2007;26(5):663–70.

53. Wolfe RM, Peacock JE Jr. Pneumocystis pneumonia and the rheumatologist: which patients are at risk and how can PCP Be prevented? Curr Rheumatol Rep 2017;19(6):35.

54. Faisal A, Alghamdi BJ, Ciavaglia CE, et al. Common mechanisms of dyspnea in chronic interstitial and obstructive lung disorders. Am J Respir Crit Care Med 2016;193(3):299–309.

55. Flaherty KR, Mumford JA, Murray S, et al. Prognostic implications of physiologic and radiographic changes in idiopathic interstitial pneumonia. Am J Respir Crit Care Med 2003;168(5):543–8.

56. Lama VN, Flaherty KR, Toews GB, et al. Prognostic value of desaturation during a 6-minute walk test in idiopathic interstitial pneumonia. Am J Respir Crit Care Med 2003;168(9):1084–90.

57. Sanges S, Giovannelli J, Sobanski V, et al. Factors associated with the 6-minute walk distance in patients with systemic sclerosis. Arthritis Res Ther 2017;19(1):279.

58. Kafaja S, Clements PJ, Wilhalme H, et al. Reliability and minimal clinically important differences of forced vital capacity: results from the Scleroderma Lung Studies (SLS-I and SLS-II). Am J Respir Crit Care Med 2018;197(5):644–52.

59. Winstone TA, Assayag D, Wilcox PG, et al. Predictors of mortality and progression in scleroderma-associated interstitial lung disease: a systematic review. Chest 2014;146(2):422–36.

60. Goh NS, Hoyles RK, Denton CP, et al. Short-term pulmonary function trends are predictive of mortality in interstitial lung disease associated with systemic sclerosis. Arthritis Rheumatol 2017;69(8):1670–8.

61. Solomon JJ, Chung JH, Cosgrove GP, et al. Predictors of mortality in rheumatoid arthritis-associated interstitial lung disease. Eur Respir J 2016;47(2): 588–96.

62. Ryerson CJ, Vittinghoff E, Ley B, et al. Predicting survival across chronic interstitial lung disease: the ILD-GAP model. Chest 2014;145(4): 723–8.

63. Showalter K, Hoffmann A, Rouleau G, et al. Performance of forced vital capacity and lung diffusion cutpoints for associated radiographic interstitial lung disease in systemic sclerosis. J Rheumatol 2018;45(11):1572–6.

64. Goh NS, Desai SR, Veeraraghavan S, et al. Interstitial lung disease in systemic sclerosis: a simple staging system. Am J Respir Crit Care Med 2008; 177(11):1248–54.

65. Khanna D, Nagaraja V, Tseng CH, et al. Predictors of lung function decline in scleroderma-related interstitial lung disease based on high-resolution computed tomography: implications for cohort enrichment in systemic sclerosis-associated interstitial lung disease trials. Arthritis Res Ther 2015; 17:372.

66. Jacob J, Hirani N, van Moorsel CHM, et al. Predicting outcomes in rheumatoid arthritis related interstitial lung disease. Eur Respir J 2019;53(1) [pii: 1800869].

67. Golden MR, Katz RS, Balk RA, et al. The relationship of preexisting lung disease to the development of methotrexate pneumonitis in patients with rheumatoid arthritis. J Rheumatol 1995;22(6): 1043–7.

68. Chartrand S, Fischer A. Management of connective tissue disease-associated interstitial lung disease. Rheum Dis Clin North Am 2015;41(2):279–94.

69. Volkmann ER, Tashkin DP, Sim M, et al. Cyclophosphamide for systemic sclerosis-related interstitial lung disease: a comparison of scleroderma lung study I and II. J Rheumatol 2019. [Epub ahead of print].

70. Kabia A, Lettieri G, Vital EM, et al. Effect of rituximab on the progression of rheumatoid arthritis–related interstitial lung disease: 10 years' experience at a single centre. Rheumatology 2017; 56(8):1348–57.

71. Robles-Perez A, Molina-Molina M. Treatment considerations of lung involvement in rheumatologic disease. Respiration 2015;90(4):265–74.

72. Barba T, Fort R, Cottin V, et al. Treatment of idiopathic inflammatory myositis associated interstitial lung disease: a systematic review and meta-analysis. Autoimmun Rev 2019;18(2):113–22.

73. Adler S, Huscher D, Siegert E, et al. Systemic sclerosis associated interstitial lung disease - individualized immunosuppressive therapy and course of lung function: results of the EUSTAR group. Arthritis Res Ther 2018;20(1):17.

74. Steen VD, Medsger TA Jr. Case-control study of corticosteroids and other drugs that either precipitate or protect from the development of scleroderma renal crisis. Arthritis Rheum 1998;41(9): 1613–9.

75. Ha YJ, Lee YJ, Kang EH. Lung involvements in rheumatic diseases: update on the epidemiology, pathogenesis, clinical features, and treatment. Biomed Res Int 2018;2018:6930297.

76. Maltzman JS, Koretzky GA. Azathioprine: old drug, new actions. J Clin Invest 2003;111(8):1122–4.

77. Lennard L, Van Loon JA, Weinshilboum RM. Pharmacogenetics of acute azathioprine toxicity: relationship to thiopurine methyltransferase genetic polymorphism. Clin Pharmacol Ther 1989;46(2): 149–54.

78. Jensen ML, Lokke A, Hilberg O, et al. Clinical characteristics and outcome in patients with antisynthetase syndrome associated interstitial lung disease: a retrospective cohort study. Eur Clin Respir J 2019;6(1):1583516.

79. Kundu S, Paul S, Hariprasath K, et al. Effect of Sequential intravenous pulse cyclophosphamide-azathioprine in systemic sclerosis-interstitial lung disease: an open-label study. Indian J Chest Dis Allied Sci 2016;58(1):7–10.

80. Iudici M, Cuomo G, Vettori S, et al. Low-dose pulse cyclophosphamide in interstitial lung disease associated with systemic sclerosis (SSc-ILD): efficacy of maintenance immunosuppression in responders and non-responders. Semin Arthritis Rheum 2015; 44(4):437–44.

81. Paone C, Chiarolanza I, Cuomo G, et al. Twelve-month azathioprine as maintenance therapy in early diffuse systemic sclerosis patients treated for 1-year with low dose cyclophosphamide pulse therapy. Clin Exp Rheumatol 2007;25(4): 613–6.

82. Berezne A, Ranque B, Valeyre D, et al. Therapeutic strategy combining intravenous cyclophosphamide followed by oral azathioprine to treat worsening interstitial lung disease associated with systemic sclerosis: a retrospective multicenter open-label study. J Rheumatol 2008;35(6): 1064–72.

83. Pavlov-Dolijanovic S, Vujasinovic Stupar N, Zugic V, et al. Long-term effects of immunosuppressive therapy on lung function in scleroderma patients. Clin Rheumatol 2018;37(11):3043–50.

84. Dheda K, Lalloo UG, Cassim B, et al. Experience with azathioprine in systemic sclerosis associated with interstitial lung disease. Clin Rheumatol 2004;23(4):306–9.

85. Nadashkevich O, Davis P, Fritzler M, et al. A randomized unblinded trial of cyclophosphamide versus azathioprine in the treatment of systemic sclerosis. Clin Rheumatol 2006;25(2):205–12.

86. Oldham JM, Lee C, Valenzi E, et al. Azathioprine response in patients with fibrotic connective tissue disease-associated interstitial lung disease. Respir Med 2016;121:117–22.

87. Villarroel MC, Hidalgo M, Jimeno A. Mycophenolate mofetil: an update. Drugs Today (Barc) 2009; 45(7):521–32.

88. Fischer A, Brown KK, Du Bois RM, et al. Mycophenolate mofetil improves lung function in connective tissue disease-associated interstitial lung disease. J Rheumatol 2013;40(5):640–6.

89. Morganroth PA, Kreider ME, Werth VP. Mycophenolate mofetil for interstitial lung disease in dermatomyositis. Arthritis Care Res 2010;62(10):1496–501.

90. Brito Y, Glassberg MK, Ascherman DP. Rheumatoid arthritis-associated interstitial lung disease: current concepts. Curr Rheumatol Rep 2017; 19(12):79.

91. Tashkin DP, Roth MD, Clements PJ, et al. Mycophenolate mofetil versus oral cyclophosphamide in scleroderma-related interstitial lung disease (SLS II): a randomised controlled, double-blind, parallel group trial. Lancet Respir Med 2016;4(9):708–19.

92. Fu Q, Wang L, Li L, et al. Risk factors for progression and prognosis of rheumatoid arthritis-associated interstitial lung disease: single center study with a large sample of Chinese population. Clin Rheumatol 2019;38(4):1109–16.

93. Mecoli CA, Christopher-Stine L. Management of interstitial lung disease in patients with myositis specific autoantibodies. Curr Rheumatol Rep 2018;20(5):27 (1534-6307 [Electronic]).

94. Sullivan KM, Goldmuntz EA, Keyes-Elstein L, et al. Myeloablative autologous stem-cell transplantation for severe scleroderma. N Engl J Med 2018;378(1): 35–47.

95. Burt RK, Shah SJ, Dill K, et al. Autologous non-myeloablative haemopoietic stem-cell transplantation compared with pulse cyclophosphamide once per month for systemic sclerosis (ASSIST): an open-label, randomised phase 2 trial. Lancet 2011;378(9790):498–506.

96. van Laar JM, Farge D, Sont JK, et al. Autologous hematopoietic stem cell transplantation vs intravenous pulse cyclophosphamide in diffuse cutaneous systemic sclerosis: a randomized clinical trial. JAMA 2014;311(24):2490–8.

97. Tashkin DP, Elashoff R, Clements PJ, et al. Cyclophosphamide versus placebo in scleroderma lung disease. N Engl J Med 2006;354(25):2655–66.

98. Muangchan C, van Vollenhoven RF, Bernatsky SR, et al. Treatment algorithms in systemic lupus erythematosus. Arthritis Care Res (Hoboken) 2015; 67(9):1237–45.

99. Matsuda S, Koyasu S. Mechanisms of action of cyclosporine. Immunopharmacology 2000;47(2–3):119–25.

100. Thompson G, McLean-Tooke A, Wrobel J, et al. Sjogren syndrome with associated lymphocytic interstitial pneumonia successfully treated with tacrolimus and abatacept as an alternative to rituximab. Chest 2018;153(3):e41–3.

101. Sharma N, Putman MS, Vij R, et al. Myositis-associated interstitial lung disease: predictors of failure of conventional treatment and response to tacrolimus in a US cohort. J Rheumatol 2017;44(11):1612–8 (0315-162X [Print]).

102. Witt LJ, Demchuk C, Curran JJ, et al. Benefit of adjunctive tacrolimus in connective tissue disease-interstitial lung disease. Pulm Pharmacol Ther 2016;36:46–52 (1522-9629 [Electronic]).

103. Hanaoka HA, Iida H, Kiyokawa T, et al. Mycophenolate mofetil treatment with or without a calcineurin inhibitor in resistant inflammatory myopathy. Clin Rheumatol 2019;38(2):585–90 (1434-9949 [Electronic]).

104. Kawasumi H, Gono T, Kawaguchi Y, et al. Recent treatment of interstitial lung disease with idiopathic inflammatory myopathies. Clin Med Insights Circ Respir Pulm Med 2015;9(Suppl 1):9–17 (1179-5484 [Print]).

105. Shimojima Y, Ishii W, Matsuda M, et al. Effective use of calcineurin inhibitor in combination therapy for interstitial lung disease in patients with dermatomyositis and polymyositis. J Clin Rheumatol 2017; 23(2):87–93 (1536-7355 [Electronic]).

106. Filaci G, Cutolo M, Scudeletti M, et al. Cyclosporin A and iloprost treatment of systemic sclerosis: clinical results and interleukin-6 serum changes after 12 months of therapy. Rheumatology (Oxford) 1999;38(10):992–6.

107. Konma J, Kotani T, Shoda T, et al. Efficacy and safety of combination therapy with prednisolone and oral tacrolimus for progressive interstitial pneumonia with systemic sclerosis: a retrospective study. Mod Rheumatol 2018;28(6):1009–15.

108. Matsui A, Ikeuchi H, Shimizu A, et al. Case report: posterior reversible encephalopathy syndrome and scleroderma renal crisis developed in a patient with overlap syndrome after treatment with high-dose steroids and tacrolimus. Nihon Naika Gakkai Zasshi 2012;101(7):2051–4 [in Japanese].

109. Nunokawa T, Akazawa M, Yokogawa N, et al. Late-onset scleroderma renal crisis induced by tacrolimus and prednisolone: a case report. Am J Ther 2014;21(5):e130–3.

110. Doyle TJ, Dhillon N, Madan R, et al. Rituximab in the treatment of interstitial lung disease associated with antisynthetase syndrome: a multicenter retrospective case review. J Rheumatol 2018;45(6): 841–50.

111. So H, Wong VTL, Lao VWN, et al. Rituximab for refractory rapidly progressive interstitial lung disease related to anti-MDA5 antibody-positive amyopathic

dermatomyositis. Clin Rheumatol 2018;37(7): 1983–9.

112. Fraticelli P, Fischetti C, Salaffi F, et al. Combination therapy with rituximab and mycophenolate mofetil in systemic sclerosis. A single-centre case series study. Clin Exp Rheumatol 2018;36 Suppl 113(4): 142–5.

113. Sircar G, Goswami RP, Sircar D, et al. Intravenous cyclophosphamide vs rituximab for the treatment of early diffuse scleroderma lung disease: open label, randomized, controlled trial. Rheumatology (Oxford) 2018;57(12):2106–13.

114. Thiebaut M, Launay D, Riviere S, et al. Efficacy and safety of rituximab in systemic sclerosis: French retrospective study and literature review. Autoimmun Rev 2018;17(6):582–7.

115. Ebata S, Yoshizaki A, Fukasawa T, et al. Unprecedented success of rituximab therapy for prednisolone- and immunosuppressant-resistant systemic sclerosis-associated interstitial lung disease. Scand J Rheumatol 2017;46(3):247–52.

116. Sari A, Guven D, Armagan B, et al. Rituximab experience in patients with long-standing systemic sclerosis-associated interstitial lung disease: a series of 14 patients. J Clin Rheumatol 2017;23(8): 411–5.

117. Ogawa Y, Kishida D, Shimojima YA-O, et al. Effective administration of rituximab in anti-MDA5 antibody-positive dermatomyositis with rapidly progressive interstitial lung disease and refractory cutaneous involvement: a case report and literature review. Case Rep Rheumatol 2017;2017:5386797 (2090-6889 [Print]).

118. Roofeh D, Jaafar S, Vummidi D, et al. Management of systemic sclerosis-associated interstitial lung disease. Curr Opin Rheumatol 2019;31(3): 241–9.

119. Roden AC, Camus P. Iatrogenic pulmonary lesions. Semin Diagn Pathol 2018;35(4):260–71.

120. Saunders P, Tsipouri V, Keir GJ, et al. Rituximab versus cyclophosphamide for the treatment of connective tissue disease-associated interstitial lung disease (RECITAL): study protocol for a randomised controlled trial. Trials 2017;18(1):275.

121. Koch AE, Kronfeld-Harrington LB, Szekanecz Z, et al. In situ expression of cytokines and cellular adhesion molecules in the skin of patients with systemic sclerosis. Their role in early and late disease. Pathobiology 1993;61(5–6):239–46.

122. Nishimoto N, Kishimoto T, Yoshizaki K. Anti-interleukin 6 receptor antibody treatment in rheumatic disease. Ann Rheum Dis 2000;59(Suppl 1):i21–7.

123. Akiyama M, Kaneko Y, Yamaoka K, et al. Association of disease activity with acute exacerbation of interstitial lung disease during tocilizumab treatment in patients with rheumatoid arthritis: a

retrospective, case-control study. Rheumatol Int 2016;36(6):881–9.

124. Roubille C, Haraoui B. Interstitial lung diseases induced or exacerbated by DMARDS and biologic agents in rheumatoid arthritis: a systematic literature review. Semin Arthritis Rheum 2014;43(5): 613–26.

125. Kawashiri SY, Kawakami A, Sakamoto N, et al. A fatal case of acute exacerbation of interstitial lung disease in a patient with rheumatoid arthritis during treatment with tocilizumab. Rheumatol Int 2012;32(12):4023–6.

126. Curtis JR, Sarsour K, Napalkov P, et al. Incidence and complications of interstitial lung disease in users of tocilizumab, rituximab, abatacept and anti-tumor necrosis factor alpha agents, a retrospective cohort study. Arthritis Res Ther 2015;17: 319 (1478-6362 [Electronic]).

127. Kurata I, Tsuboi H, Terasaki M, et al. Effect of biological disease-modifying anti-rheumatic drugs on airway and interstitial lung disease in patients with rheumatoid arthritis. Intern Med 2019;58(12): 1703–12.

128. Khanna D, Denton CP, Lin CJF, et al. Safety and efficacy of subcutaneous tocilizumab in systemic sclerosis: results from the open-label period of a phase II randomised controlled trial (faSScinate). Ann Rheum Dis 2018;77(2):212–20.

129. Moroncini G, Calogera G, Benfaremo D, et al. Biologics in inflammatory immune-mediated systemic diseases. Curr Pharm Biotechnol 2017;18(12): 1008–16.

130. Bruni C, Praino E, Allanore Y, et al. Use of biologics and other novel therapies for the treatment of systemic sclerosis. Expert Rev Clin Immunol 2017; 13(5):469–82.

131. Koguchi-Yoshioka H, Okiyama N, Iwamoto K, et al. Intravenous immunoglobulin contributes to the control of antimelanoma differentiation-associated protein 5 antibody-associated dermatomyositis with palmar violaceous macules/papules. Br J Dermatol 2017;177(5):1442–6 (1365-2133 [Electronic]).

132. Takai M, Katsurada N, Nakashita T, et al. Rapidly progressive interstitial lung disease associated with dermatomyositis treated with combination of immunosuppressive therapy, direct hemoperfusion with a polymyxin B immobilized fiber column and intravenous immunoglobulin. Intern Med 2015; 54(17):2225–9.

133. Gomes JP, Santos L, Shoenfeld Y. Intravenous immunoglobulin (IVIG) in the vanguard therapy of Systemic Sclerosis. Clin Immunol 2019;199:25–8.

134. Hallowell RW, Amariei D, Danoff SK. Intravenous immunoglobulin as potential adjunct therapy for interstitial lung disease. Ann Am Thorac Soc 2016;13(10):1682–8.

135. Denton CP, Merkel PA, Furst DE, et al. Recombinant human anti-transforming growth factor beta1 antibody therapy in systemic sclerosis: a multicenter, randomized, placebo-controlled phase I/II trial of CAT-192. Arthritis Rheum 2007;56(1): 323–33.

136. Gordon JK, Spiera RF. Targeting tyrosine kinases: a novel therapeutic strategy for systemic sclerosis. Curr Opin Rheumatol 2010;22(6):690–5.

137. Gordon JK, Martyanov V, Magro C, et al. Nilotinib (Tasigna) in the treatment of early diffuse systemic sclerosis: an open-label, pilot clinical trial. Arthritis Res Ther 2015;17:213.

138. Martyanov V, Kim GJ, Hayes W, et al. Novel lung imaging biomarkers and skin gene expression subsetting in dasatinib treatment of systemic sclerosis-associated interstitial lung disease. PLoS One 2017;12(11):e0187580.

139. Go SI, Lee WS, Lee GW, et al. Nilotinib-induced interstitial lung disease. Int J Hematol 2013;98(3): 361–5.

140. Zhang P, Huang J, Jin F, et al. Imatinib-induced irreversible interstitial lung disease: a case report. Medicine 2019;98(8):e14402.

141. Hinchcliff ME, Lomasney J, Johnson JA, et al. Fulminant capillary leak syndrome in a patient with systemic sclerosis treated with imatinib mesylate. Rheumatology (Oxford) 2016;55(10):1916–8.

142. Pope J, McBain D, Petrlich L, et al. Imatinib in active diffuse cutaneous systemic sclerosis: results of a six-month, randomized, double-blind, placebo-controlled, proof-of-concept pilot study at a single center. Arthritis Rheum 2011;63(11): 3547–51.

143. Kakuwa T, Izumi S, Sakamoto K, et al. A successful treatment of rheumatoid arthritis-related interstitial pneumonia with nintedanib. Respir Med Case Rep 2019;26:50–2.

144. Flaherty KR, Brown KK, Wells AU, et al. Design of the PF-ILD trial: a double-blind, randomised, placebo-controlled phase III trial of nintedanib in patients with progressive fibrosing interstitial lung disease. BMJ Open Respir Res 2017;4(1): e000212.

145. Kolb M, Bonella F, Wollin L. Therapeutic targets in idiopathic pulmonary fibrosis. Respir Med 2017; 131:49–57.

146. Huang H, Feng RE, Li S, et al. A case report: the efficacy of pirfenidone in a Chinese patient with progressive systemic sclerosis-associated interstitial lung disease: a CARE-compliant article. Medicine 2016;95(27):e4113.

147. Udwadia ZF, Mullerpattan JB, Balakrishnan C, et al. Improved pulmonary function following pirfenidone treatment in a patient with progressive interstitial lung disease associated with systemic sclerosis. Lung India 2015;32(1):50–2.

148. Khanna D, Albera C, Fischer A, et al. An open-label, phase II study of the safety and tolerability of pirfenidone in patients with scleroderma-associated interstitial lung disease: the LOTUSS trial. J Rheumatol 2016;43(9):1672–9.

149. Li T, Guo L, Chen Z, et al. Pirfenidone in patients with rapidly progressive interstitial lung disease associated with clinically amyopathic dermatomyositis. Sci Rep 2016;6:33226.

150. Elhai M, Meune C, Boubaya M, et al. Mapping and predicting mortality from systemic sclerosis. Ann Rheum Dis 2017;76(11):1897–905.

151. De Cruz S, Ross D. Lung transplantation in patients with scleroderma. Curr Opin Rheumatol 2013; 25(6):714–8.

152. Shah RJ, Boin F. Lung transplantation in patients with systemic sclerosis. Curr Rheumatol Rep 2017;19(5):23.

153. Crespo MM, Bermudez CA, Dew MA, et al. Lung transplant in patients with scleroderma compared with pulmonary fibrosis. Short- and long-term outcomes. Ann Am Thorac Soc 2016;13(6):784–92.

154. Pradere P, Tudorache I, Magnusson J, et al. Lung transplantation for scleroderma lung disease: an international, multicenter, observational cohort study. J Heart Lung Transplant 2018;37(7): 903–11.

155. Courtwright AM, El-Chemaly S, Dellaripa PF, et al. Survival and outcomes after lung transplantation for non-scleroderma connective tissue-related interstitial lung disease. J Heart Lung Transplant 2017;36(7):763–9.

156. Eberlein M, Mathai SC. Lung transplantation in scleroderma. Time for the pendulum to swing? Ann Am Thorac Soc 2016;13(6):767–9.

157. Bissell LA, Md Yusof MY, Buch MH. Primary myocardial disease in scleroderma-a comprehensive review of the literature to inform the UK Systemic Sclerosis Study Group cardiac working group. Rheumatology (Oxford) 2017;56(6):882–95.

158. Agusti AG, Roca J, Gea J, et al. Mechanisms of gas-exchange impairment in idiopathic pulmonary fibrosis. Am Rev Respir Dis 1991;143(2):219–25.

159. Ryerson CJ, Berkeley J, Carrieri-Kohlman VL, et al. Depression and functional status are strongly associated with dyspnea in interstitial lung disease. Chest 2011;139(3):609–16.

160. Strange C, Highland KB. Pulmonary hypertension in interstitial lung disease. Curr Opin Pulm Med 2005;11(5):452–5.

161. Schaeffer MR, Ryerson CJ, Ramsook AH, et al. Effects of hyperoxia on dyspnoea and exercise endurance in fibrotic interstitial lung disease. Eur Respir J 2017;49(5).

162. Visca D, Montgomery A, de Lauretis A, et al. Ambulatory oxygen in interstitial lung disease. Eur Respir J 2011;38(4):987–90.

163. Edvardsen A, Jarosch I, Grongstad A, et al. A randomized cross-over trial on the direct effects of oxygen supplementation therapy using different devices on cycle endurance in hypoxemic patients with Interstitial Lung Disease. PLoS One 2018; 13(12):e0209069.

164. Visca D, Mori L, Tsipouri V, et al. Effect of ambulatory oxygen on quality of life for patients with fibrotic lung disease (AmbOx): a prospective, open-label, mixed-method, crossover randomised controlled trial. Lancet Respir Med 2018;6(10): 759–70.

165. Khor YH, Goh NSL, McDonald CF, et al. Oxygen therapy for interstitial lung disease. A mismatch between patient expectations and experiences. Ann Am Thorac Soc 2017;14(6):888–95.

166. McDonald CF. Exercise desaturation and oxygen therapy in ILD and COPD: similarities, differences and therapeutic relevance. Respirology 2018; 23(4):350–1.

167. Bell EC, Cox NS, Goh N, et al. Oxygen therapy for interstitial lung disease: a systematic review. Eur Respir Rev 2017;26(143) [pii:160080].

168. Page DB, Thannickal VJ. Ambulatory oxygen and quality of life in interstitial lung disease. Lancet Respir Med 2018;6(10):730–1.

169. Ryerson CJ, Camp PG, Eves ND, et al. High oxygen delivery to preserve exercise capacity in patients with idiopathic pulmonary fibrosis treated with nintedanib. Methodology of the HOPE-IPF study. Ann Am Thorac Soc 2016; 13(9):1640–7.

170. Morisset J, Ryerson CJ, Johannson KA. Oxygen prescription in interstitial lung disease: 2.5 billion years in the making. Ann Am Thorac Soc 2017; 14(12):1755–6.

171. Swigris JJ. Supplemental oxygen for patients with interstitial lung disease: managing expectations. Ann Am Thorac Soc 2017;14(6):831–2.

172. Ramadurai D, Riordan M, Graney B, et al. The impact of carrying supplemental oxygen on exercise capacity and dyspnea in patients with interstitial lung disease. Respir Med 2018;138:32–7.

173. Jacobs SS, Lederer DJ, Garvey CM, et al. Optimizing home oxygen therapy. An official American Thoracic Society workshop report. Ann Am Thorac Soc 2018;15(12):1369–81.

174. Holland AE, Dowman LM, Hill CJ. Principles of rehabilitation and reactivation: interstitial lung disease, sarcoidosis and rheumatoid disease with respiratory involvement. Respiration 2015;89(2): 89–99.

175. Lindell KO, Collins EG, Catanzarite L, et al. Equipment, access and worry about running short of oxygen: key concerns in the ATS patient supplemental oxygen survey. Heart Lung 2019; 48(3):245–9.

176. Fischer A, Antoniou KM, Brown KK, et al. An official European Respiratory Society/American Thoracic Society research statement: interstitial pneumonia with autoimmune features. Eur Respir J 2015; 46(4):976–87.

177. Dowman LM, McDonald CF, Hill CJ, et al. The evidence of benefits of exercise training in interstitial lung disease: a randomised controlled trial. Thorax 2017;72(7):610–9.

178. Sciriha A, Lungaro-Mifsud S, Fsadni P, et al. Pulmonary rehabilitation in patients with interstitial lung disease: the effects of a 12-week programme. Respir Med 2019;146:49–56.

179. Perez-Bogerd S, Wuyts W, Barbier V, et al. Short and long-term effects of pulmonary rehabilitation in interstitial lung diseases: a randomised controlled trial. Respir Res 2018;19(1):182.

180. Deniz S, Sahin H, Yalniz E. Does the severity of interstitial lung disease affect the gains from pulmonary rehabilitation? Clin Respir J 2018;12(6): 2141–50.

181. Rochester CL, Vogiatzis I, Powell P, et al. Patients' perspective on pulmonary rehabilitation: experiences of European and American individuals with chronic respiratory diseases. ERJ Open Res 2018;4(4) [pii:00085-2018].

182. Braga BP, Prieto-Gonzalez S, Hernandez-Rodriguez J. Pneumocystis jirovecii pneumonia prophylaxis in immunocompromised patients with systemic autoimmune diseases. Med Clin (Barc) 2019;152(12):502–7.

183. Ognibene FP, Shelhamer JH, Hoffman GS, et al. Pneumocystis carinii pneumonia: a major complication of immunosuppressive therapy in patients with Wegener's granulomatosis. Am J Respir Crit Care Med 1995;151(3 Pt 1):795–9.

184. Rizzoli R. Bone: towards a better management of glucocorticoid-induced osteoporosis? Nat Rev Rheumatol 2017;13(11):635–6.

185. Buckley L, Guyatt G, Fink HA, et al. 2017 American College of Rheumatology guideline for the prevention and treatment of glucocorticoid-induced osteoporosis. Arthritis Care Res (Hoboken) 2017; 69(8):1095–110.

186. Rizzoli R, Biver E. Glucocorticoid-induced osteoporosis: who to treat with what agent? Nat Rev Rheumatol 2015;11(2):98–109.

187. Lin D, Kramer JR, Ramsey D, et al. Oral bisphosphonates and the risk of Barrett's esophagus: case-control analysis of US veterans. Am J Gastroenterol 2013;108(10):1576–83.

188. Rubin LG, Levin MJ, Ljungman P, et al. 2013 IDSA clinical practice guideline for vaccination of the immunocompromised host. Clin Infect Dis 2014; 58(3):309–18.

189. Simonneau G, Montani D, Celermajer DS, et al. Haemodynamic definitions and updated clinical

classification of pulmonary hypertension. Eur Respir J 2019;53(1) [pii:1801913].

190. Allanore Y, Meune C, Vonk MC, et al. Prevalence and factors associated with left ventricular dysfunction in the EULAR Scleroderma Trial and Research group (EUSTAR) database of patients with systemic sclerosis. Ann Rheum Dis 2010; 69(1):218–21.

191. Young A, Vummidi D, Visovatti S, et al. Prevalence, treatment and outcomes of coexistent pulmonary hypertension and interstitial lung disease in systemic sclerosis. Arthritis Rheumatol 2019. [Epub ahead of print].

192. Young A, Nagaraja V, Basilious M, et al. Update of screening and diagnostic modalities for connective tissue disease-associated pulmonary arterial hypertension. Semin Arthritis Rheum 2019;48(6): 1059–67.

193. Margaritopoulos GA, Antoniou KM, Wells AU. Comorbidities in interstitial lung diseases. Eur Respir Rev 2017;26(143) [pii:160027].

194. Strek ME. Systemic sclerosis-associated interstitial lung disease: role of the oesophagus in outcomes. Respirology 2018;23(10):885–6.

195. Denaxas K, Ladas SD, Karamanolis GP. Evaluation and management of esophageal manifestations in systemic sclerosis. Ann Gastroenterol 2018;31(2): 165–70.

196. Khanna NN, Jamthikar AD, Gupta D, et al. Rheumatoid arthritis: atherosclerosis imaging and cardiovascular risk assessment using machine and deep learning-based tissue characterization. Curr Atheroscler Rep 2019;21(2):7.

197. Ozen G, Inanc N, Unal AU, et al. Subclinical atherosclerosis in systemic sclerosis: not less frequent than rheumatoid arthritis and not detected with cardiovascular risk indices. Arthritis Care Res (Hoboken) 2016;68(10):1538–46.

198. Tektonidou MG, Kravvariti E, Konstantonis G, et al. Subclinical atherosclerosis in systemic lupus erythematosus: comparable risk with diabetes mellitus and rheumatoid arthritis. Autoimmun Rev 2017; 16(3):308–12.

199. Naccache JM, Gibiot Q, Monnet I, et al. Lung cancer and interstitial lung disease: a literature review. J Thorac Dis 2018;10(6):3829–44.

200. Troy LK, Young IH, Lau EMT, et al. Nocturnal hypoxaemia is associated with adverse outcomes in interstitial lung disease. Respirology 2019. [Epub ahead of print].

201. Ungprasert P, Srivali N, Kittanamongkolchai W. Risk of venous thromboembolism in patients with

Sjogren's syndrome: a systematic review and meta-analysis. Clin Exp Rheumatol 2015;33(5): 746–50.

202. Ungprasert P, Srivali N, Kittanamongkolchai W. Systemic sclerosis and risk of venous thromboembolism: a systematic review and meta-analysis. Mod Rheumatol 2015;25(6):893–7.

203. Yusuf HR, Hooper WC, Grosse SD, et al. Risk of venous thromboembolism occurrence among adults with selected autoimmune diseases: a study among a U.S. cohort of commercial insurance enrollees. Thromb Res 2015;135(1):50–7.

204. Carvajalino S, Reigada C, Johnson MJ, et al. Symptom prevalence of patients with fibrotic interstitial lung disease: a systematic literature review. BMC Pulm Med 2018;18(1):78.

205. Kreuter M, Bendstrup E, Russell AM, et al. Palliative care in interstitial lung disease: living well. Lancet Respir Med 2017;5(12):968–80.

206. Bajwah S, Koffman J, Higginson IJ, et al. 'I wish I knew more …' the end-of-life planning and information needs for end-stage fibrotic interstitial lung disease: views of patients, carers and health professionals. BMJ Support Palliat Care 2013; 3(1):84–90.

207. Lindell KO, Nouraie M, Klesen MJ, et al. Randomised clinical trial of an early palliative care intervention (SUPPORT) for patients with idiopathic pulmonary fibrosis (IPF) and their caregivers: protocol and key design considerations. BMJ Open Respir Res 2018;5(1):e000272.

208. Bajwah S, Davies JM, Tanash H, et al. Safety of benzodiazepines and opioids in interstitial lung disease: a national prospective study. Eur Respir J 2018;52(6) [pii:1801278].

209. Matsuda Y, Morita T, Miyaji T, et al. Morphine for refractory dyspnea in interstitial lung disease: a phase I study (JORTC-PAL 05). J Palliat Med 2018. [Epub ahead of print].

210. Mintz S, Lee JK. Gabapentin in the treatment of intractable idiopathic chronic cough: case reports. Am J Med 2006;119(5):e13–5.

211. Lindell KO, Kavalieratos D, Gibson KF, et al. The palliative care needs of patients with idiopathic pulmonary fibrosis: a qualitative study of patients and family caregivers. Heart Lung 2017;46(1):24–9.

212. Barratt SL, Morales M, Spiers T, et al. Specialist palliative care, psychology, interstitial lung disease (ILD) multidisciplinary team meeting: a novel model to address palliative care needs. BMJ Open Respir Res 2018;5(1):e000360.

Lung Transplant in Patients with Connective Tissue Diseases

Tanmay S. Panchabhai, MD[a,b,*], Hesham A. Abdelrazek, MD[a,b],
Ross M. Bremner, MD, PhD[b,c]

KEYWORDS

- Scleroderma • Connective tissue disease • Lung transplant • Lung allocation score
- Esophageal dysmotility • Gastroesophageal reflux after lung transplant

KEY POINTS

- Lung transplant can be considered for patients with connective tissue diseases with extensive pulmonary involvement (parenchymal or pulmonary vascular) that progress despite immunosuppressive therapy.
- Reports from high-volume transplant centers suggest similar 1-year, 3-year, and 5-year survival in patients with connective tissue diseases (especially scleroderma) compared with patients diagnosed with other common indications, such as idiopathic pulmonary fibrosis and chronic obstructive pulmonary disease, with the caveat that these patients with connective tissue diseases are carefully selected for transplant.
- Management of gastroesophageal reflux and esophageal dysmotility before and after lung transplant in patients with connective tissue disease requires a multidisciplinary approach that often involves proton pump inhibitors, nasojejunal tube feeding to minimize aspiration risk, elevation of the head to 45°, and antireflux procedures such as fundoplication and Roux-en-Y esophagojejunostomy.
- Increased anti–human leukocyte antigen antibody levels (measured as calculated panel-reactive antibodies) have been thought to be more prevalent in patients diagnosed with connective tissue disease, although this has not been consistently reflected in single-center reports (perhaps because of a selection bias). Increased panel-reactive antibody levels in this patient group can narrow the potential donor pool and prolong waitlist time. Early referral to lung transplant programs is recommended.

INTRODUCTION

Lung transplant has become an accepted treatment modality for patients diagnosed with end-stage lung disease refractory to medical treatment or that progresses despite maximal medical therapy.[1] An overview of the history of lung transplant is shown in **Fig. 1**.[2] A major milestone in the evolution of lung transplant was the introduction of the lung allocation score (LAS) in 2005, which has changed the way donor lungs are allocated in the United States.[2] The LAS measures clinical acuity

Disclosure: The authors have nothing to disclose.
[a] Lung Transplant Program, John and Doris Norton Thoracic Institute, St. Joseph's Hospital and Medical Center, 500 West Thomas Road, Suite 500, Phoenix, AZ 85013, USA; [b] Creighton University School of Medicine (Phoenix Campus), Omaha, NE, USA; [c] Thoracic Diseases and Transplantation, John and Doris Norton Thoracic Institute, Norton Thoracic Institute, St. Joseph's Hospital and Medical Center, 500 West Thomas Road, Suite 500, Phoenix, AZ 85013, USA
* Corresponding author. Lung Transplant Program, John and Doris Norton Thoracic Institute, St. Joseph's Hospital and Medical Center, 500 West Thomas Road, Suite 500, Phoenix, AZ 85013.
E-mail address: tspanchabhai@gmail.com

Clin Chest Med 40 (2019) 637–654
https://doi.org/10.1016/j.ccm.2019.05.009

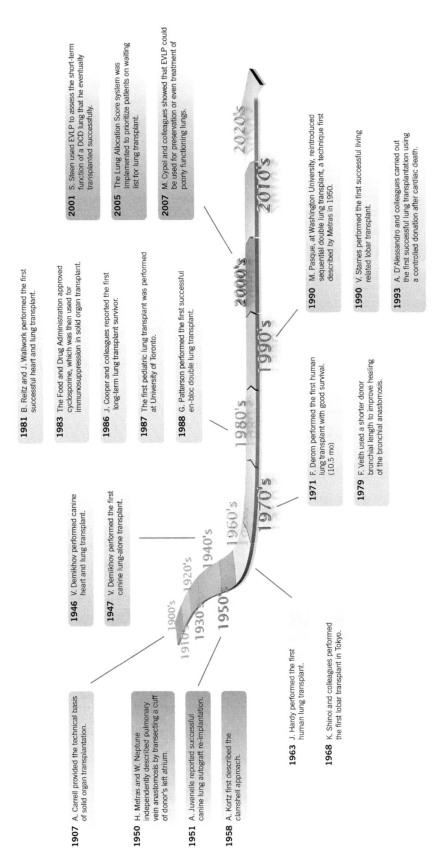

Fig. 1. History of lung transplant. (*Courtesy of Norton Thoracic Institute, Phoenix, Arizona.*)

on a scale of 1 to 100, using a complex algorithm that accounts for medical urgency (ie, waitlist mortality or predicted survival without transplant) and net transplant benefit (ie, predicted survival with or without transplant).[3,4] A significant effect of the LAS is that the proportion of patients undergoing transplant for interstitial lung disease (ILD), especially idiopathic pulmonary fibrosis (IPF), has increased compared with the number undergoing transplant for chronic obstructive pulmonary disease (COPD), which was the predominant indication for lung transplant in the pre-LAS era.[5,6] The most common indications for lung transplant include IPF, COPD, cystic fibrosis (CF), and pulmonary hypertension (PH). A much smaller proportion of patients undergo lung transplant for other rare lung diseases, such as pulmonary involvement from connective tissue diseases (CTDs) such as ILD and PH, lymphangioleiomyomatosis, sarcoidosis, non-CF bronchiectasis, and redo lung transplant.[5,7]

Pulmonary involvement with either ILD or PH remains a significant cause of morbidity and mortality in patients with CTDs.[8] Patients may be evaluated for lung transplant for CTD with pulmonary involvement refractory to conventional medical therapy or that progresses despite conventional medical therapy. No separate guidelines exist for referral and listing of patients with CTDs for lung transplant. At present, guidelines published by the International Society for Heart and Lung Transplantation (ISHLT) that specify criteria for referral and listing for IPF and PH are extrapolated to patients with CTDs, depending on the predominant pulmonary involvement (ie, ILD or PH).[2,4] This article outlines the specific challenges of evaluating patients with CTDs for lung transplant, and describes practices in high-volume lung transplant centers for pretransplant and posttransplant management of lung transplant candidates with CTDs.

This article classifies CTDs into the following groups:

A. Pulmonary involvement from scleroderma (SSc)
   1. SSc-related ILD
   2. SSc-related pulmonary arterial hypertension
B. Pulmonary involvement (ILD and PH) from non-SSc CTDs
   1. Rheumatoid arthritis (RA)
   2. Dermatomyositis and polymyositis (DM/PM)
   3. Sjögren syndrome (SJS)
   4. Systemic lupus erythematosus (SLE)
   5. Mixed connective tissue disease (MCTD)
   6. Overlap syndromes
   7. Interstitial pneumonia with autoimmune features/lung-dominant CTD/autoimmune-featured ILD

INDICATIONS FOR LUNG TRANSPLANT

Of the 55,795 lung transplants performed in the United States through June 2015, only 0.7% were performed for patients with pulmonary involvement from CTDs.[7]

Scleroderma

SSc is a chronic autoimmune disease characterized by vasculopathy of the small vessels and fibrosis of the skin and internal organs. SSc-ILD affects nearly 40% of patients diagnosed with SSc.[9] Radiographic abnormalities are seen in almost 90% of patients with SSc, whereas physiologic abnormalities occur in around 60% of patients.[8,10] The predominant pattern in most patients with SSc-ILD is that of nonspecific interstitial pneumonia (NSIP) (**Fig. 2**), although a usual interstitial pneumonia (UIP) pattern can also be seen. Other forms of pulmonary involvement in SSc that are not indications for lung transplant (but their evaluation during lung transplant assessment is critical) include constrictive bronchiolitis, pleural effusions, neuromuscular findings (including diaphragmatic weakness), and aspiration-related lung injury.[11]

Pulmonary Involvement (Interstitial Lung Disease and Pulmonary Hypertension) from Nonscleroderma Connective Tissue Diseases

ILD is the most common pulmonary manifestation in patients with RA, and it is the only CTD in which UIP-patterned involvement is more common than NSIP.[11] Lung involvement in the form of pleural effusions is the most common manifestation of pleurisy, although lupus pneumonitis with diffuse alveolar hemorrhage can progress to fibrotic lung disease. ILD patterns such as UIP, NSIP, and organizing pneumonia have been described in SLE, but are uncommon. Restrictive lung disease from shrinking lung syndrome (thought to result from diaphragmatic inflammation) needs to be excluded during pretransplant testing.[12] Along with restrictive lung involvement from ILD (UIP, NSIP), lung involvement in SJS is also characterized by constrictive bronchiolitis (obstructive pattern on pulmonary function tests) and lymphocytic interstitial pneumonia.[11,13] NSIP is the more common form of progressive lung disease, and it eventually leads to lung transplant referral in patients with mixed CTD as well as DM/PM, although all pathologic patterns have been reported. The classic antisynthetase syndrome often presents with rapidly progressing respiratory failure caused by ILD in the setting of inflammatory myositis, and many cases of emergent listing and successful

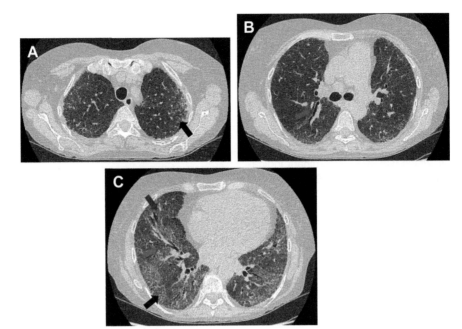

Fig. 2. Computed tomogram of the chest in a patient undergoing lung transplant evaluation for SSc-ILD showing a nonspecific interstitial pneumonia pattern with reticulation (*black arrows* [*A,C*]), traction bronchiectasis (*red arrows* [*B, C*]), and ground-glass opacities (*purple arrow* [*C*]).

lung transplant have been reported (**Fig. 3**).[14,15] However, it is common for patients to present for lung transplant evaluation without one or more of the following: a clear CTD phenotype, an overlapping phenotype, or the more recently described entity of interstitial pneumonia with autoimmune features (or lung-dominant CTD or autoimmune-featured ILD).

FEATURES OF CONNECTIVE TISSUE DISEASES THAT MAY COMPLICATE LUNG TRANSPLANT OUTCOMES

Although no specific guidelines exist for pre–lung transplant evaluation of patients with CTDs, the following clinical features are commonly associated with CTDs and should be carefully evaluated before lung transplant, because they can affect lung transplant outcomes:

1. Dysfunction of the gastrointestinal tract
   a. Gastroesophageal reflux disease (GERD) (both gastroesophageal and esophagoesophageal reflux)
   b. Esophageal dysmotility
   c. Delayed gastric emptying
   d. Small intestinal bacterial overgrowth
   e. Malabsorption syndromes
2. Renal dysfunction
   a. History of SSc renal crisis
   b. Chronic kidney disease associated with prior immunosuppression

3. Cardiac dysfunction
   a. Left ventricular dysfunction (myocardial involvement)
   b. Diastolic dysfunction
4. Neuromuscular involvement
   a. Active myositis
   b. Diaphragmatic involvement
5. Vascular involvement
   a. Raynaud phenomenon
   b. Antiphospholipid antibody syndrome
6. Anti–human leukocyte antigen (HLA) antibodies

These challenges are covered in greater detail later, in relation to the referral, evaluation, listing, surgical procedure, and postoperative management of patients undergoing lung transplant.

PRETRANSPLANT CONSIDERATIONS
Referral for Lung Transplant

Criteria set forth by ISHLT for referring patients with CTD-ILD are the same as those for patients with IPF (and other non–CTD-ILDs) (**Box 1**). Similarly, criteria for referring patients with CTD-PH and those with non–CTD-PH are the same (see **Box 1**).[16] In patients with ILD, histologic or radiographic evidence of UIP or NSIP; abnormal lung function (forced vital capacity <80% or diffusing capacity for carbon monoxide <40%); dyspnea or functional limitation; any oxygen requirement (even with exertion only); and lack of improvement

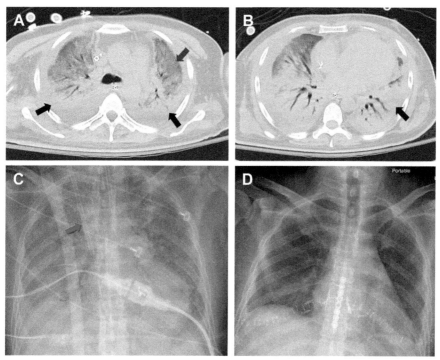

Fig. 3. Rapidly progressive respiratory failure in a patient with Jo-1–positive antisynthetase syndrome. Computed tomogram of the chest (*A, B*) with dense consolidations (*black arrow*) and ground-glass opacities (*purple arrow*) consistent with ILD flare-up. (*C*) Chest radiograph of the same patient when placed on venovenous extracorporeal membrane oxygenation through a single cannula (*red arrow*). (*D*) Chest radiograph of the same patient at day 30 after lung transplant with no parenchymal infiltrates.

in dyspnea, pulmonary function, or supplemental oxygen requirement despite medical therapy should prompt a referral for lung transplant consideration.[16] In patients with PH, New York Heart Association (NYHA) class III or IV symptoms despite escalating vasodilator treatment, rapidly progressive disease, use of parenteral vasodilator therapy, or known or suspected pulmonary venoocclusive disease or pulmonary capillary hemangiomatosis should prompt a referral for lung transplant consideration.[16] At our center, we recommend early referral, because other conditions (eg, concurrent GERD or increased antibody levels that might limit the potential donor pool) are likely to complicate listing, although no specific guidelines dictate which factors should indicate a need for early referral. Close multidisciplinary management involving the pulmonologists, rheumatologists, and the lung transplant team is essential to ensure appropriate medical optimization (eg, nutrition, rehabilitation, immunosuppression).

Lung Transplant Evaluation

Because of the systemic nature of CTDs, lung transplant evaluation focuses on ensuring that there is minimal or no evidence of nonpulmonary organ involvement that may limit survival posttransplant. This evaluation requires a multidisciplinary team to uphold the following general criteria:

1. Greater than 50% risk of death within 2 years from lung disease, if lung transplant is not offered
2. Greater than 80% likelihood of survival 90 days after lung transplant
3. Greater than 80% chance of 5-year survival after lung transplant, assuming stable allograft function[16]

A detailed history and physical examination in patients with CTDs is required to look for skin ulcers, calcinosis, and evidence of peripheral neuropathy and/or autonomic dysfunction (common in patients with SSc).[17] History of orthopnea should be explored to assess any diaphragmatic dysfunction. Issues that need to be discussed in detail include history of SSc renal crisis (although this is rare), history of symptomatic GERD, use of aspiration precautions (especially in patients with SSc), history and severity of episodes of Raynaud phenomenon, history of malignancies (especially

---

Box 1
Criteria for referral for lung transplant evaluation

ILD

- Evidence of UIP or nonspecific interstitial pneumonia (histologic or radiographic)
- Forced vital capacity less than 80% or diffusing capacity for carbon monoxide less than less than 40%
- Dyspnea or functional limitation
- Any oxygen requirement
- Failure to improve (dyspnea, pulmonary function, or oxygen requirement) despite therapy

PH

- New York Heart Association (NYHA) class III or IV symptoms despite vasodilator therapy
- Rapidly progressive disease
- Use of parenteral vasodilator therapy
- Known or suspected pulmonary venoocclusive disease or pulmonary capillary hemangiomatosis

Adapted from Weill D, Benden C, Corris PA, et al. A consensus document for the selection of lung transplant candidates: 2014–an update from the pulmonary transplantation council of the international society for heart and lung transplantation. J Heart Lung Transplant 2015;34(1):1–15.

---

in patients with DM/PM), and history of venous thromboembolism (particularly in patients with SLE). **Box 2** provides a detailed list of testing performed at most lung transplant centers; other evaluations may be omitted or performed after transplant, depending on disease severity. Tests to evaluate organ system dysfunction in patients with CTDs that may not be otherwise indicated are detailed in **Box 3**.

Box 2
Lung transplant evaluation

Consultations

- Transplant pulmonologist
- Transplant surgeon
- Transplant psychiatrist
- Social worker
- Financial adviser
- Physical therapist
- Pharmacist
- Nutritionist

Laboratory testing

- Complete blood count
- Complete metabolic profile
- Coagulation profile
- Creatinine clearance
- Serology (human immunodeficiency virus [HIV], hepatitis B, hepatitis C, cytomegalovirus, Epstein-Barr virus, toxoplasmosis, syphilis)
- Urine drug screen
- Vaccination history/titers
- Panel-reactive antibodies

Physiologic testing

- Spirometry, lung volumes, diffusion capacity
- Arterial blood gas
- Six-minute walk test

Imaging

- Computed tomogram of the chest
- Ventilation-perfusion scan
- SNIFF test
- Carotid Doppler test
- Femoral ultrasonography

Cardiac testing

- Left heart catheterization
- Right heart catheterization
- Two-dimensional echocardiogram

Age-related and sex-related screening

- Mammogram
- Papanicolaou test
- Colonoscopy
- Dual energy x-ray absorptiometry scan for osteoporosis

Gastroesophageal reflux testing

- Esophagogastroduodenoscopy
- Manometry
- pH probe
- Esophagram
- Gastric emptying study

The ISHLT has specified both absolute (**Box 4**) and relative (**Box 5**) contraindications for lung transplant.[16] Patients with many of the relative contraindications (see **Box 5**) can still be considered at experienced lung transplant centers on a case-by-case basis. For example, patients with

Box 3
Additional testing for patients with connective tissue diseases

- Upper gastrointestinal barium swallow (if patient has a history of swallowing problems)
- Transesophageal echocardiogram
  - To evaluate cardiac function in patients with CTDs, especially SSc
- Cardiac MRI
  - To evaluate cardiac involvement patients with in CTDs, especially SSc
- Laboratory testing
  - CTD serology tests, including myositis panel (especially in patients without a clearly established diagnosis)
  - RNA polymerase III testing (because of higher risk of SSc renal crisis)
  - Myositis markers, such as creatinine phosphokinase and aldolase
- Assessment of diaphragmatic function
  - Sitting-supine spirometry
  - Maximal inspiratory pressure
  - Maximal expiratory pressure
  - Diaphragmatic ultrasonography/electromyography

Box 4
Absolute contraindications to lung transplant

- Recent history of malignancy
  - Two-year disease-free survival for nonmelanoma skin cancer
  - Five-year disease-free survival for other solid organ tumors
- Untreatable dysfunction of another major organ system (heart, kidney, liver, or brain)
- Acute medical instability
- Uncorrectable bleeding diathesis
- Chronic infection with highly virulent or resistant microorganisms
- Infection with *Mycobacterium tuberculosis*
- Chest wall or spinal deformity
- Class II or III obesity (ie, body mass index $\geq$35 kg/m^2)
- Chronic nonadherence to medical therapy
- Psychiatric or psychological conditions resulting in inability to cooperate with medical care
- Poor rehabilitation potential
- Ongoing substance abuse

Adapted from Weill D, Benden C, Corris PA, et al. A consensus document for the selection of lung transplant candidates: 2014–an update from the pulmonary transplantation council of the international society for heart and lung transplantation. J Heart Lung Transplant 2015;34(1):1–15.

hepatitis B or C without evidence of cirrhosis or portal hypertension and who are stable on medical therapy (or treated completely) can be considered for lung transplant. Although the details of program-specific considerations with regard to relative contraindications are beyond the scope of this article, patients diagnosed with CTDs who also have GERD and increased panel-reactive antibody (PRA) levels are increasingly being considered for lung transplant on a case-by-case basis at experienced centers. The diagnosis and management of GERD is the major challenge in treating patients with CTDs, especially SSc. This approach is detailed later.

Listing for Lung Transplant

Criteria for listing
There are no disease-specific criteria for listing patients with CTDs for lung transplant. The ISHLT criteria used for listing patients with ILD and PH are the same as those used for listing patients with CTDs (**Box 6**). Timing of listing depends on the assessment of natural history of disease, the likelihood of complications affecting survival, and ISHLT guidelines.

Timing of listing
It is the responsibility of the lung transplant team to determine each patient's disease stability. Patients with CTDs may show clinical stability despite meeting only several criteria recommended by ISHLT. In such cases, close multidisciplinary monitoring is recommended to ensure that the patient is listed while in the lung transplant "window." If the patient is clinically stable for more than 1 year, most transplant programs require updated testing at the time of listing (especially cardiac work-up with heart catheterization, echocardiograms, and so forth), depending on each individual scenario.

Anti–human leukocyte antigen antibodies and desensitization
Patients with CTDs frequently have increased HLA class I and class II antibody levels.[18] Determining single HLA antibody specificity allows a calculated PRA value from which the donor pool can be estimated. Depending on the percentage of PRAs present, a significant number of donor organs may be

Box 5
Relative contraindications to lung transplant
• Advanced age (determined by individual transplant program)
• Class I obesity (body mass index 30–34.9 kg/m²), particularly truncal obesity
• Severe malnutrition
• Severe symptomatic osteoporosis
• Prior extensive chest surgery
• Mechanical ventilation or extracorporeal life support
• Colonization with highly resistant or virulent bacteria
• Infection with hepatitis B or C
• Infection with HIV
• Infection with *Burkholderia cenocepacia*, *Burkholderia gladiola*, or multidrug-resistant *Mycobacterium abscessus*
• Coronary artery disease not amenable to pretransplant percutaneous coronary intervention or coronary artery bypass graft surgery
• Medical conditions that cannot be optimally treated (eg, diabetes mellitus, hypertension, gastroesophageal reflux disease, peptic ulcer disease, central venous obstruction)
Adapted from Weill D, Benden C, Corris PA, et al. A consensus document for the selection of lung transplant candidates: 2014–an update from the pulmonary transplantation council of the international society for heart and lung transplantation. J Heart Lung Transplant 2015;34(1):1–15.

Box 6
Listing criteria for lung transplant
ILD
• Decline in forced vital capacity greater than or equal to 10% in 6 months
• Decline in diffusing capacity for carbon monoxide greater than or equal to 15% in 6 months
• Desaturation to less than 88%, or 6-minute walking distance less than 250 m, or greater than 50 m decline in 6-minute walking distance in 6 months
• Evidence of PH on right heart catheterization or echocardiogram
• Hospitalization caused by declining pulmonary status, pneumothorax, or exacerbation of ILD
PH
• NYHA class III or IV symptoms despite a minimum of 3-month trial of combination therapy, including prostanoids
• Cardiac index less than 2 L/min/m²
• Mean right atrial pressure greater than 15 mm Hg
• Six-min walking distance less than 250 m
• Development of hemoptysis, pericardial effusion, or signs of right heart failure
Adapted from Weill D, Benden C, Corris PA, et al. A consensus document for the selection of lung transplant candidates: 2014–an update from the pulmonary transplantation council of the international society for heart and lung transplantation. J Heart Lung Transplant 2015;34(1):1–15.

unusable for patients listed for lung transplant for CTDs. Waitlist times for such individuals may be longer than center-specific waitlist times for age-matched, sex-matched, and disease-matched candidates. Anti-HLA antibodies against donor antigens can predispose recipients to hyperacute rejection, acute cellular rejection, and chronic rejection of the allograft.[19–21]

Depending on the level of PRAs, some HLA antigens in the donor pool need to be avoided in order to prevent hyperacute rejection and other complications that have been listed earlier. A prospective crossmatch, in which donor and recipient blood samples are tested for cross reactivity before the organ is procured and implanted, is sometimes required. Multidisciplinary management involving an immunologist is key in determining which HLA antigens need to be avoided and which are related to background activity. If a prospective crossmatch is deemed necessary, donor blood is stored at a regional HLA laboratory in the donor catchment area for the transplant center. As mentioned earlier, the presence of increased PRA levels can significantly prolong waitlist time for patients with CTDs.

Desensitization is an approach to suppress and remove anti-HLA antibodies in sensitized lung transplant candidates; the goal of desensitization is to broaden the donor pool. Several approaches for desensitization are used at experienced centers across the United States (**Box 7**). Desensitization outcomes have been mixed in terms of overall survival compared with outcomes in unsensitized patients or sensitized patients who did not undergo desensitization,[22,23] and center-specific experience plays a major role in decision making about whether to pursue desensitization.

SURGICAL PROCEDURE CONSIDERATIONS

Most patients diagnosed with CTDs (especially SSc-ILD) are young and have some degree of

Box 7
Approaches used for desensitization

Antibodies

- Alemtuzumab (monoclonal)
- Eculizumab (monoclonal)
- Rituximab (monoclonal)
- Antithymocyte globulin (polyclonal)
- Intravenous immunoglobulin (polyclonal)

Drugs

- Bortezomib
- Cyclophosphamide

Procedures

- Plasma exchange
- Splenectomy

PH. The outcomes of bilateral sequential lung transplant have been better than outcomes after single-lung transplant, especially in patients with PH (**Fig. 4**).[24] An important consideration is that the waitlist time for patients with increased PRA levels may be longer than those of recipients without increased PRA levels. Patients with normal pulmonary pressures at initial evaluation may have PH that has worsened by the time of transplant. In patients with SSc, the left ventricular involvement is evaluated with heart catheterization (left and right) and cardiac MRI in select patients. Diastolic dysfunction in such patients is often underestimated because of concurrent right ventricular dysfunction. Although diastolic dysfunction is not a contraindication to lung transplant, it can be associated with challenges postoperatively.

Extracorporeal support is being increasingly used in the management of lung transplant recipients. Extracorporeal membrane oxygenation (ECMO) can be either used via a venovenous route (mainly for oxygenation; **Fig. 5**) or a venoarterial method (mainly for cardiac support). At high-volume lung transplant centers, outcomes of patients who received ECMO as a bridge therapy to lung transplant had comparable survival and functional status at 1 year posttransplant.[25,26] ECMO as bridge to transplant needs to be carefully evaluated as an option in patients with CTDs with high PRA levels because of the likely long waitlist time. Rapid progressive respiratory failure in patients with antisynthetase syndrome has been successfully managed with ECMO as a bridge to lung transplant (see **Fig. 3**).[14,15] Intraoperative ECMO (with either central or peripheral cannulation) is considered when patients have severe PH and need significant hemodynamic support. Vasopressors should be judiciously monitored if they are used, especially in patients with history of Raynaud phenomenon, and radial arterial lines should be avoided. In patients with severe PH with right ventricular dysfunction, use of extended awake postoperative venoarterial ECMO (with groin cannulation) has shown benefit in decreasing postoperative mortality and favors better cardiac function.[27] Other approaches that have been used in patients diagnosed with CTDs (mainly SSc) and Raynaud phenomenon include sympathectomy at the time of transplant (for patients with Raynaud phenomenon) and intraoperative plasma exchange for patients with a very high PRA burden.

POSTTRANSPLANT MANAGEMENT OF PATIENTS DIAGNOSED WITH CONNECTIVE TISSUE DISEASES
Management of Gastroesophageal Reflux Disease

The risks of aspiration and GERD have been associated with poor outcomes after lung transplant, mainly as they relate to chronic lung allograft dysfunction (CLAD).[28,29] The prevalence of GERD in patients with end-stage lung disease who undergo evaluation for lung transplant can be as high as 50%.[28,30] The presence of a patulous esophagus or air fluid level on chest computed tomography can suggest poor esophageal peristalsis on initial evaluation.[31] At our institution, a detailed evaluation of GERD (whether symptomatic or asymptomatic) during transplant evaluation

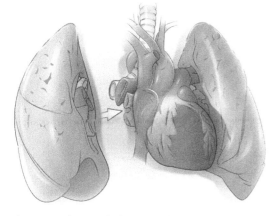

Fig. 4. Fundamental elements of lung transplant procedure that involves surgical anastomosis of the donor bronchus, pulmonary artery, and pulmonary veins respectively to the recipient bronchus, pulmonary artery, and pulmonary veins. (*Courtesy of* Norton Thoracic Institute, Phoenix, Arizona.)

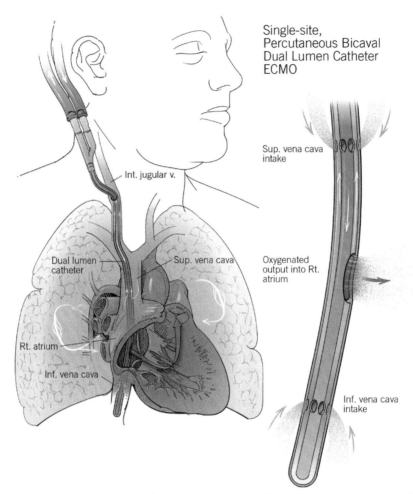

Single-site,
Percutaneous Bicaval
Dual Lumen Catheter
ECMO

Int. jugular v.

Sup. vena cava
intake

Dual lumen
catheter

Sup. vena cava

Oxygenated
output into Rt.
atrium

Rt. atrium

Inf. vena cava

Inf. vena cava
intake

Fig. 5. Venovenous extracorporeal membrane oxygenation can be used to augment oxygenation in patients for whom other respiratory assistance strategies fail, and can be used to bridge patients to transplant. This figure shows a cannulation strategy in which blood is removed from the superior (Sup.) vena cava and inferior (Inf.) vena cava, is oxygenated, and is returned to the right (Rt.) atrium directed to the right ventricle. Int., internal; v., vein. (*Courtesy of* Norton Thoracic Institute, Phoenix, Arizona.)

includes ambulatory 24-hour pH monitoring, a barium esophagram, manometry, and esophago-gastroduodenoscopy with biopsies to assess for changes suggestive of Barrett esophagus or high-grade dysplasia.

Ambulatory pH testing is performed after patients have ceased taking antireflux medications for at least 10 days. For this testing, a standard catheter-based dual-electrode probe is used. Normal values for acid contact times in the distal probe are total greater than 4.2%, upright less than 6.3%, and supine less than 1.2%. All studies are interpreted after clinical correlation by a thoracic surgeon. The DeMeester score is then calculated using standard variables (reference score <14.72). The overall GERD evaluation is examined at length during lung transplant selection committee meetings, at which time the

care team discusses all patients being considered for lung transplant. The esophagram and manometry data are used to assess the motility of the esophagus and to determine whether esophageal reflux is present. If Barrett esophagus is diagnosed on esophageal biopsies, our protocol is surveillance esophagogastroduodenoscopy every 2 years, because of the risk of transformation to high-grade dysplasia and esophageal adenocarcinoma.[32]

The effects of GERD in patients with CTDs who have undergone lung transplant has resulted in the adoption of a conservative approach when considering transplant candidacy at many institutions. However, data from experienced, large-volume centers indicate that lung transplant can be performed in patients with CTDs and GERD with outcomes comparable with those of patients who are not diagnosed with CTD or GERD (discussed later). However, this group of patients is likely carefully selected, because patients with end-stage SSc with extensive esophageal involvement represent the highest-risk subset for severe GERD, stricture, and aspiration. The authors have recently shown that a dilated aperistaltic esophagus is unlikely to improve after transplant, and that these patients are at greater risk of aspiration than a matched cohort.[33]

The principles of GERD management in patients with CTDs who are being evaluated for lung transplant remain similar, although the specifics may vary depending on the individual experience of each lung transplant program. The authors think it is important to perform complete foregut testing both before and after transplant. Management strategies may include:

1. Objective GERD should be treated with aggressive medical management with proton pump inhibitors beginning in the pretransplant stage and continued posttransplant.
2. Conservative measures, including head of bed elevation to 45° in the pretransplant stage.
3. In patients with GERD in which the natural history indicates slower progression, an antireflux procedure can be considered in the pre–lung transplant period. The authors prefer to perform a partial fundoplication, understanding that disease progression may be associated with deterioration in esophageal peristalsis.
4. In patients with GERD and abnormal esophageal motility (typical for patients with SSc with so-called aperistaltic esophagus; **Fig. 6**), our

recommendation is to consider placing a gastrojejunostomy tube and initiating jejunal feedings to avoid the risk of aspiration and allograft dysfunction after lung transplant. The timing of gastrojejunostomy tube placement depends on the severity of pulmonary disease; however, in most instances it is placed posttransplant to avoid pretransplant complications. These patients cannot have any oral intake via the mouth for 3 months posttransplant. However, in most cases we let them have pleasure feeds in the morning and afternoon only, depending on their posttransplant progress. Patients are then assessed for changes in esophageal motility in the posttransplant period by foregut testing.
5. Patients deemed high risk based on pretransplant GERD evaluation are required to undergo early GERD testing posttransplant. Based on the results of this testing, a decision is made regarding the need for antireflux procedure. Decision making for antireflux procedures is discussed later.

Ineffective esophageal motility is common in patients with CTDs. For this reason, the authors prefer to perform a partial fundoplication such as a Toupet procedure for patients who require surgery (**Fig. 7**). We are reluctant to perform even a 270° fundoplication in patients with complete aperistalsis because of the risk of esophageal outlet obstruction. We consider a hiatal hernia repair (if a hernia is present) and an anterior fundoplication in this situation, but with the knowledge that these patients may still have some reflux postprocedure.

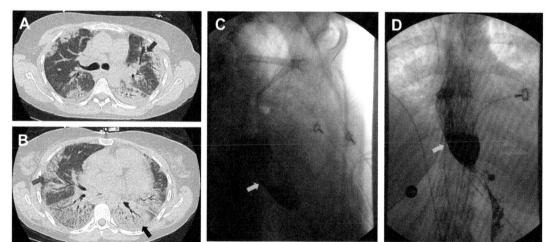

Fig. 6. Computed tomogram of the chest (*A, B*) in a patient undergoing lung transplant evaluation for flare-up of SSc-ILD showing a nonspecific interstitial pneumonia pattern with reticulation (*red arrow*), traction bronchiectasis (*purple arrow*), and dense consolidation (*black arrow*). (*C, D*) An esophagram of the same patient with poor esophageal motility (*yellow arrow*). The patient was ultimately diagnosed with aperistaltic esophagus and managed with jejunal feeds (postpyloric) posttransplant.

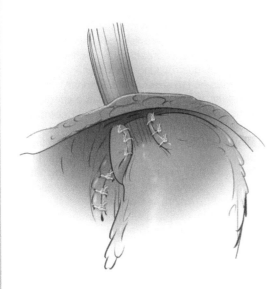

270 ° Toupet

Fig. 7. Toupet fundoplication involves an approximately 270° fundoplication thought to provide less of an outflow obstruction to the esophagus in patients who have ineffective esophageal motility. (*Courtesy of* Norton Thoracic Institute, Phoenix, Arizona.)

Another option for patients with severe reflux and a dilated esophagus is a Roux-en-Y esophagojejunostomy. In this situation, the alimentary limb should not measure more than 60 cm in length, because of the implications of immunosuppressive drug absorption. This procedure is much more invasive than a fundoplication, and it can have a dramatic physiologic impact on the patient, so its use should be carefully considered. Nonetheless, it is the ultimate antireflux procedure, because it eliminates continuity between the acid and reservoir function of the stomach and the esophagus. Esophageal dysmotility remains, but gastroesophageal reflux is no longer a problem.[34]

Survival and Outcomes

Because of the smaller proportion of patients who undergo lung transplant for CTD compared with other lung diseases (eg, IPF, CF, COPD),[18] studies of recipients with CTDs are largely limited to case series and single-center or multicenter experiences. Because the overall number of lung transplants performed every year is increasing, the clinical experience in management of patients with CTDs (pretransplant and posttransplant) is also increasing.[2] Within CTDs, SSc-related ILD and PH have been more extensively studied than non-SSc CTDs, possibly because of their low prevalence and/or better response to conventional

immunosuppressive therapy. **Table 1** summarizes various studies that compared outcomes of patients with CTDs after lung transplant. Although other case series or case reports have been published,[14,15,35–37] studies of outcomes are mainly included in this table.

Scleroderma
Over the past 2 decades, 11 studies have described institutional or multicenter outcomes after lung transplant in patients with SSc (see **Table 1**).[31,38–47] Issues surrounding GERD have been studied in detail only in a few studies.[31,40,43] Short-term and long-term survival (1-year, 3-year, and 5-year survival) in patients with SSc (ie, ILD, ILD-PH, or PH) seem to be comparable with those of lung transplant recipients for non-SSc-ILD, PH, or COPD (see **Table 1**).[31,38–47] The overall prevalence of GERD and esophageal dysmotility was higher in patients with SSc than in control groups, but this did not seem to affect clinical outcomes (eg, mortality and freedom from bronchiolitis obliterans syndrome). There was only 1 study in which posttransplant survival in patients with CTDs (mainly SSc) was lower than in patients with COPD after 5 years and lower than in patients with IPF at 1 year.[47] With the exception of this study, no difference in survival between SSc and non-SSc lung diseases was observed. Other clinical outcomes, such as the incidence of primary graft dysfunction, number of days on mechanical ventilation, number of hospitalizations, incidence of acute cellular rejection, and freedom from bronchiolitis obliterans syndrome have also been reported as comparable between patients with SSc and non-SSc lung disease across multiple studies (see **Table 1**).[31,38–47] Autoantibodies and anti-HLA antibodies are thought to be more prevalent in patients with CTDs. Although few studies have explored this in detail, the number of patients with increased PRA levels was similar in SSc and non-SSc groups in 2 studies.[39,42]

Nonscleroderma connective tissue diseases
Fewer reports have studied patients with non-SSc CTDs (see **Table 1**),[48–50] although individual case reports have described successful outcomes.[14,15,36] One-year, 3-year, and 5-year survival in patients with non-SSc CTDs is similar to survival in patients with IPF or non-CTD ILDs. Neither autoimmunity nor GERD has been evaluated in detail in these studies, and the number of patients in the CTD group was consistently small.[48,50] Posttransplant complications caused by the native CTD were infrequently reported.

Table 1
Outcomes of patients with connective tissue diseases after lung transplant

Study Type Time Period	Number of Patients	GERD	Increased PRAs	Survival	Freedom from BOS
SSc					
Massad et al,[42] 2005 UNOS database, multicenter 1987–2004	47 pts with SSc vs 10,117 pts with other lung diseases	NR	4.3% in SSc vs 4.5% in others (PRA>10%)	1 y 68% (SSc). 756% (control) 3 y 45% (SSc) 59% (control)	1 y 89% (SSc) 91 (control)
Schachna et al,[45] 2006 Two centers 1989–2002	29 pts with SSc vs 70 pts with IPF vs 38 pts with IPAH	NR	NR	2 y 61% (SSc) 64% (IPF) 63% (IPAH)	NR
Saggar et al,[44] 2010 Single center 2003–2007	15 pts with SSc vs 38 pts with IPF	DS = 42 (SSc)	NR	1 y 93% (SSc) 87% (IPF)	1 y 70% (SSc) 80% (IPF) 3 y 52% (SSc) 60% (IPF)
Takagishi et al,[47] 2012 UNOS database, multicenter 1991–2009	284 pts with CTD vs 9720 pts with COPD vs 4190 pts with IPF Distribution within the pts with CTDs: SSc (61.2%), RA (12.7%), DM/PM (12.0%), MCTD (7.7%), SLE (4%), and SJS (2.5%)	NR	NR	1 y 73% (CTD) 83% (COPD)[a] 78% (IPF)[b] 3 y 59% (CTD) 65% (COPD)[b] 61% (IPF) 5 y 46% (CTD) 50% (COPD)[b] 47% (IPF)	NR

(continued on next page)

Table 1
(continued)

Study Type Time Period	Number of Patients	GERD	Increased PRAs	Survival	Freedom from BOS
Sottile et al,[46] 2013 Single center 1998–2010	23 pts with SSc vs 46 pts with ILD	DS 65 (SSc) 31 (ILD)	NR	1 y 83% (SSc) 91% (ILD) 3 y 83% (SSc) 77% (ILD) 5 y 76% (SSc) 64% (ILD)	1 y 100% (SSc) 98% (ILD) 3 y 74% (SSc) 77% (ILD) 5 y 74% (SSc) 69% (ILD)
Bernstein et al,[38] 2015 UNOS database, multicenter 2005–2012	229 pts with SSc vs 201 pts with PAH vs 3333 pts with ILD	NR	NR	1 y 81% (SSc) 84% (PAH) 84 (ILD) 3 y 72% (SSc) 68% (PAH) 70% (ILD)	NR
Miele et al,[31] 2016 Single center 2000–2012	35 pts with SSc vs 264 pts with fibrotic ILD vs 527 non-SSc	Severe esophageal dysfunction[c] 54% (SSc) 8% (matched cohort ILD)[d]	NR	1 y 94% (SSc) 88% (ILD) 84% (non-SSc) 3 y 70% (SSc) 54% (ILD) 49% (non-SSc) 5 y 70% (SSc) 54% (ILD) 49% (non-SSc)	3 y 71% (SSc) 62% (ILD) 59% (non-SSc) 5 y 56% (SSc) 47% (ILD) 49% (non-SSc)
Crespo et al,[40] 2016 Single center 2005–2013	72 pts with SSc vs 311 pts with ILD (pulmonary fibrosis)	Moderate to severe esophageal dysmotility	NR	1 y 81% (SSc) 79% (ILD)	1 y 81% (SSc) 76% (ILD)

		60% (SSc) 20% (ILD)[e]		3 y 54% (SSc) 53% (ILD) 5 y 21% (SSc) 26% (ILD)	3 y 72% (SSc)[f] 55% (ILD) 5 y 49% (SSc)[f] 38% (ILD)
Chan et al,[39] 2018 Single center 2008–2014	26 pts with SSc vs 155 pts with restrictive lung disease (ILD)	NR	Class I >20% 12% (SSc) 9% (ILD) Class II >20% 12% (SSc) 14% (ILD)	1 y 73% (SSc) 80% (ILD) 3 y 69% (SSc) 70% (ILD) 5 y 65% (SSc) 67% (ILD)	NR
Gadre et al,[41] 2017 Single center 1992–2013	9 pts with SSc-PAH vs 42 pts with non-SSc-PAH	NR	NR	1 y 100% (SSc-PAH) 87% (non-SSc-PAH) 2 y 71% (SSc-PAH) 76% (non-SSc-PAH) 5 y 14% (SSc-PAH) 47% (non-SSc-PAH)[g]	NR
Pradère et al,[43] 2018 Multicenter 1993–2016	40 pts with SSc-PH-ILD vs 30 pts with SSc-ILD vs 20 pts with SSc-PAH	Severe GERD 4% (SSc-ILD-PH) 7% (SSc-ILD) 5% (SSc-PAH) Aperistaltic esophagus 17% (SSc-ILD-PH) 18% (SSc-ILD) 0% (SSc-PAH)	NR	1 y 79% (SSc-ILD-PH) 75% (SSc-ILD) 71% (SSc-PAH) 3 y 93% (SSc-ILD-PH) 76% (SSc-ILD) 60% (SSc-PAH) 5 y 70% (SSc-ILD-PH) 50% (SSc-ILD) 43% (SSc-PAH)	NS

(continued on next page)

Table 1
(continued)

Study Type Time Period	Number of Patients	GERD	Increased PRAs	Survival	Freedom from BOS
Non-SSc CTDs					
Ameye et al,[48] 2014 Single center 2004–2013	5 pts with DM/PM vs 49 pts with IPF vs 37 pts with non-IPF non-IIM ILD	NR	NR	1 y 100% (DM/PM) 86% (IPF) 86% (ILD) 5 y 75% (DM/PM) 58% (IPF) 57% (ILD)	NR
Yazdani et al,[50] 2014 Single center 1989–2011	10 pts with RA-ILD vs 53 pts with IPF vs 17 pts with SSc-ILD	NR	NR	1 y 67% (RA-ILD) 69% (IPF) 82% (SSc-ILD)	NR
Courtwright et al,[49] 2017 SRTR, multicenter 2005–2016	275 pts with non–SSC-ILD vs 6346 pts with IPF	NR	NS	NS	NS

Abbreviations: BOS, bronchiolitis obliterans syndrome (now grouped under CLAD); DS, DeMeester score; IPAH, idiopathic pulmonary arterial hypertension; NR, not reported; NS, nonsignificant; PAH, pulmonary arterial hypertension; pts, patients; UNOS, United Network for organ sharing.

[a] $P<.001$ versus CTD.

[b] $P<.05$ versus CTD.

[c] Severe esophageal dysfunction was defined as either aperistalsis by manometry or the combination of maximum esophageal diameter on computed tomography chest greater than 20 mm and air fluid level.

[d] $P<.001$ versus control.

[e] $P<.001$ versus control.

[f] $P<.05$ versus ILD.

[g] No statistically significant difference, but 5-year survival is numerically much less in SSc–pulmonary arterial hypertension group and the lack of statistical significance may be caused by the small sample size.

SUMMARY

Lung transplant for CTDs (both SSc and non-SSc) is feasible, with posttransplant survival similar to outcomes in patients with IPF or COPD. However, this historical cohort of patients with CTDs was likely carefully selected for transplant and may represent a selection bias. The low overall prevalence of this disease pool makes it more challenging to study their outcomes. Further studies should focus on management of GERD and the levels of PRAs in detail to determine how these should be incorporated in selection algorithms of lung transplant programs.

ACKNOWLEDGMENTS

The authors wish to express their gratitude to Clare Sonntag, for providing editorial expertise, and to Marco Marchionni, for the original artwork that accompanies this article.

REFERENCES

1. Kotloff RM, Thabut G. Lung transplantation. Am J Respir Crit Care Med 2011;184(2):159–71.

2. Panchabhai TS, Chaddha U, McCurry KR, et al. Historical perspectives of lung transplantation: connecting the dots. J Thorac Dis 2018;10(7):4516–31.

3. Egan TM, Murray S, Bustami RT, et al. Development of the new lung allocation system in the United States. Am J Transplant 2006;6(5 Pt 2):1212–27.

4. Tsuang WM. Contemporary issues in lung transplant allocation practices. Curr Transplant Rep 2017;4(3): 238–42.

5. Egan TM, Edwards LB. Effect of the lung allocation score on lung transplantation in the United States. J Heart Lung Transplant 2016;35(4):433–9.

6. Panchabhai TS, Arrossi AV, Highland KB, et al. A single-institution study of concordance of pathological diagnoses for interstitial lung diseases between pre-transplantation surgical lung biopsies and lung explants. BMC Pulm Med 2019; 19(1):20.

7. Yusen RD, Edwards LB, Dipchand AI, et al. The registry of the international society for heart and lung transplantation: thirty-third adult lung and heart-lung transplant report-2016; focus theme: primary diagnostic indications for transplant. J Heart Lung Transplant 2016;35(10):1170–84.

8. Jablonski R, Dematte J, Bhorade S. Lung transplantation in scleroderma: recent advances and lessons. Curr Opin Rheumatol 2018;30(6):562–9.

9. Highland KB, Garin MC, Brown KK. The spectrum of scleroderma lung disease. Semin Respir Crit Care Med 2007;28(4):418–29.

10. Solomon JJ, Olson AL, Fischer A, et al. Scleroderma lung disease. Eur Respir Rev 2013;22(127):6–19.

11. Mira-Avendano I, Abril A, Burger CD, et al. Interstitial lung disease and other pulmonary manifestations in connective tissue diseases. Mayo Clin Proc 2019; 94(2):309–25.

12. Panchabhai TS, Bandyopadhyay D, Highland KB, et al. A 26-year-old woman with systemic lupus erythematosus presenting with orthopnea and restrictive lung impairment. Chest 2016;149(1):e29–33.

13. Panchabhai TS, Farver C, Highland KB. Lymphocytic interstitial pneumonia. Clin Chest Med 2016; 37(3):463–74.

14. Broome M, Palmer K, Schersten H, et al. Prolonged extracorporeal membrane oxygenation and circulatory support as bridge to lung transplant. Ann Thorac Surg 2008;86(4):1357–60.

15. Delplanque M, Gatfosse M, Ait-Oufella H, et al. Bilung transplantation in anti-synthetase syndrome with life-threatening interstitial lung disease. Rheumatology (Oxford) 2018;57(9):1688–9.

16. Weill D, Benden C, Corris PA, et al. A consensus document for the selection of lung transplant candidates: 2014–an update from the pulmonary transplantation council of the international society for heart and lung transplantation. J Heart Lung Transplant 2015;34(1):1–15.

17. Amaral TN, Peres FA, Lapa AT, et al. Neurologic involvement in scleroderma: a systematic review. Semin Arthritis Rheum 2013;43(3):335–47.

18. Lee JC, Ahya VN. Lung transplantation in autoimmune diseases. Clin Chest Med 2010;31(3): 589–603.

19. Dragun D. Humoral responses directed against non-human leukocyte antigens in solid-organ transplantation. Transplantation 2008;86(8):1019–25.

20. Hadjiliadis D, Chaparro C, Reinsmoen NL, et al. Pre-transplant panel reactive antibody in lung transplant recipients is associated with significantly worse post-transplant survival in a multicenter study. J Heart Lung Transplant 2005;24(7 Suppl):S249–54.

21. Lau CL, Palmer SM, Posther KE, et al. Influence of panel-reactive antibodies on posttransplant outcomes in lung transplant recipients. Ann Thorac Surg 2000;69(5):1520–4.

22. Snyder LD, Gray AL, Reynolds JM, et al. Antibody desensitization therapy in highly sensitized lung transplant candidates. Am J Transplant 2014;14(4): 849–56.

23. Tinckam KJ, Keshavjee S, Chaparro C, et al. Survival in sensitized lung transplant recipients with perioperative desensitization. Am J Transplant 2015;15(2):417–26.

24. Bando K, Armitage JM, Paradis IL, et al. Indications for and results of single, bilateral, and heart-lung transplantation for pulmonary hypertension. J Thorac Cardiovasc Surg 1994;108(6):1056–65.

25. Biscotti M, Gannon WD, Agerstrand C, et al. Awake extracorporeal membrane oxygenation as bridge to

lung transplantation: a 9-year experience. Ann Thorac Surg 2017;104(2):412–9.

26. Todd EM, Biswas Roy S, Hashimi AS, et al. Extracorporeal membrane oxygenation as a bridge to lung transplantation: a single-center experience in the present era. J Thorac Cardiovasc Surg 2017; 154(5):1798–809.

27. Salman J, Ius F, Sommer W, et al. Mid-term results of bilateral lung transplant with postoperatively extended intraoperative extracorporeal membrane oxygenation for severe pulmonary hypertension. Eur J Cardiothorac Surg 2017;52(1):163–70.

28. Biswas Roy S, Elnahas S, Serrone R, et al. Early fundoplication is associated with slower decline in lung function after lung transplantation in patients with gastroesophageal reflux disease. J Thorac Cardiovasc Surg 2018;155(6):2762–71.e1.

29. Murthy SC, Nowicki ER, Mason DP, et al. Pretransplant gastroesophageal reflux compromises early outcomes after lung transplantation. J Thorac Cardiovasc Surg 2011;142(1):47–52.e3.

30. D'Ovidio F, Singer LG, Hadjiliadis D, et al. Prevalence of gastroesophageal reflux in end-stage lung disease candidates for lung transplant. Ann Thorac Surg 2005;80(4):1254–60.

31. Miele CH, Schwab K, Saggar R, et al. Lung transplant outcomes in systemic sclerosis with significant esophageal dysfunction. A comprehensive single-center experience. Ann Am Thorac Soc 2016; 13(6):793–802.

32. Biswas Roy S, Banks P, Kunz M, et al. Prevalence and natural history of Barrett's esophagus in lung transplant: a single-center experience. Ann Thorac Surg 2019;107(4):1017–23.

33. Masuda T, Mittal SK, Kovacs B, et al. Esophageal aperistalsis and lung transplant: recovery of peristalsis after transplant is associated with improved long-term outcomes. Western Thoracic Surgical Association Annual Meeting, Olympic Valley, California, June 26-29, 2019.

34. Kent MS, Luketich JD, Irshad K, et al. Comparison of surgical approaches to recalcitrant gastroesophageal reflux disease in the patient with scleroderma. Ann Thorac Surg 2007;84(5):1710–5 [discussion: 1715–6].

35. Gasper WJ, Sweet MP, Golden JA, et al. Lung transplantation in patients with connective tissue disorders and esophageal dysmotility. Dis Esophagus 2008;21(7):650–5.

36. Kim J, Kim YW, Lee SM, et al. Successful lung transplantation in a patient with dermatomyositis and acute form of interstitial pneumonitis. Clin Exp Rheumatol 2009;27(1):168–9.

37. Shitrit D, Amital A, Peled N, et al. Lung transplantation in patients with scleroderma: case series, review of the literature, and criteria for transplantation. Clin Transplant 2009;23(2):178–83.

38. Bernstein EJ, Peterson ER, Sell JL, et al. Survival of adults with systemic sclerosis following lung transplantation: a nationwide cohort study. Arthritis Rheumatol 2015;67(5):1314–22.

39. Chan EY, Goodarzi A, Sinha N, et al. Long-term survival in bilateral lung transplantation for scleroderma-related lung disease. Ann Thorac Surg 2018;105(3):893–900.

40. Crespo MM, Bermudez CA, Dew MA, et al. Lung transplant in patients with scleroderma compared with pulmonary fibrosis. Short- and long-term outcomes. Ann Am Thorac Soc 2016;13(6):784–92.

41. Gadre SK, Minai OA, Wang XF, et al. Lung or heart-lung transplant in pulmonary arterial hypertension: what is the impact of systemic sclerosis? Exp Clin Transplant 2017;15(6):676–84.

42. Massad MG, Powell CR, Kpodonu J, et al. Outcomes of lung transplantation in patients with scleroderma. World J Surg 2005;29(11):1510–5.

43. Pradère P, Tudorache I, Magnusson J, et al. Lung transplantation for scleroderma lung disease: an international, multicenter, observational cohort study. J Heart Lung Transplant 2018;37(7):903–11.

44. Saggar R, Khanna D, Furst DE, et al. Systemic sclerosis and bilateral lung transplantation: a single centre experience. Eur Respir J 2010;36(4): 893–900.

45. Schachna L, Medsger TA Jr, Dauber JH, et al. Lung transplantation in scleroderma compared with idiopathic pulmonary fibrosis and idiopathic pulmonary arterial hypertension. Arthritis Rheum 2006;54(12): 3954–61.

46. Sottile PD, Iturbe D, Katsumoto TR, et al. Outcomes in systemic sclerosis-related lung disease after lung transplantation. Transplantation 2013;95(7):975–80.

47. Takagishi T, Ostrowski R, Alex C, et al. Survival and extrapulmonary course of connective tissue disease after lung transplantation. J Clin Rheumatol 2012; 18(6):283–9.

48. Ameye H, Ruttens D, Benveniste O, et al. Is lung transplantation a valuable therapeutic option for patients with pulmonary polymyositis? Experiences from the Leuven transplant cohort. Transplant Proc 2014;46(9):3147–53.

49. Courtwright AM, El-Chemaly S, Dellaripa PF, et al. Survival and outcomes after lung transplantation for non-scleroderma connective tissue-related interstitial lung disease. J Heart Lung Transplant 2017;36(7):763–9.

50. Yazdani A, Singer LG, Strand V, et al. Survival and quality of life in rheumatoid arthritis-associated interstitial lung disease after lung transplantation. J Heart Lung Transplant 2014;33(5):514–20.

Imaging of the Thoracic Manifestations of Connective Tissue Disease

Brett M. Elicker, MD*, Kimberly G. Kallianos, MD, Travis S. Henry, MD

KEYWORDS

- Diffuse lung disease • Connective tissue disease • Interstitial pneumonia with autoimmune features
- Computed tomography • Nonspecific interstitial pneumonia • Organizing pneumonia
- Lymphoid interstitial pneumonia

KEY POINTS

- The primary role of imaging in patients with connective tissue disease (CTD)-related diffuse lung disease is to determine the pattern of injury present.
- Imaging plays a limited role in the diagnosis of CTD, except in cases in which the lung disease is the primary presenting feature. These cases are termed interstitial pneumonia with autoimmune features.
- Although CTD can present with any pattern of injury, the computed tomography (CT) patterns most closely associated with CTD include nonspecific interstitial pneumonia (NSIP), organizing pneumonia, and lymphoid interstitial pneumonia.
- Subpleural sparing is the most specific CT sign of nonspecific interstitial pneumonia.
- Usual interstitial pneumonia is most commonly due to idiopathic pulmonary fibrosis; however, when seen in the setting of CTD it is most closely associated with rheumatoid arthritis.

INTRODUCTION

Diffuse lung disease (DLD) is an important cause of pulmonary symptoms and is associated with significant morbidity and mortality. The most common causes of DLD include idiopathic disorders, exposures, and connective tissue diseases (CTDs). Distinguishing these various etiologies is critical in directing a patient's treatment and determining prognosis. Diagnosis, treatment, and follow-up of patients with DLD are performed using a multidisciplinary approach that incorporates clinical information, radiologic findings, and pathologic data. Each of these brings unique information to the table, and diagnosis is most accurate when at least 2, but often 3, are integrated.

CTD is one of the most common etiologies of DLD and should always be investigated as a potential etiology. In one institution's cohort, 30% of patients presenting with DLD met the criteria for CTD, and a subset of 15% were newly diagnosed with CTD as a consequence of their DLD diagnosis.[1] Given their systemic nature, diagnosis in CTD differs somewhat from other causes of DLD given the reliance on clinical symptoms, physical examination findings, and serologic data. Radiology, and specifically high-resolution chest computed tomography (HRCT), provides a global anatomic visualization of lung anatomy

Disclosures: None.
Department of Radiology and Biomedical Imaging, University of California San Francisco, 505 Parnassus Avenue, Box 0628, San Francisco, CA 94143, USA
* Corresponding author.
E-mail address: brett.elicker@ucsf.edu

Clin Chest Med 40 (2019) 655–666
https://doi.org/10.1016/j.ccm.2019.05.010

and provides unique information not found in the clinical presentation or pathologic findings. The goal of this article was to provide an overview of the use of HRCT in patients with suspected or known lung disease related to CTD and to delineate the key roles of HRCT in these patients. The extrapulmonary manifestations of CTD are also discussed, as they often represent important additional clues to diagnosis.

GENERAL IMAGING CONSIDERATIONS

Chest radiographs have a limited role in the evaluation of DLD. Although they are often the first diagnostic imaging test obtained in patients with pulmonary symptoms, they demonstrate limited sensitivity and specificity for CTD-related lung disease.[2] Chest radiographs may be obtained in patients with acute symptoms in search for pneumonia, pulmonary edema, or other acute processes. It is important to note that in the setting of preexisting DLD, acute chest radiographic abnormalities may be difficult to interpret, and thus HRCT is the imaging test of choice in most patients.

HRCT is highly sensitive for most manifestations of CTD and may detect early abnormalities before pulmonary function tests (PFTs) become abnormal. In a study of 11 children with scleroderma, 91% had interstitial lung disease on HRCT, and of those patients, 78% had normal PFTs.[3] Although treatment may be withheld in those with early manifestations, the presence of DLD necessitates close follow-up to monitor for progression over time.

CTDs may result in a variety of different manifestations within the chest, including interstitial lung disease, airways diseases, vascular manifestations, and serositis. It is important to note that the patterns of DLD seen in CTD and its treatment show significant overlap with other etiologies of DLD, particularly idiopathic disorders, thus a multidisciplinary approach incorporating all available data allows for the highest accuracy in diagnosis. The specific roles of HRCT in the diagnosis and management of CTD are discussed as follows. A summary of the key roles of imaging is also presented in **Table 1**.

DIAGNOSIS OF CONNECTIVE TISSUE DISEASE

Diagnosis in CTD is primarily made using clinical and serologic criteria. Imaging and pathology play limited roles in most cases. In addition, lung disease is not part of the diagnostic criteria of any of the CTDs with the exception of scleroderma. There is, however, an increased

recognition of lung disease presenting as one of the initial manifestations of CTD, before the development of other typical clinical features. In one investigation, 19% of patients initially diagnosed with an idiopathic interstitial pneumonia subsequently developed CTD over a mean 3.4-year follow-up period.[3]

Many patients with a combination of DLD and a clinical suspicion for CTD do not meet the strict diagnostic criteria of any specific CTD. This occurrence has been labeled by several names, including undifferentiated CTD, lung dominant CTD, and interstitial pneumonia with autoimmune features (IPAF). In these cases, imaging plays a key role in diagnosis. Diagnostic criteria recently have been developed for IPAF[4] and include having at least 1 positive finding in 2 of the following 3 domains: (1) clinical, (2) serologic, and (3) anatomic, with the anatomic domain including data from either imaging or pathology.

The patterns of lung disease on HRCT that satisfy the anatomic criteria are those that are most closely associated with CTD, including (1) nonspecific interstitial pneumonia (NSIP), (2) organizing pneumonia (OP), (3) NSIP and OP overlap, and (4) lymphoid interstitial pneumonia. When one of these patterns is present, a careful search for clinical and serologic findings to support the diagnosis of CTD should be undertaken. If at least 1 clinical or serologic finding is also present, a diagnosis of IPAF can be made at a minimum. The patterns of lung disease included in the anatomic criteria are those that are most closely associated with CTD; however, it is important to remember that CTD may present with any pattern of lung injury or DLD. For instance, rheumatoid arthritis commonly presents with usual interstitial pneumonia (UIP). On the other hand, UIP is much more likely to be caused by idiopathic pulmonary fibrosis as opposed to CTD, which is why it is not included in the anatomic domain for IPAF.

The anatomic criteria for IPAF also may be met in the presence of multicompartmental disease. Specifically, the presence of any type of DLD in association with unexplained pleural effusion(s) or thickening, pericardial effusion or thickening, airways disease, or pulmonary vasculopathy meets this criterion.

DETERMINING THE PATTERN OF INJURY

Although HRCT does not often contribute to diagnosis in CTD, except in cases of IPAF, its primary role is to define the pattern of lung injury present in known CTD. This is particularly relevant given that pathology is not typically obtained in patients

Table 1
Roles of high-resolution chest computed tomography in the setting of connective tissue disease (CTD)-related diffuse lung disease

Role of Imaging	Notes
Diagnosis of CTD	• Diagnosis usually made by clinical symptoms/signs and serologic markers • Computed tomography (CT) important in diagnosis when lung disease is the primary manifestation of CTD: interstitial pneumonia with autoimmune features (IPAF) • IPAF needs 2 of 3 domains: 1. Clinical 2. Serologic 3. Anatomic • CT patterns in the anatomic domain: 1. Nonspecific interstitial pneumonia (NSIP) 2. Organizing pneumonia (OP) 3. NSIP and OP overlap 4. Lymphoid interstitial pneumonia
Determining the pattern of injury in established CTD	• Pattern of lung injury is important in directing treatment and determining prognosis • Pathology usually not obtained • CTDs can present with any pattern of injury but associations exist • Most common patterns include the following: 1. Scleroderma: NSIP, pulmonary hypertension 2. Rheumatoid: unusual interstitial pneumonia, NSIP 3. Sjögren's syndrome: NSIP, lymphoid interstitial pneumonia, airways disease 4. Myositis: NSIP, OP 5. Systemic lupus erythematosus: serositis, pulmonary hypertension 6. Mixed CTD: NSIP, OP
Follow-up of diffuse lung disease (DLD) over time	• Pulmonary function test (PFTs) are typically used to follow patients over time • CT may be used when PFTs might be inaccurate, including in the setting of the following: 1. Early DLD 2. Multicompartmental disease (interstitial, airways, pleura, and/or vascular disease) 3. Patient unable to cooperate with PFTs
Evaluation of acute symptoms	• Acute symptoms may be due to worsening of the known DLD or a new process • CT is superior to PFTs in distinguishing these etiologies • Helpful findings on CT include the following: 1. Tree-in-bud opacities: highly suggestive of infection or aspiration 2. Small, centrilobular nodules: infection or follicular bronchiolitis 3. Larger nodules: infection, organizing pneumonia, rheumatoid nodules 4. Ground glass opacity and consolidation: these findings are nonspecific
Monitoring for complications of treatment	• Drugs also may cause a variety of different patterns of injury • Pneumotox is an online resource (https://www.pneumotox.com/) that describes the most common patterns of injury associated with each drug • Temporal relationship between the onset of symptoms and starting the medication is important • Immunosuppressive drugs also may predispose to infection

with CTD, thus HRCT provides the only anatomic information. The pattern present has a significant impact on treatment and prognosis. Certain patterns of injury, such as organizing pneumonia (OP), are expected to be highly responsive to immunosuppressive therapy with improvement or resolution of symptoms and radiologic abnormalities. Other patterns of injury, such as UIP, are characterized by irreversible fibrosis that is unresponsive to most treatments.

Determining the pattern of injury on HRCT involves 3 steps: (1) identifying the predominant finding, (2) assessing the distribution of findings in the axial and craniocaudal plane, and (3) evaluating for the presence of other associated findings that may increase specificity for the main pattern.

A list of the most common patterns of injury in CTD and their HRCT findings is shown in **Table 2**. In some cases, HRCT may have a high specificity for the pattern of injury, whereas in others the HRCT findings may be relatively nonspecific. The imaging findings of the most common CTDs are detailed below, each of which is paired with a pattern of injury that is most closely tied to that specific CTD. Keep in mind that each CTD may manifest with one of several different patterns, and the archetypal pattern with which they are associated is not always the most common manifestation.

Scleroderma and Nonspecific Interstitial Pneumonia

Lung disease has a higher prevalence in scleroderma compared with other CTDs, seen in more than 70% of patients on autopsy.[5] DLD and pulmonary hypertension, the 2 most common patterns of lung disease in scleroderma, account for

Table 2
Patterns of injury in connective tissue disease (CTD) and their high-resolution computed tomography (HRCT) findings

Pattern of Injury	HRCT Findings	Most Common CTD(s) with Which It Is Associated
Nonspecific interstitial pneumonia (NSIP)	• Ground glass opacity • Irregular reticulation • Traction bronchiectasis • Honeycombing (usually absent or limited in distribution) • Distribution: basilar predominant • Subpleural sparing (most specific finding)	• Common with all CTDs except systemic lupus erythematosus
Usual interstitial pneumonia (UIP)	• Irregular reticulation • Traction bronchiectasis • Honeycombing • Distribution: basilar and subpleural • Absence of findings atypical for UIP, including ground glass opacity, consolidation, mosaic perfusion, air trapping, nodules, cysts, subpleural sparing	• Rheumatoid arthritis
Follicular bronchiolitis (FB)	• Small nodules: ground glass attenuation, centrilobular distribution • Findings overlap with lymphoid interstitial pneumonia (see next section)	• Sjögren's syndrome • Rheumatoid arthritis
Lymphoid interstitial pneumonia	• Ground glass opacity • Consolidation • Cysts (most suggestive) • Findings overlap with FB (see preceding section)	• Sjögren's syndrome • Rheumatoid arthritis
Organizing pneumonia	• Consolidation: often rounded with irregular margins • Distribution: peribronchovascular and subpleural • Often present in association with NSIP	• Myositis
Diffuse alveolar damage	• Ground glass opacity • Consolidation • Distribution: bilateral, extensive or diffuse	• Systemic lupus erythematosus • Myositis
Constrictive bronchiolitis	• Geographic areas of lucent lung (mosaic perfusion) • Air trapping on expiratory computed tomography • Bronchiectasis	• Rheumatoid arthritis • Sjögren's syndrome

approximately 60% of scleroderma-related deaths.[6] In a study of the patterns of interstitial lung disease in scleroderma, 64% had NSIP and 36% had UIP.[7]

NSIP is the most common pattern of injury seen in CTD. Other diseases that may result in an NSIP pattern include drug toxicity, hypersensitivity pneumonitis, and idiopathic NSIP. There are 3 forms of NSIP: cellular, fibrotic, or mixed. The typical finding of cellular NSIP is ground glass opacity, whereas fibrotic NSIP demonstrates reticulation and traction bronchiectasis. These usually demonstrate a basilar predominance. Unfortunately, CT is limited in its ability to predict the predominant form of NSIP, as a significant overlap of findings occurs.[8] Honeycombing is uncommon in NSIP, but when present is typically very limited in extent. The most predictive finding of NSIP is the presence of subpleural sparing (**Fig. 1**) in which the lung directly adjacent to the pleura is not as severely affected compared with the more central lung.[9]

Rheumatoid Arthritis and Usual Interstitial Pneumonia

DLD in rheumatoid arthritis is often asymptomatic. In one study of rheumatoid arthritis, HRCT abnormalities were present in 27% of patients but only 10% of those had pulmonary symptoms.[10] The presence of symptomatic DLD, however, is associated with significant mortality. Five-year mortality in patients with rheumatoid arthritis with DLD in one cohort was 39% compared with 18% in those without DLD.[11] Rheumatoid arthritis has approximately an equal distribution of UIP and NSIP.[12,13] Airways disease, including bronchiectasis, and OP are less common manifestations of rheumatoid arthritis.[14]

UIP is most commonly seen as a manifestation of idiopathic pulmonary fibrosis (IPF); however, when seen with CTD it is most often associated with rheumatoid arthritis.[12] Although CTD-related UIP has a worse prognosis than NSIP, there have been mixed results when comparing CTD-UIP with IPF.[15,16] The radiologic criteria for UIP were defined around a diagnosis of IPF[17]; however, the criteria are also accurate in distinguishing rheumatoid arthritis–UIP from other patterns of injury.[18] A confident diagnosis of UIP (**Fig. 2**) can be made when the following 4 HRCT criteria are met:

1. Presence of honeycombing
2. Presence of reticulation with or without traction bronchiectasis
3. Subpleural and basilar distribution of findings
4. Lack of features that are atypical for UIP, including ground glass opacity, mosaic perfusion, air trapping, nodules, cysts, consolidation, and subpleural sparing

Sjögren Syndrome, Lymphoid Interstitial Pneumonia and Other Lymphoproliferative Diseases

Lung abnormalities in Sjögren syndrome are seen in approximately 16% of patients. In an investigation of the CT findings of 35 patients with Sjögren syndrome, the most common patterns were airways disease (54% of patients), lung fibrosis (20% patients), and findings suggestive of lymphoid interstitial pneumonia (14% of patients).[19] The most common patterns of DLD in Sjögren's syndrome include NSIP and lymphoid interstitial pneumonia (LIP).[20,21]

Sjögren syndrome may be associated with a variety of non-neoplastic or neoplastic lymphoproliferative diseases. The proliferation of non-neoplastic collections of lymphocytes within the

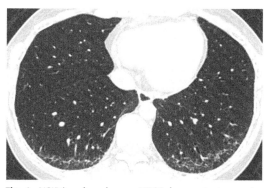

Fig. 1. NSIP in scleroderma. HRCT demonstrates posterior and peripheral interstitial lung disease characterized by irregular reticulation and mild traction bronchiectasis. Note that the disease relatively spares the immediate subpleural lung. This subpleural sparing is highly suggestive of NSIP.

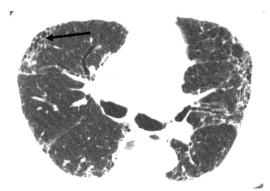

Fig. 2. UIP in rheumatoid arthritis. This HRCT shows a peripheral distribution of fibrosis with honeycombing (*arrow*). No other significant findings, such as nodules, are seen. This combination of findings is compatible with UIP.

lung interstitium is termed follicular bronchiolitis (FB) when the collections are localized around bronchioles or LIP when more diffuse lung involvement is present. FB and LIP are a spectrum of disease, and thus clinical, radiologic, and pathologic overlap is common. These patterns are most commonly seen in association with Sjögren's syndrome, but also may be present in rheumatoid arthritis. The most characteristic HRCT feature of FB is centrilobular nodules, reflecting the bronchiolocentric nature of the disease.[22] A lack of subpleural nodules on HRCT is a characteristic feature of a centrilobular distribution.

LIP, on the other hand, usually shows bilateral ground glass opacity or consolidation, both relatively nonspecific findings. The presence of cysts, often perivascular in distribution, is more suggestive of LIP.[23] These cysts may be seen in isolation or associated with other findings (**Fig. 3**). It is important to note that FB and LIP may be seen in combination with other patterns in CTD, particularly NSIP. FB and LIP also may be secondary to immunosuppressive states (eg, acquired immunodeficiency syndrome and common variable immunodeficiency) or rarely idiopathic. Other pulmonary lymphoproliferative processes in Sjögren syndrome include benign lymphoid hyperplasia and pulmonary lymphoma, which typically present with lymphadenopathy, one or multiple lung nodules, or patchy bilateral consolidation.

Myositis and Organizing Pneumonia

The prevalence of DLD in myositis is variable and ranges from 23% to 78% in different centers.[24,25] Mortality is significantly higher in patients with DLD compared with those without, with a hazard ratio of 2.13.[26] The most common patterns of DLD in patients with myositis includes NSIP, organizing pneumonia, and an overlap of NSIP and OP. In a recent analysis of 33 patients with myositis, these 3 patterns accounted for 90% of cases of DLD.[24] Diffuse alveolar damage also may be seen occasionally in this patient population.[27] It is important to note that respiratory muscle weakness and aspiration events also may contribute to pulmonary symptoms and PFT abnormalities.

OP is an immune reaction characterized pathologically by the formation of plugs of granulation tissue within the respiratory bronchioles and alveolar spaces. It may be seen as an isolated pattern in CTD; however, it more commonly presents in combination with other patterns, particularly NSIP. Polymyositis, dermatomyositis, and the anti-synthetase syndrome are the most common CTDs to present with OP. On HRCT, the most characteristic finding of OP is consolidation. Although consolidation by itself is a nonspecific HRCT finding, it has a characteristic appearance in OP (**Fig. 4**) that includes focal, often rounded, areas of peribronchovascular and subpleural consolidation with irregular borders and associated with architectural distortion.[28] When OP is associated with another pattern of injury, there will be overlap in the HRCT findings. For instance, OP/NSIP (**Fig. 5**) overlap often shows uniform peripheral and basilar consolidation, in contrast to the focal, patchy nature of OP in isolation.[24] After treatment, consolidation typically shows improvement or resolution; however, residual or progressive fibrosis is common and often resembles NSIP.[24] Other potential causes of OP include drugs, toxic inhalations, and cryptogenic OP. OP also may be seen as a minor component of

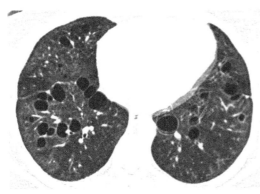

Fig. 3. LIP in Sjögren syndrome. Patchy bilateral ground glass opacity is seen on HRCT. This finding, by itself, is nonspecific, but the presence of associated cysts in this clinical setting is very suggestive of LIP.

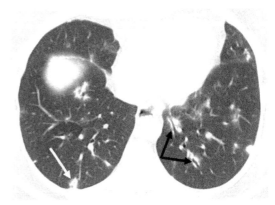

Fig. 4. OP in myositis. Bilateral, rounded areas of consolidation with irregular margins are seen on HRCT. Note the patchy distribution and predominance in the subpleural (*white arrow*) and peribronchovascular (*black arrows*) regions. This constellation is compatible with OP.

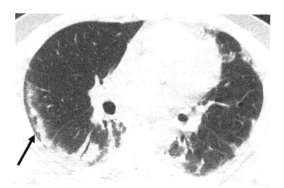

Fig. 5. NSIP and OP overlap in myositis. On this HRCT consolidation is present in a posterior and subpleural distribution. Note the focal areas of subpleural sparing (*arrow*). The distribution and subpleural sparing is compatible with NSIP, and consolidation as the predominant finding is compatible with OP.

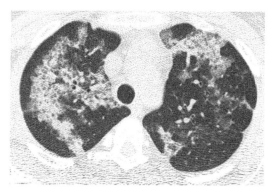

Fig. 6. DAD in SLE. HRCT demonstrates bilateral ground glass opacity and consolidation in a patient with acute symptoms. These findings are nonspecific and the differential diagnosis includes edema, infection, and hemorrhage. DAD was diagnosed on lung biopsy.

another lung disease, such as infection or aspiration.

Systemic Lupus Erythematosus and Diffuse Alveolar Damage

The patterns of lung involvement in systemic lupus erythematosus (SLE) differ compared with other CTDs. Lung fibrosis is rare in SLE, seen in only 4% of patients.[29] More typical findings include serositis and pulmonary hypertension. When lung disease is seen it may represent a chronic fibrotic process, such as NSIP or UIP, or an acute process, such as diffuse alveolar hemorrhage and diffuse alveolar damage. Lupus pneumonitis, a rare complication, likely represents a combination of diffuse alveolar damage and hemorrhage. Chronic airways disease and OP also may be rarely seen.

Diffuse alveolar damage (DAD) in association with CTD may occur as an isolated abnormality or may represent an acute exacerbation of preexisting interstitial lung disease. In a study of 58 consecutive patients with DAD on surgical biopsy, 16% had CTD.[30] DAD may occur as the initial manifestation of CTD, particularly in myositis,[27] or years after a diagnosis of CTD is made. The imaging findings of DAD include bilateral, often symmetric, ground glass opacity and consolidation (**Fig. 6**). These findings are indistinguishable from pulmonary edema, infection (particularly viral infection), diffuse alveolar hemorrhage, and DAD from other causes (eg, sepsis). On serial CT, findings of fibrosis (reticulation and traction bronchiectasis) start to develop within the first 1 to 3 weeks after the onset of symptoms. These findings of fibrosis may persist and worsen over time, particularly in patients with preexisting interstitial lung disease, or may improve over several months.

Mixed Connective Tissue Disease

The HRCT patterns associated with mixed CTD show the most significant overlap with scleroderma and myositis.[31] Thus, the most common patterns include NSIP, OP, and NSIP/OP overlap.

Other Lung Findings

Involvement of the airways is most closely associated with rheumatoid arthritis, Sjögren's syndrome, and SLE. Both the large and the small airways may be involved, and the mechanisms by which airway disease occurs varies. In some cases, constrictive bronchiolitis induces concentric fibrosis within and around bronchiolar walls inducing small airways stenosis. Small airways disease manifests on imaging as geographic areas of mosaic perfusion (lucent lung) due to regional hypoxia and reflex vasoconstriction. Expiratory CT increases the sensitivity for airways disease; however, good quality images are dependent on ideal patient cooperation (**Fig. 7**). Direct injury to the large airways may result in central airway dilation and/or inflammation.

A variety of other, less common patterns may be seen in association with CTD. Diffuse alveolar hemorrhage is most commonly associated with SLE. Pulmonary edema may be associated with a cardiomyopathy from direct insult to the myocardium or due to coronary arterial vasculitis. Scattered cavitary nodules may be seen in rheumatoid arthritis, often subpleural in distribution.

Extrapulmonary Findings

Multicompartmental disease is typical of CTD. Other compartments of the chest that may be involved include the pulmonary vasculature,

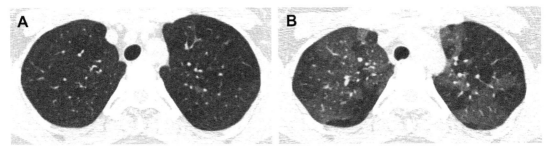

Fig. 7. Airways disease in rheumatoid arthritis. Inspiratory CT (*A*) shows subtle geographic, sharply defined areas of lucent lung reflecting airways obstruction with reflex vasoconstriction. On expiratory CT (*B*) air trapping is present in the lucent lung regions, whereas the normal lung shows an expected, normal increase in attenuation.

pleura, pericardium, and esophagus. The combination of DLD and involvement of one of these other compartments should prompt an investigation into the possibility of an undiagnosed CTD.

Pulmonary hypertension is most commonly associated with scleroderma, specifically its CREST (calcinosis, Raynaud phenomenon, esophageal dysmotility, sclerodactyly, telangiectasias) variant, and SLE. Typical findings of pulmonary hypertension include enlargement of the main pulmonary artery and right ventricle; however, these findings are not consistently present. In a comparison of pulmonary artery size on CT and the presence of pulmonary hypertension on right heart catheterization in patients with scleroderma, a pulmonary artery diameter threshold of greater than 3.0 cm was 81% sensitive and 88% specific.[4] Centrilobular nodules of ground glass attenuation may be seen in association with pulmonary hypertension. These likely represent focal areas of edema or prior hemorrhage (cholesterol granulomas). This finding is not highly specific for pulmonary hypertension, however, as it also may be seen in FB.

Serositis is most commonly associated with SLE. Pleural disease will manifest as effusions, commonly exudative, and/or pleural thickening (**Fig. 8**). Extensive pleural thickening may result in a significant restrictive defect on PFTs. Pericardial effusions or thickening may have physiologic effects on impaired diastolic relaxation of the ventricles resulting in constrictive pericarditis. Esophageal dilation because of impaired contractility is most commonly seen in scleroderma and may be associated with aspiration pneumonitis or pneumonia.

FOLLOW-UP OF LUNG DISEASE OVER TIME

In patients with known DLD, PFTs are the standard modality used in the serial evaluation of the severity of lung disease over time. PFTs may detect significant changes, even in patients with stable symptoms, allowing for the ability to intervene earlier. Although PFTs are sensitive to the serial worsening of DLD, they are not specific as to the etiology, thus CT is often obtained as a complementary modality to distinguish the potential etiologies for these changes.

There are several situations in which PFTs may be less accurate, and thus CT may be superior in the longitudinal evaluation of changes over time. First, CT is often more sensitive for early DLD and may detect significant abnormalities before the development of PFT abnormalities. Significant progression of disease, that was mild to begin with, may go undetected using PFTs. Second, PFTs are limited in their evaluation of multicompartmental disease. For instance, a combination of interstitial and airways disease may give a pseudo-normalization of the lung volumes on PFTs. In addition, a restrictive defect on PFTs may be a result of disease in different compartments: lung, pleura, or musculoskeletal. CT may

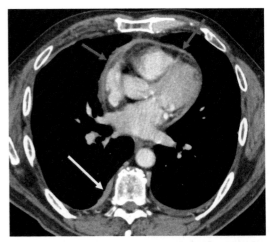

Fig. 8. Serositis in SLE. A combination of right-sided pleural thickening (*yellow arrow*), left-sided pleural effusion, and pericardial thickening (*red arrows*) is compatible with a serositis in a patient with SLE.

be superior, in these situations, in distinguishing the origin of the abnormality and its change in severity over time. Finally, some patients may not be able to cooperate with PFTs.

The expected evolution of DLD over time is dependent on the primary pattern of injury present. Different patterns will demonstrate varying responses to treatment, ranging from complete resolution to continued progression. OP is, arguably, the pattern that is most likely to respond to treatment with a significant improvement in clinical symptoms and CT abnormalities in more than 90% of patients after treatment,[32] although recurrence may occur after treatment. Symptomatic fibrosis after treatment of OP is not common, and when present it often resembles NSIP. LIP and FB are predominantly infiltrative/inflammatory disorders, thus also typically show significant improvement following treatment.

NSIP, the most common pattern associated with CTD, shows different trajectories depending on whether the predominant pathologic findings are cellular or fibrotic. In a longitudinal study of patients with NSIP, 38% demonstrated improvement, 22% demonstrated worsening, and 40% showed no change.[33] Unfortunately, the findings seen on the initial CT are not highly predictive of whether NSIP has potentially reversible changes.[8] The presence of ground glass opacity, typically thought to correspond to more inflammatory changes, in the setting of NSIP not uncommonly represents microscopic fibrosis. UIP is a pattern characterized entirely by fibrosis that will not improve with immunosuppression. However, although not well studied, there is the suggestion that CTD-related UIP may not show the same rate of progression as UIP related to IPF. Airways disease, particularly when due to bronchiolitis obliterans, is not usually a reversible process.

EVALUATION OF ACUTE SYMPTOMS

There are several potential causes of acute or new symptoms in patients with CTD-related DLD. CT is one of the most accurate modalities used to distinguish these various etiologies. The causes may be divided into 2 broad categories: worsening or exacerbation of preexisting lung disease and superimposed processes unrelated to DLD, such as infection.

On pathology, acute exacerbation of DLD is characterized by one or more of the following patterns: (1) progressive fibrosis, (2) DAD, (3) OP. When seen in this context, the findings of DAD and OP (discussed previously) are superimposed on preexisting fibrosis.[34] DAD due to an acute exacerbation typically has a very poor prognosis.

Infection is a common cause of acute symptoms that often has characteristic CT findings that distinguish it from DLD. Tree-in-bud opacities are small, branching, tubular opacities associated with nodules that are highly specific for infection or aspiration (**Fig. 9**). Small (<10 mm), clustered centrilobular nodules also are suggestive of infection, although they may be occasionally associated with FB. Larger nodules are a common feature of infection, particularly fungal and mycobacterial infection, but also may be seen in patients with OP or rheumatoid nodules. Ground glass opacity and consolidation are both nonspecific findings in which the clinical presentation is paramount in formulating a differential diagnosis.

MONITORING FOR COMPLICATIONS OF TREATMENT

The drugs used to treat CTD have potential toxicity in their own right. Similar to CTD-related DLD, each drug can manifest with different patterns of

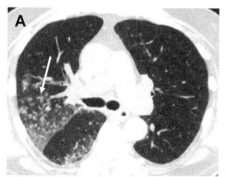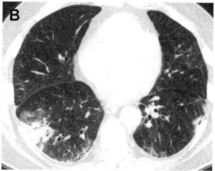

Fig. 9. Infection in rheumatoid arthritis. A patient with rheumatoid arthritis presents with acute symptoms. HRCT through the upper lung (*A*) shows right-sided small clustered nodules with tree-in-bud opacities (*arrow*). An image through the lower lung (*B*) shows rounded areas of consolidation. Although the consolidation has an appearance that resembles OP, the presence of tree-in-bud strongly suggests infection as opposed to CTD-related DLD as a cause of symptoms.

lung injury. Some of these patterns overlap with those of CTD, making diagnosis complicated. Understanding the most common pattern(s) associated with each drug is critical in determining the likelihood of medication-induced lung toxicity. Pneumotox (https://www.pneumotox.com/) is an excellent online resource for the patterns that are most commonly associated with specific drugs. The temporal relationship between starting the medication and the onset of symptoms is also important in determining the likelihood of drug-induced lung disease. Although this temporal relationship demonstrates a wide range, from minutes to years after starting the medication, most patients with drug-induced lung injury develop symptoms weeks to months after the start of the medication. It is important to note that the data on drug-induced lung disease are, in general, poor. Most of the literature has focused on case reports and small case series. In addition, a diagnosis of drug-induced lung disease is often difficult to make with confidence given that there are no firm criteria and the patterns overlap with those of CTD.

Methotrexate is a common treatment for CTD that is a well-established cause of lung injury. Most cases of methotrexate-induced lung injury resemble hypersensitivity pneumonitis. The typical findings of methotrexate toxicity include ground glass opacity, irregular reticulation, and traction bronchiectasis. The distribution of these findings typically involves the mid-upper lung in the craniocaudal plane with central or diffuse involvement in the axial plane (**Fig. 10**). This distribution is in distinction to the basilar and often peripheral distribution of many cases of CTD-related NSIP. In addition, centrilobular nodules, mosaic perfusion, and air trapping are typical features of methotrexate toxicity, but not usually seen in NSIP.

Many of the agents used to treat CTD function by suppressing the immune system. These include corticosteroids, cyclophosphamide, and others. The primary adverse effect of these medications is an increased risk of infections, including those that affect the lungs. Although organisms that affect immunocompetent patients are also common in patients with CTD on immunosuppressive treatment, the differential diagnosis of specific organisms needs to be broadened to include others, such as *Pneumocystis jiroveci* (particularly common in patients with myositis), fungal infections such as aspergillus, mycobacterial infections (tuberculous or nontuberculous), and nocardia.

SUMMARY

HRCT plays an important role in the multidisciplinary evaluation of patients with CTD in conjunction with clinical assessment and sometimes pathologic analysis. The most important role of HRCT is to determine the predominant pattern of lung injury in patients with known CTD. Identification of this pattern then directs appropriate treatment and helps to determine a patient's prognosis. CT is also critical in the subsequent evaluation of patients with worsening or new symptoms. It is also helpful in being able to distinguish worsening of DLD from superimposed processes, such as infection, pulmonary edema, or drug toxicity. Although a diagnosis of CTD is typically made using clinical and serologic criteria, there is an increased recognition of lung disease manifesting as the initial presentation of CTD, in which case anatomic assessment is important in suggesting the diagnosis. CT patterns that should prompt an intensive evaluation for possible CTD include NSIP, OP, NSIP and OP overlap, and LIP.

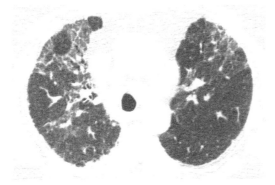

Fig. 10. Methotrexate toxicity in rheumatoid arthritis. HRCT shows fibrosis that is mid-lung predominant. Note there is involvement of both the subpleural and central lung. This distribution is unusual for CTD-related NSIP. This patient developed dyspnea a few months after starting methotrexate therapy.

REFERENCES

1. Mittoo S, Gelber AC, Christopher-Stine L, et al. Ascertainment of collagen vascular disease in patients presenting with interstitial lung disease. Respir Med 2009;103:1152–8.
2. Schurawitzki H, Stiglbauer R, Graninger W, et al. Interstitial lung disease in progressive systemic sclerosis: high-resolution CT versus radiography. Radiology 1990;176:755–9.
3. Homma Y, Ohtsuka Y, Tanimura K, et al. Can interstitial pneumonia as the sole presentation of collagen vascular diseases be differentiated from idiopathic interstitial pneumonia? Respiration 1995;62:248–51.

4. Fischer A, Antoniou KM, Brown KK, et al. An official European Respiratory Society/American Thoracic Society research statement: interstitial pneumonia with autoimmune features. Eur Respir J 2015;46: 976–87.

5. D'Angelo WA, Fries JF, Masi AT, et al. Pathologic observations in systemic sclerosis (scleroderma). A study of fifty-eight autopsy cases and fifty-eight matched controls. Am J Med 1969;46:428–40.

6. Steen VD, Medsger TA. Changes in causes of death in systemic sclerosis, 1972-2002. Ann Rheum Dis 2007;66:940–4. BMJ Publishing Group Ltd.

7. Fischer A, Swigris JJ, Groshong SD, et al. Clinically significant interstitial lung disease in limited scleroderma: histopathology, clinical features, and survival. Chest 2008;134:601–5.

8. Screaton NJ, Hiorns MP, Lee KS, et al. Serial high resolution CT in non-specific interstitial pneumonia: prognostic value of the initial pattern. Clin Radiol 2005;60:96–104.

9. Silva CI, Müller NL, Lynch DA, et al. Chronic hypersensitivity pneumonitis: differentiation from idiopathic pulmonary fibrosis and nonspecific interstitial pneumonia by using thin-section CT. Radiology 2008;246:288–97.

10. Habib HM, Eisa AA, Arafat WR, et al. Pulmonary involvement in early rheumatoid arthritis patients. Clin Rheumatol 2011;30:217–21.

11. Hyldgaard C, Bendstrup E, Pedersen AB, et al. Increased mortality among patients with rheumatoid arthritis and COPD: a population-based study. Respir Med 2018;140:101–7.

12. Lee H-K, Kim DS, Yoo B, et al. Histopathologic pattern and clinical features of rheumatoid arthritis-associated interstitial lung disease. Chest 2005; 127:2019–27.

13. Tanaka N, Kim JS, Newell JD, et al. Rheumatoid arthritis-related lung diseases: CT findings. Radiology 2004;232:81–91.

14. Mori S, Cho I, Koga Y, et al. Comparison of pulmonary abnormalities on high-resolution computed tomography in patients with early versus longstanding rheumatoid arthritis. J Rheumatol 2008;35:1513–21.

15. Moua T, Zamora Martinez AC, Baqir M, et al. Predictors of diagnosis and survival in idiopathic pulmonary fibrosis and connective tissue disease-related usual interstitial pneumonia. Respir Res 2014;15: 154.

16. Kim EJ, Elicker BM, Maldonado F, et al. Usual interstitial pneumonia in rheumatoid arthritis-associated interstitial lung disease. Eur Respir J 2010;35: 1322–8.

17. Raghu G, Remy-Jardin M, Myers JL, et al. Diagnosis of idiopathic pulmonary fibrosis. An official ATS/ERS/JRS/ALAT clinical practice guideline. Am J Respir Crit Care Med 2018;198:e44–68.

18. Assayag D, Elicker BM, Urbania TH, et al. Rheumatoid arthritis-associated interstitial lung disease: radiologic identification of usual interstitial pneumonia pattern. Radiology 2014;270: 583–8.

19. Taouli B, Brauner MW, Mourey I, et al. Thin-section chest CT findings of primary Sjögren's syndrome: correlation with pulmonary function. Eur Radiol 2002;12:1504–11. Springer-Verlag.

20. Parambil JG, Myers JL, Lindell RM, et al. Interstitial lung disease in primary Sjögren syndrome. Chest 2006;130:1489–95.

21. Ito I, Nagai S, Kitaichi M, et al. Pulmonary manifestations of primary Sjogren's syndrome: a clinical, radiologic, and pathologic study. Am J Respir Crit Care Med 2005;171:632–8.

22. Howling SJ, Hansell DM, Wells AU, et al. Follicular bronchiolitis: thin-section CT and histologic findings. Radiology 1999;212:637–42.

23. Lynch DA, Travis WD, Müller NL, et al. Idiopathic interstitial pneumonias: CT features. Radiology 2005;236:10–21.

24. Debray M-P, Borie R, Revel M-P, et al. Interstitial lung disease in anti-synthetase syndrome: initial and follow-up CT findings. Eur J Radiol 2015;84: 516–23.

25. Fathi M, Vikgren J, Boijsen M, et al. Interstitial lung disease in polymyositis and dermatomyositis: longitudinal evaluation by pulmonary function and radiology. Arthritis Rheum 2008;59:677–85. John Wiley & Sons, Ltd.

26. Johnson C, Pinal-Fernandez I, Parikh R, et al. Assessment of mortality in autoimmune myositis with and without associated interstitial lung disease. Lung 2016;194:733–7. Springer US.

27. Matsuki Y, Yamashita H, Takahashi Y, et al. Diffuse alveolar damage in patients with dermatomyositis: a six-case series. Mod Rheumatol 2012;22:243–8. Taylor & Francis.

28. Kim SJ, Lee KS, Ryu YH, et al. Reversed halo sign on high-resolution CT of cryptogenic organizing pneumonia: diagnostic implications. AJR Am J Roentgenol 2003;180:1251–4.

29. Haupt HM, Moore GW, Hutchins GM. The lung in systemic lupus erythematosus. Analysis of the pathologic changes in 120 patients. Am J Med 1981;71: 791–8.

30. Parambil JG, Myers JL, Aubry M-C, et al. Causes and prognosis of diffuse alveolar damage diagnosed on surgical lung biopsy. Chest 2007;132: 50–7.

31. Yamanaka Y, Baba T, Hagiwara E, et al. Radiological images of interstitial pneumonia in mixed connective tissue disease compared with scleroderma and polymyositis/dermatomyositis. Eur J Radiol 2018; 107:26–32.

32. Bonnefoy O, Ferretti G, Calaque O, et al. Serial chest CT findings in interstitial lung disease associated with polymyositis-dermatomyositis. Eur J Radiol 2004;49:235–44.

33. Akira M, Inoue Y, Arai T, et al. Long-term follow-up high-resolution CT findings in non-specific interstitial pneumonia. Thorax 2011;66:61–5. BMJ Publishing Group Ltd and British Thoracic Society.

34. Silva CIS, Müller NL, Fujimoto K, et al. Acute exacerbation of chronic interstitial pneumonia: high-resolution computed tomography and pathologic findings. J Thorac Imaging 2007;22:221–9.

Pulmonary Pathology in Rheumatic Disease

Andrea V. Arrossi, MD

KEYWORDS

- Pathology • Histopathologic patterns of injury • Connective tissue disorders • Pulmonary vasculitis
- IgG4-related disease • Interstitial lung disease • Pulmonary hypertension

KEY POINTS

- Rheumatic disorders may show histopathologic alterations involving any of the compartments of the respiratory system.
- The pulmonary and pleural histopathologic patterns of injury are not specific for rheumatic disorders, because they overlap with the findings seen in other clinical scenarios, such as, but not limited to, the idiopathic forms of interstitial lung disease, drug reactions, infections, or environmental exposures.
- The histopathology of interstitial lung disease associated with connective tissue disorders follows similar diagnostic criteria to the classification of idiopathic interstitial pneumonias.

INTRODUCTION

Pulmonary pathologic manifestations are commonly present in patients with rheumatic autoimmune disorders and may be the initial presentation of the disease, preceding systemic manifestations.

Although pleural disease and interstitial pneumonias, in particular nonspecific interstitial pneumonia, are the most common manifestations of connective tissue disorders (CTDs) in the respiratory system, any compartment, including large airways, small airways, parenchymal interstitium, vessels, and pleura may be involved, either in isolation or as combined disease. Some histologic patterns are more commonly associated with certain disorders than others, such as pulmonary hypertension (PH) in scleroderma (SSc), or usual interstitial pneumonia (UIP) in rheumatoid arthritis (RA).

Furthermore, histopathologic changes associated with rheumatic disease overlap with those resulting from complications of therapy, including drug reactions and/or infections.

This article covers the histopathologic characteristics of rheumatic diseases involving the respiratory system, divided by anatomic compartments.

The most common histopathologic patterns occurring in association with defined CTDs are shown in **Tables 1–5**. Vasculitides more commonly associated with pulmonary involvement are described within the discussion of vascular patterns of disease. I addition, the histopathology of Ig G4–related lung disease (IgG4-RD) is outlined.

HISTOPATHOLOGIC PATTERNS BY ANATOMIC COMPARTMENTS

Airways

Airway inflammation and/or fibrosis may occur in various degrees of severity, and, when present in the setting of CTD, are associated, in decreasing order of frequency, with Sjögren syndrome (SS), RA, systemic lupus erythematosus (SLE), and polymyositis/dermatomyositis (PM/DM).[1]

On histology, airway disease can be classified based on the presence of predominant inflammation or predominant fibrosis (**Box 1**).

Cellular bronchitis/bronchiolitis and follicular bronchiolitis

In cellular bronchitis/bronchiolitis (CB), lymphoplasmacytic infiltrates with variable degrees of

Disclosures: No disclosures or financial conflicts of interest.
Cleveland Clinic, 9500 Euclid Avenue, Cleveland, OH 44195, USA
E-mail address: arrossa@ccf.org

Clin Chest Med 40 (2019) 667–677
https://doi.org/10.1016/j.ccm.2019.05.011

Table 1
Histopathologic patterns in rheumatoid arthritis

Compartment	Pattern	Selected Relevant Points
Pleura	Pleuritis Pleural effusion Empyema (sterile or septic) Necrobiotic nodules Bronchopulmonary fistula, or pyopneumothorax	—

Parenchyma/
  interstitium
	Usual interstitial pneumonia
	
	Nonspecific interstitial pneumonia
	Organizing pneumonia
	DAD
	Necrobiotic nodules (rheumatoid nodules)
		40%–60%
		Increased inflammation and/or lymphoid
		  follicular hyperplasia commonly present
		10%–30%
		Up to 6%
		Rare (1.5%)
		Detected radiologically in up to 22%

Airways	FB Obliterative bronchiolitis Bronchiectasis	— — —
Vascular	PH	—

Data from Refs.[1–8]

severity involve the walls of the terminal bronchioles and respiratory bronchioles, and, less frequently, bronchi. In follicular bronchiolitis (FB), numerous lymphoid follicles predominate, which can extend into the peribronchiolar alveolar interstitium[19] (**Fig. 1A**).

Obliterative (constrictive) bronchiolitis

Obliterative (constrictive) bronchiolitis (OB) is characterized by the presence of fibrosis in various stages affecting terminal and respiratory bronchioles and leading to partial or complete obliteration of the bronchiolar lumina. Chronic inflammatory lymphoplasmacytic infiltrates may be present, especially in earlier stages. In early lesions, the fibrosis is rich in myofibroblasts embedded in a myxoid stroma that expands the submucosa concentrically or eccentrically. As the lesions progress, the airways become obliterated by hypocellular collagen-rich fibrosis, leaving only an area of scar. OB might be patchy and subtle in lung biopsies, and surgical lung biopsies are often needed if there is a clinical indication to obtain a histopathologic diagnosis. The use of connective tissue stains, such as pentachrome Movat stain, can help in the recognition of the scarred airways that may not be evident with routine hematoxylin-eosin–stained sections (**Fig. 1B**). Histologic changes secondary to airway obliteration, such as postobstructive pneumonia, air trapping, and bronchiolectasis are usually present.

Table 2
Histopathologic patterns in scleroderma

Compartment	Pattern	Selected Relevant Points

Interstitium	Nonspecific interstitial
	  pneumonia
	UIP
	
	OP
		Most frequent pattern (up to 70% of cases)
		
		Second most frequent pattern. Chronic inflammation
		  with lymphoid follicles may be prominent
		—

Vascular	PH	Highest prevalence among CTDs Plexiform lesions and fibrinoid necrosis not common
Airways	Bronchiolitis	Mostly associated with aspiration and gastroesophageal reflux disease
Pleura	Pleural effusion	Rare

Data from Refs.[1,2,9–13]

Table 3
Histopathologic patterns in systemic lupus erythematosus

Compartment	Pattern	Selected Relevant Points
Pleura	Pleural effusions, pleuritis	Most common manifestation (30%–50%)
Interstitium	Nonspecific interstitial pneumonia	Most frequent pattern of ILD
	UIP	—
	OP	—
	DAD (acute lupus pneumonitis)	Rare, up to 50% mortality
Airways	Cellular bronchiolitis	Rare
	FB	
	Obliterative bronchiolitis	
Vascular	Vasculitis/alveolar hemorrhage	0.6%–5.4%
	Pulmonary thromboembolism	Increased risk with lupus anticoagulant
	PH	0.5%–14%
		Similar morphology to primary PH (plexogenic lesions and fibrinoid necrosis may be present)
		Chronic thromboembolic PH (in cases with lupus anticoagulant)

Data from Refs.[1,2,9,13–15]

Table 4
Histopathologic patterns in polymyositis/dermatomyositis

Compartment	Pattern	Selected Relevant Points
Interstitium Histologic patterns vary with serologic type and onset of presentation	Nonspecific interstitial pneumonia	Common in acute and insidious presentations
	OP	Most common in cases with acute onset
	DAD	—
—	UIP	—
Airways	Obliterative bronchiolitis	—
Vascular	PH	Rare
Pleura	Pleuritis, pleural effusion	Exceedingly rare

Data from Refs.[1,2,9,16–17]

Table 5
Histopathologic patterns in Sjögren syndrome

Compartment	Pattern	Selected Relevant Points
Airways	FB	Most common pattern
Interstitium	Nonspecific interstitial pneumonia	Most frequent pattern of ILD
	OP	—
	LIP	May be associated with cystic lung disease
	UIP	—
	Amyloidosis, light chain deposition disease	May be associated with cystic lung disease
Vascular	PH	Rare
Pleural	Pleuritis, pleural effusion	Exceedingly rare

Data from Refs.[1,2,9,18]

Box 1
Key histologic features of connective tissue disorder–related airway disease

Cellular bronchiolitis

- Lymphoplasmacytic infiltrates centered on bronchioles

FB

- Predominance of lymphoid follicles with germinal centers

Obliterative constrictive bronchiolitis

- Early lesions: concentric or eccentric fibroblastic tissue with partial obliteration
- Late lesions: scarring collagen fibrosis with complete luminal collapse

---

Bronchiectasis

Bronchiectasis refers to the permanent dilatation of the airways caused by chronic recurrent episodes of inflammation. The architecture of the bronchial and bronchiolar walls is altered with varying degrees of fibrosis and inflammation.

Interstitium

RA, SSc, and PM/DM are disorders that commonly present with interstitial lung disease (ILD) when the lung is involved. The interstitium is involved by various degrees of inflammation and/or fibrosis.

The histologic patterns of ILD are classified according to the American Thoracic Society and European Respiratory Society classifications, and include UIP, nonspecific interstitial pneumonia (NSIP), organizing pneumonia (OP), lymphocytic interstitial pneumonia (LIP), and diffuse alveolar damage (DAD).[20] CTDs may involve the lung, showing any of the histologic patterns of ILD, either isolated or in combination. Furthermore,

histologic interstitial patterns of injury are part of the criteria for the classification of interstitial pneumonia with autoimmune features (IPAF), a recently proposed term for cases of interstitial pneumonia that have clinical, radiologic, and histologic features suggestive of an underlying systemic autoimmune disorder but that do not meet the criteria for a classifiable CTD.

Usual interstitial pneumonia

UIP is a fibrosing interstitial pneumonia characterized by temporal and spatial heterogeneity, patchy distribution, architectural destruction, fibrosis including honeycombing, and fibroblastic foci.[20–22] The temporal heterogeneity is recognized by the presence of scarring, irreversible, collagen-rich fibrosis, and foci of early fibrosis composed of a cellular myofibroblastic proliferation in a myxoid background, referred to as "fibroblastic foci" foci. The spatial heterogeneity refers to the patchy configuration of the fibrosis, with involvement of the subpleural, paraseptal, and peribronchial regions, alternating with areas of normal to near-normal lung (**Fig. 2**A, B). Disease progression leads to parenchymal destruction and collapse with development of honeycomb changes, defined as cystically dilated air spaces, lined by bronchiolar metaplastic epithelium, luminal mucin, and fibrino-inflammatory debris (**Box 2**).

Nonspecific interstitial pneumonia

In contrast with UIP, NSIP is a diffuse process that may be inflammatory-predominant or fibrotic-predominant. NSIP is recognized by its diffuse and homogeneous appearance at low magnification. The alveolar septa are involved by mononuclear infiltrates rich in lymphocytes and plasma cells (**Fig. 2**C). The fibrosis in NSIP is temporally homogeneous and consists mostly of collagen-rich fibrosis. Fibroblastic foci are absent or scarce. Honeycomb changes, or OP, if present, are focal

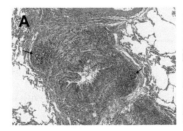 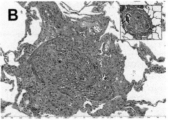

Fig. 1. Bronchiolitis. (*A*) FB with prominent bronchiolar lymphoplasmacytic infiltrates with lymphoid follicles (*arrows*) (hematoxylin-eosin [H&E], original magnification ×4.4). (*B*) Obliterative bronchiolitis with almost complete obliteration of the lumen (*asterisk*) (H&E, original magnification ×14.8). Inlet: Luminal fibromyoid tissue (*asterisk*) residual muscularis mucosae (*short arrow*), and epithelium (*long arrows*) (Movat, original magnification ×6.8).

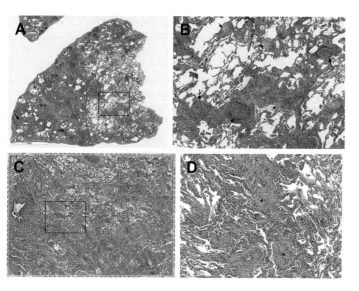

Fig. 2. ILD. (*A*) UIP in RA shows patchy fibrosis (*double asterisk*), alternating areas of normal lung (*asterisk*), and focal microscopic honeycombing (*arrow*) (H&E, original magnification ×1.2); inlet is presented in (*B*) showing lymphoid follicles (*long arrows*) and fibroblastic foci (*short arrows*) (H&E, original magnification ×2.8). (*C*) Nonspecific interstitial pneumonia showing expansion of alveolar septae by lymphocytic infiltrates (*arrow* in inlet) (H&E, original magnification ×1.4). (*D*) OP showing plugs of luminal fibromyxoid tissue (*asterisk*) (H&E, original magnification ×10).

and not prominent.[20,21,23] (**Box 3**) NSIP has been proposed as a histologic criterion within the morphologic domain for the classification of IPAF. The presence of interstitial lymphoid aggregates with germinal centers or diffuse lymphoplasmacytic infiltration (with or without lymphoid follicles) without features of a defined histologic pattern are also criteria included within the morphologic domain.[24]

Diffuse alveolar damage

DAD is a manifestation of acute lung injury. It constitutes the histologic pattern of acute interstitial pneumonia and acute respiratory distress syndrome (ARDS).[21,25] The morphologic features of DAD depend on the stage of the process. Early DAD shows only subtle changes, such as interstitial edema/inflammation and reactive type II pneumocytes. As the process progresses, fibrin leaks from the capillaries and is distributed along the alveolar septa forming hyaline membranes, the hallmark of the active phase of DAD. In the organizing stage, there is reabsorption of the hyaline membranes and remaining fibrin, followed by diffuse fibromyxoid interstitial organization and regenerative/reparative type II pneumocyte

---

Box 2
Key features of connective tissue disorder–related usual interstitial pneumonia

Histology

- Temporally heterogeneous fibrosis
- Fibroblastic foci
- Honeycomb changes
- Chronic interstitial pneumonitis with prominent lymphoid follicles

Most common associations in order of frequency

- RA
- Scleroderma
- PM/DM
- Systemic lupus erythematosus
- IPAF

Box 3
Key histologic features of connective tissue disorder–related nonspecific interstitial pneumonia

Histology

- Variable degrees of chronic inflammation and/or fibrosis
- Diffuse lymphoplasmacytic interstitial infiltrates
- Diffuse homogeneous interstitial fibrosis

Most common associations in order of frequency

- Scleroderma
- IPAF
- PM/DM
- RA
- IPAF
- Sjögren syndrome
- Systemic lupus erythematosus

hyperplasia. DAD may progress to interstitial fibrosis, leading to NSIP or interstitial fibrosis without a specific pattern (**Box 4**).[21,25]

Organizing pneumonia

OP is also a pattern of organizing acute lung injury.[25] The process is mostly patchy, centered on the alveolar ducts and alveoli, with or without small airway involvement. The morphologic hallmark of OP is the presence of alveolar polypoid fibromyxoid tissue formed by myofibroblasts embedded in a myxoid stroma within airspaces.[21,25] Although the morphology and characteristics of the fibromyxoid tissue in OP resembles the fibroblastic foci seen in UIP, the former is recognized by its intraluminal location (so-called Masson bodies), and its centrilobular-predominant distribution (**Fig. 2**D), whereas the latter represents organizing fibromyxoid tissue within the alveolar interstitium in the interface between collagen-type fibrosis and preserved lung parenchyma. Numerous postobstructive foamy alveolar macrophages may be present.[21,25] (**Box 5**) OP is also one of the proposed criteria within the morphologic domain for the classification of IPAF.[24]

Lymphoid interstitial pneumonia

LIP is a diffuse inflammatory process with involvement of the alveolar septa by prominent lymphoplasmacytic infiltrates.[20,21] Overlapping histologic features may be encountered between LIP and NSIP; however, the interstitial infiltrates of the former are more profuse and usually accompanied by scattered lymphoid follicles, and sometimes referred to as diffuse lymphoid hyperplasia. In addition to interstitial alveolar inflammation, FB may be present (**Box 6**). Although not the most common pattern, LIP constitutes a feature almost unique to Sjögren syndrome. LIP is also included

as a histologic criterion within the morphologic domain for the classification of IPAF.[24]

Unclassifiable histologic pattern

ILD may be histologically unclassifiable because of overlap and coexistence of 2 or more patterns.[21] Biopsies with areas of patchy fibrosis resembling UIP may alternate with areas of diffuse interstitial pneumonitis and fibrosis resembling NSIP. Likewise, prominent OP may be present in cases that are otherwise NSIP. Unclassifiable ILD occurs less frequently in idiopathic ILD, therefore, when present, it strongly suggests an alternative cause, including CTD-related ILD. Coexistence of alterations involving different compartments is also a feature of CTDs, such as a combination of interstitial pneumonia and FB in RA. Furthermore, overlap of OP and NSIP, as well as the presence of interstitial lymphoid aggregates with germinal centers, and diffuse lymphoplasmacytic infiltration (with or without lymphoid follicles) without features of a

---

Box 4
Key features of connective tissue disorder–related diffuse alveolar damage

Histology

- Diffuse interstitial edema and mild inflammation
- Hyaline membranes
- Interstitial fibroblastic organization

Most common associations in order of frequency

- PM/DM
- Systemic lupus erythematosus

Box 5
Key features of connective tissue disorder–related organizing pneumonia

Histology

- Patchy centrilobular distribution
- Airspace plugs of fibromyxoid tissue

Most common associations in order of frequency

- PM/DM
- Systemic lupus erythematosus
- RA
- Sjögren syndrome
- IPAF
- Scleroderma

Box 6
Key features of connective tissue disorder–related lymphoid interstitial pneumonia

Histology

- Diffuse inflammation
- Profuse lymphoplasmacytic infiltrates
- Minor features of FB

Most common associations in order of frequency

- Sjögren syndrome
- IPAF

classifiable pattern, constitute histologic criteria within the morphologic domain for the classification of IPAF.[24]

Necrobiotic nodules

Necrobiotic nodules are seen in RA, and are histologically similar to the subcutaneous rheumatoid nodules. Morphologically, the nodules consist of chronic and granulomatous inflammation with palisading epithelioid histiocytes surrounding a necrotic center. The nodules may have similar morphology to necrotizing granulomas of other causes, including granulomatosis with polyangiitis (discussed later).

Pleura

Serosal involvement is one of the most common compartments involved in collagen vascular disorders.[2] Pleural and/or pericardial effusions, pleuritis, fibrosis, and necrobiotic nodules, with or without bronchopleural fistulae, may be present. Pleuritis and/or pericarditis may be acute or chronic. Acute pleuritis has predominantly neutrophilic infiltrates with fibrinonecrotic debris along the surface, with underlying granulation tissue. In contrast, in chronic pleuritis, lymphoplasmacytic infiltrates predominate with or without fibrosis.

Vascular

The vascular changes in CTDs include mostly PH and vascular inflammation or vasculitis. Rarely, pulmonary embolism may occur secondary to CTD, particularly in patients with SLE.

Vasculitis

Vasculitides are classified according to the 2012 Revised International Chapel Hill Consensus Conference on the Nomenclature of Vasculitides.[26] Antineutrophil cytoplasmic antibodies (ANCA)–associated small vessel vasculitis, which includes granulomatosis with polyangiitis (GPA), formerly Wegener granulomatosis, eosinophilic granulomatosis with polyangiitis (EGPA), formerly Churg Strauss syndrome; and microscopic polyangiitis (MPA) comprise the group of vasculitides that most frequently affect the lung. Rarely, other types of vasculitides may involve the lung, including vasculitis secondary to systemic disease, vasculitis associated with a specific cause (infection, drug reactions), and other large, medium, and small vessel vasculitides, such as immune complex vasculitis, necrotizing sarcoid granulomatosis, polyarteritis nodosa, Takayasu arteritis, Behçet syndrome, cryoglobulinemic vasculitis, hypocomplementemic vasculitis, or giant cell arteritis.[27]

Capillaritis, which consists of acute neutrophilic/fibrinoid infiltrates within alveolar septa with damage to the alveolar capillary endothelium, is a common finding in most small vessel vasculitides (**Fig. 3**A). Apoptotic bodies and small capillary luminal fibrin thrombi are usually present. In more severe cases, the inflammation may spill into the alveolar spaces.

Pulmonary hemorrhage is usually seen in the setting of vasculitides and is recognized by the presence of hemosiderin-laden macrophages and organizing blood and fibrinoid exudates. Epithelial injury leading to reactive type II pneumocytes hyperplasia is usually present.

Granulomatosis with polyangiitis

GPA is characterized by consolidated nodular areas of inflammation and necrosis. Distinctive features include necrotizing granulomatous

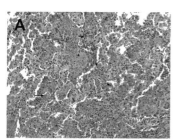
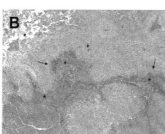
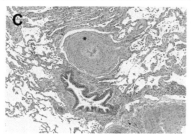

Fig. 3. Vascular pathology. (*A*) Capillaritis showing alveolar septal neutrophilic infiltrates (*short arrows*), organizing blood (*asterisk*), and hemosiderin-laden macrophages (*long arrow*) (H&E, original magnification ×20). (*B*) Granulomatosis with polyangiitis: necrotizing granulomas with geographic basophilic necrosis (*asterisks*), palisading histiocytes (*long arrows*), and multinucleated giant cells (*short arrow*) (H&E, original magnification ×4). (*C*) PH. Pulmonary artery with intimal fibroplasia and medial hypertrophy (*asterisk*) (H&E, original magnification ×10).

inflammation with atypical multinucleated giant cells, vascular changes, and microabscesses.[27,28]

Vascular changes constitute a major manifestation of GPA, present in more than 96% of the cases[27,28] and may involve small vessels, including arteritis, phlebitis/venulitis, and capillaritis. Acute, chronic, or granulomatous inflammation may be seen. When capillaritis is prominent, the presence of distinctive features of GPA is helpful to differentiate it from other small vessel vasculitis to establish the diagnosis.

The granulomas have central basophilic necrosis with so-called geographic or serpiginous borders, surrounded by epithelioid histiocytes. Multinucleated giant cells with dense eosinophilic cytoplasm are a common finding (**Fig. 3**B). This morphology of the granulomas is suggestive of GPA, however, some infections may have a similar pattern. Furthermore, while, the borders of rheumatoid nodules are usually regular and round, their morphology may overlap with the necrotizing granulomas of GPA.

In addition to the vascular alterations, alveolar hemorrhage, and necrotizing granulomas, minor pathologic changes may be present such as OP, FB interstitial lymphoid aggregates, bronchocentric granulomatosis, or tissue eosinophilia.[27,28]

Eosinophilic granulomatosis with polyangiitis
EGPA is an eosinophil-rich granulomatous process with small to medium vessel necrotizing vasculitis, associated with asthma and eosinophilia. EGPA is primarily a clinical entity and, in most cases, is diagnosed from clinical findings. Lung involvement occurs in about 30% to 60% of the ANCA-positive cases, and in 60% to 80% of the ANCA-negative cases.[29]

Histopathologic abnormalities in EGPA involve the vessels, airways, and parenchyma. The airways commonly have features of reactive airway disease (asthma). Eosinophilic infiltrates may involve bronchial/bronchiolar walls, the alveolar interstitium, or aggregate within alveolar spaces, resulting in frank eosinophilic pneumonia.

The granulomas in EGPA have central eosinophilic necrotic debris surrounded by a rim of palisading epithelioid histiocytes and multinucleated giant cells. Although necrotizing eosinophilic granulomas are not included as a criterion for the classification of EGPA, their presence should raise high levels of suspicion for this diagnosis[30]

Arteries, veins, and/or capillaries have variable degrees of necrotizing eosinophilic infiltration, which may be admixed with lymphocytes, plasma cells, multinucleated giant cells, and/or neutrophils. Features of pulmonary hemorrhage may also be present. Extravascular accumulations of eosinophils along with the vascular necrotizing

inflammation was included as one of the criteria for the classification of EGPA by the American College of Rheumatology.[30] Likewise, necrotizing vasculitis is included within the definition of EGPA by the International Chapel Hill Consensus Conference on the Nomenclature Of Vasculitides.[26] However, pulmonary (or systemic) vasculitis may be absent in about 50% of the cases and proposals for revisions of the diagnostic criteria are ongoing.[31]

For the diagnosis of EGPA, it is important that other causes of eosinophilic pneumonia or eosinophilic vasculitis need to be excluded, particularly in cases with eosinophilic pneumonia as the predominant feature.

Microscopic polyangiitis
MPA is a nongranulomatous small vessel vasculitis that involves arterioles, venules, and capillaries. Necrotizing arteritis involving small and medium arteries may be present.[26] Capillaritis is seen in association with pulmonary hemorrhage, with or without features of DAD. Lung samples from areas of chronic or inactive MPA may have only features of chronic hemorrhage with hemosiderin-laden macrophages. ILD, including UIP and NSIP, has also been observed in association with MPA[32,33] (**Box 7**).

Box 7
Key features of vasculitis

Granulomatosis with polyangiitis

- Arteritis, phlebitis, venulitis, capillaritis
- Granulomas with geographic basophilic necrosis
- Multinucleated giant cells
- Microabscesses
- Alveolar hemorrhage

Eosinophilic granulomatosis with polyangiitis

- Arteritis, phlebitis, venulitis, capillaritis
- Granulomas with eosinophilic necrosis
- Airway features of asthma
- Eosinophilic airway and parenchyma infiltrates
- Alveolar hemorrhage

Microscopic polyangiitis

- Capillaritis
- Small arteries and veins less frequently involved
- Alveolar hemorrhage

Pulmonary hypertension

PH refers to the chronic remodeling of the pulmonary vessels with a subsequent increase in the pulmonary vascular resistance leading to progressive right ventricular dysfunction. PH in CTD may be classified within any of the 5 groups of the clinical classification of PH due to the various possible physiologic mechanisms involved in its development. PH may constitute an isolated form of vascular disease (pulmonary arterial hypertension [PAH]–associated with CTD [group 1.4]), or it may be the result of heart disease (group 2), chronic ILD (group 3), thromboembolism (group 4), or multifactorial (group 5).[9,34]

On histology, features of vascular remodeling in PAH include concentric intimal proliferation and medial hypertrophy with muscularization of the arterioles (**Fig. 3**C). Plexiform lesions and in situ thrombosis are less frequent.

PATHOLOGY OF COMPLICATIONS OF THERAPY

Lung disorders in patients with CTD may be a primary manifestation of the disease but may also be secondary to the therapies these patients may receive, resulting from drug lung toxicity or oportunistic infections.

Drug reactions and infections may have histologic patterns similar to those observed in pulmonary involvement by the rheumatic disorder. Therefore, a careful search for clues using special histochemical or immunohistochemical stains may be helpful in identifying specific features, such as microorganisms, to suggest possible causes.

PULMONARY INVOLVEMENT WITH IMMUNOGLOBULIN G4–RELATED DISEASE

IgG4-RD is a recently described entity.[35] Its histologic diagnosis, in any affected organ, is based on the presence of characteristic findings, which include lymphoplasmacytic infiltrates, sclerosing fibrosis, and obliterative vasculitis, in combination with increased numbers of tissue IgG4-positive plasma cells or increased IgG4/IgG ratio.[36]

The inflammatory infiltrate in IgG4-RD has a plasma cell–rich predominant lymphoplasmacytic population with variable amounts of eosinophils.

The fibrosis consists of a fibromyoblastic proliferation with storiform areas and varying degrees of hyalinized dense collagen deposition.

Obliterative vasculitis most frequently involves veins (obliterative phlebitis); however, particularly in pulmonary lesions, arteries may also be affected.

The vessels contain dense lymphoplasmacytic infiltrates that lead to fibrosis with luminal obliteration.[36]

Four groups of pulmonary involvement have been described based on radiologic findings: the bronchovascular type, alveolar interstitial type, round-shaped ground-glass opacities, (GGOs), and solid nodular type.[37] On histology, in the bronchovascular type, the lymphoplasmacytic infiltrates expand bronchovascular bundles, and may involve the alveolar interstitium, the interlobular septa, and the pleura. In the alveolar interstitial and the nodular GGO types, the lymphoplasmacytic infiltrates involve the interstitium with a similar appearance to NSIP. In the solid nodular type, the pulmonary architecture is distorted by the presence of sclerosing fibrosis and inflammation.[37,38]

Pleural involvement may be seen as localized nodular lesions, or as diffuse serosal thickening. The sclerosing fibrosis occuring in pleural lesions may be extensive, and may extend into the soft tissues and bone of the chest wall.[38]

Because of the organ-dependent variability of the number of IgG4-positive plasma cells and extent of fibrosis at the time of diagnosis in IgG4-RD, the number of plasma cells required for diagnosis varies among different organs.[36] However, in general, an increased IgG4/IgG ratio of 40% is highly suggestive of IgG4-RD, regardless of the organ involved. In the lung, greater than 50 IgG4-positive plasma cells per high-power field defines probable IgG4-RD if 1 morphologic finding is present, or highly suggestive of IgG4-RD if 2 or more morphologic findings are present when a surgical lung biopsy is examined.[36]

It is important to note that increased numbers of IgG4-positive plasma cells per-se are not specific for IgG4-RD, Inflammatory or neoplastic conditions may have increased numbers of tissue IgG4-positive plasma cells such as ANCA–associated vasculitis, RA, inflammatory bowel disease, necrotizings granulomatous inflammation, and malignant neoplasms including various types of lymphomas and carcinomas. In these instances, the morphologic features of IgG4-RD are lacking. Therefore, interpretation of IgG4-positive plasma cell counts should always be correlated with the associated histopathologic features and the clinical findings.[39,40]

REFERENCES

1. Tansey D, Wells AU, Colby TV, et al. Variations in histological patterns of interstitial pneumonia between connective tissue disorders and their relationship to prognosis. Histopathology 2004;44(6):585–96.

2. Bouros D, Pneumatikos I, Tzouvelekis A. Pleural involvement in systemic autoimmune disorders. Respiration 2008;75(4):361–71.

3. Bongartz T, Nannini C, Medina-Velasquez YF, et al. Incidence and mortality of interstitial lung disease in rheumatoid arthritis: a population-based study. Arthritis Rheum 2010;62(6):1583–91.

4. Kim EJ, Collard HR, King TE. Rheumatoid arthritis-associated interstitial lung disease. Chest 2009; 136(5):1397–405.

5. Assayag D, Elicker BM, Urbania TH, et al. Rheumatoid arthritis–associated interstitial lung disease: radiologic Identification of usual interstitial pneumonia pattern. Radiology 2013;270(2):583–8.

6. Ryu JH, Matteson EL. Rheumatoid arthritis. In: Dellaripa PF, Fischer A, Flaherty KR, editors. Pulmonary manifestations of rheumatic disease: a comprehensive guide. New York: Springer New York; 2014. p. 25–36. https://doi.org/10.1007/978-1-4939-0770-0_3.

7. Yousem SA, Colby TV, Carrington CB. Lung biopsy in rheumatoid arthritis. Am Rev Respir Dis 1985; 131(5):770–7.

8. Cohen M, Sahn SA. Bronchiectasis in systemic diseases. Chest 1999;116(4):1063–74.

9. Mathai SC, Hummers LK. Pulmonary hypertension associated with connective tissue disease. In: Dellaripa PF, Fischer A, Flaherty KR, editors. Pulmonary manifestations of rheumatic disease: a comprehensive guide. New York: Springer New York; 2014. p. 139–66.

10. Bouros D, Wells AU, Nicholson AG, et al. Histopathologic subsets of fibrosing alveolitis in patients with systemic sclerosis and their relationship to outcome. Am J Respir Crit Care Med 2002; 165(12):1581–6.

11. Solomon JJ, Olson AL, Fischer A, et al. Scleroderma lung disease. Eur Respir Rev 2013;22(127):6–19.

12. Fujita J. Non-specific interstitial pneumonia as pulmonary involvement of systemic sclerosis. Ann Rheum Dis 2001;60(3):281–3.

13. Sasaki N, Kamataki A, Sawai T. A histopathological study of pulmonary hypertension in connective tissue disease. Allergol Int 2011;60(4):411–7.

14. Mittoo S, Swigris JJ. Pulmonary manifestations of systemic lupus erythematosus (SLE). In: Dellaripa PF, Fischer A, Flaherty KR, editors. Pulmonary manifestations of rheumatic disease: a comprehensive guide. New York: Springer New York; 2014. p. 61–72.

15. Martínez-Martínez MU, Oostdam DAH, Abud-Mendoza C. Diffuse alveolar hemorrhage in autoimmune diseases. Curr Rheumatol Rep 2017; 19(5):27.

16. Sanges S, Yelnik CM, Sitbon O, et al. Pulmonary arterial hypertension in idiopathic inflammatory myopathies: Data from the French pulmonary hypertension registry and review of the literature. Medicine (Baltimore) 2016;95(39):e4911.

17. Gutsche M, Rosen GD, Swigris JJ. Connective tissue disease-associated interstitial lung disease: a review. Curr Respir Care Rep 2012;1:224–32.

18. Parambil JG, Myers JL, Lindell RM, et al. Interstitial lung disease in primary Sjögren syndrome. Chest 2006;130(5):1489–95.

19. Yousem SA, Colby TV, Carrington CB. Follicular bronchitis/bronchiolitis. Hum Pathol 1985;16(7): 700–6.

20. Travis WD, Costabel U, Hansell DM, et al. An official American Thoracic Society/European respiratory Society statement: update of the international multidisciplinary classification of the idiopathic interstitial pneumonias. Am J Respir Crit Care Med 2013; 188(6):733–48.

21. American Thoracic Society/European respiratory Society International Multidisciplinary consensus classification of the idiopathic interstitial pneumonias: this joint statement of the American Thoracic Society (ATS), and the European respiratory Society (ERS) was adopted by the ATS board of Directors, June 2001 and by the ERS Executive Committee, June 2001. Am J Respir Crit Care Med 2002; 165(2):277–304.

22. Raghu G, Remy-Jardin M, Myers JL, et al. Diagnosis of idiopathic pulmonary fibrosis. An official ATS/ERS/JRS/ALAT clinical practice guideline. Am J Respir Crit Care Med 2018;198(5):e44–68.

23. Travis WD, Hunninghake G, King TE, et al. Idiopathic nonspecific interstitial pneumonia. Am J Respir Crit Care Med 2008;177(12):1338–47.

24. Fischer A, Antoniou KM, Brown KK, et al. An official European Respiratory Society/American Thoracic Society research statement: interstitial pneumonia with autoimmune features. Eur Respir J 2015;46(4): 976–87.

25. Katzenstein AL. Acute lung injury patterns: diffuse alveolar damage and bronchiolitis obliterans organizing pneumonia. In: Katzenstein AL, Katzenstein, Askin, editors. Surgical pathology of non-neoplastic lung disease. 4th edition. Philadelphia: Saunders Elsevier; 2006. p. 17–49.

26. Jennette JC, Falk RJ, Bacon PA, et al. 2012 Revised International Chapel Hill consensus conference nomenclature of vasculitides. Arthritis Rheum 2013; 65(1):1–11.

27. Travis WD. Pathology of pulmonary vasculitis. Semin Respir Crit Care Med 2004;25(05):475–82.

28. Travis WDMD, Hoffman GSMD, Leavitt RYMD, et al. Surgical pathology of the lung in Wegener's granulomatosis: review of 87 open lung biopsies from 67 patients. Am J Surg Pathol 1991;15(4):315–33.

29. Vaglio A, Buzio C, Zwerina J. Eosinophilic granulomatosis with polyangiitis (Churg–Strauss): state of the art. Allergy 2013;68(3):261–73.

30. Masi AT, Hunder GG, Lie JT, et al. The American College of Rheumatology 1990 criteria for the classification of churg-strauss syndrome (allergic granulomatosis and angiitis). Arthritis Rheum 1990;33(8): 1094–100.

31. Cottin V, Bel E, Bottero P, et al. Revisiting the systemic vasculitis in eosinophilic granulomatosis with polyangiitis (Churg-Strauss): a study of 157 patients by the Groupe d'Etudes et de Recherche sur les Maladies Orphelines Pulmonaires and the European Respiratory Society Taskforce on eosinophilic granulomatosis with polyangiitis (Churg-Strauss). Autoimmun Rev 2017;16(1):1–9.

32. Katsumata Y, Kawaguchi Y, Yamanaka H. Interstitial lung disease with ANCA-associated vasculitis. Clin Med Insights Circ Respir Pulm Med 2015;9(s1): 51–6.

33. Baqir M, Cox C, Yi E, et al. Radiologic and pathologic characteristics of myeloperoxidase-antineutrophil cytoplasmic antibody– associated interstitial lung disease: a retrospective analysis. Abstract #283 of the 19th International Vasculitis and ANCA Workshop. Rheumatology 2019; 58(Supplement_2):kez063.007.

34. Galiè N, Humbert M, Vachiery J-L, et al. 2015 ESC/ERS Guidelines for the diagnosis and treatment of pulmonary hypertension. The Joint Task Force for the diagnosis and Treatment of pulmonary hypertension of the European Society of Cardiology (ESC) and the European respiratory Society (ERS): Endorsed by: association for European Paediatric and Congenital Cardiology (AEPC), International Society for heart and lung Transplantation (ISHLT). Eur Heart J 2016;37(1):67–119.

35. Taniguchi T, Ko M, Seko S, et al. Interstitial pneumonia associated with autoimmune pancreatitis. Gut 2004;53(5):770–1. Available at: https://www.ncbi.nlm.nih.gov/pmc/articles/PMC1774056/. Accessed April 8, 2019.

36. Deshpande V, Zen Y, Chan JK, et al. Consensus statement on the pathology of IgG4-related disease. Mod Pathol 2012;25(9):1181–92.

37. Inoue D, Zen Y, Abo H, et al. Immunoglobulin G4–related lung disease: CT findings with pathologic correlations. Radiology 2009;251(1):260–70.

38. Zen Y, Inoue D, Kitao A, et al. IgG4-related lung and pleural disease: a clinicopathologic study of 21 cases. Am J Surg Pathol 2009;33(12):1886–93.

39. Strehl JD, Hartmann A, Agaimy A. Numerous IgG4-positive plasma cells are ubiquitous in diverse localised non-specific chronic inflammatory conditions and need to be distinguished from IgG4-related systemic disorders. J Clin Pathol 2011;64(3):237–43.

40. Yi ES, Sekiguchi H, Peikert T, et al. Pathologic manifestations of immunoglobulin(Ig)G4-related lung disease. Semin Diagn Pathol 2012;29(4):219–25.

Autoimmune Biomarkers, Antibodies, and Immunologic Evaluation of the Patient with Fibrotic Lung Disease

Argyris Tzouvelekis, MD, MSc, PhD[a], Theodoros Karampitsakos, MD, MSc[a], Evangelos Bouros, MSc, PhD[a], Vassilios Tzilas, MD, PhD[a], Stamatis-Nick Liossis, MD, PhD[b], Demosthenes Bouros, MD, PhD, FERS, FCCP, FAPSR[a],*

KEYWORDS

- Autoimmunity • Interstitial lung diseases • Connective tissue disorders • Chronic lung injury
- Biomarkers

KEY POINTS

- Pulmonary complications, including interstitial lung diseases, have a crucial impact on quality of life and mortality in patients with connective tissue diseases.
- Several biomarkers provide evidence for the role of autoimmunity in chronic lung injury.
- Autoantibodies are strongly linked with disease presentation and clinical outcomes and thus represent valuable assessment and management tools in patients with connective tissue disorders–interstitial lung diseases.
- Meticulous immunologic evaluation is mandatory to exclude autoimmune causes of interstitial lung fibrosis.

INTRODUCTION

Pulmonary complications represent an important extra-articular manifestation of connective tissue disorders (CTDs) with a negative impact on quality of life and mortality (**Table 1**).[1] Pulmonary manifestations of autoimmune disorders are mainly observed in the context of interstitial lung diseases (ILDs), airways disorders, and pleural and vascular abnormalities.[2] A possible association between ILD and autoimmunity was first reported almost 40 years ago.[3] Despite further reports linking immune deregulation and chronic lung injury, the role of autoimmunity has been largely ignored likely because of disappointing results of immunosuppressive and immunomodulatory agents in patients with idiopathic pulmonary fibrosis (IPF).[4–8]

Nonetheless, interest in autoimmunity and ILD has been recently revived by studies demonstrating the presence of highly activated CD4[+]

Disclosure Statement: None to declare.

Conflicts of Interest: None to declare.

[a] 1st Academic Department of Respiratory Medicine, Medical School, National and Kapodistrian University of Athens, Hospital for Diseases of the Chest, "Sotiria", Mesogion 152, Athens 11527, Greece; [b] Division of Rheumatology, Department of Internal Medicine, Patras University Hospital, University of Patras Medical School, Patras, Rio 26504, Greece

* Corresponding author.

E-mail address: dbouros@med.uoa.gr

Clin Chest Med 40 (2019) 679–691

https://doi.org/10.1016/j.ccm.2019.06.002

Table 1
Sensitivity and specificity of autoimmune biomarkers used in clinical practice

Antibodies	Disease	Sensitivity, %	Specificity	Reference
ANA	SLE	95	Low	Mittoo et al,[40] 2009;
	Systemic sclerosis	87	Low	Jee et al,[41] 2017
	SS	74	Low	
Anti-dsDNA	SLE	10–54	89%–99%	Vitali et al,[48] 1992
Anti-Sm	SLE	10–55	98%–100%	Janwityanuchit et al,[46] 1993
APL	APL/SLE	90	99%	Ruiz-Irastorza et al,[47] 2004
RF	RA	50–88	80%–86%	Bridges,[51] 2004; Rodriguez-Mahou et al,[52] 2006
Anti-CCP	RA	50–88	95%–99%	Bridges,[51] 2004; Rodriguez-Mahou et al,[52] 2006
Anti-Scl70	Systemic sclerosis	30–40	90%–100%	Reveille & Solomon,[69] 2003; Karampitsakos et al,[13] 2017
	Systemic sclerosis–ILD	45	81%	
ACA	Systemic sclerosis	20–40	97%	Karampitsakos et al,[71] 2018; Mehra et al,[72] 2013
Anti-RNA pol	Systemic sclerosis	20	98%–100%	Koenig et al,[73] 2008
c-ANCA/anti-PR3	GPA	85–90	95%	Brown,[86] 2006; Cornec et al,[87] 2016
p-ANCA/anti-MPO	MPA	30–75	99.4%	Choi et al,[88] 2001
	EGPA	30–50	99.4%	

Abbreviations: APL, antiphospholipid syndrome; c-ANCA/anti-PR3, cytoplasmic antineutrophil cytoplasm antibodies/anti-proteinase 3; CCP, cyclic citrullinated peptide; EGPA, eosinophilic granulomatosis with polyangiitis.

cells, circulating autoantibodies, and functionally impaired T-regulatory cells in patients with different forms of pulmonary fibrosis.[9–20] A linkage between pulmonary fibrosis and microscopic polyangiitis (MPA) highlights the role of an ongoing autoimmune process in lung fibrogenesis in a subset of patients with a phenotype compatible with IPF and/or combined pulmonary fibrosis and emphysema[21,22] (**Fig. 1**). Furthermore, the term "interstitial pneumonia with autoimmune features" (IPAF) has been proposed to describe patients with ILD and incomplete rheumatologic criteria (clinical, serologic, and morphologic),[23] suggesting an autoimmune process that may be largely confined to the lung.

Clinical observations have fueled mechanistic discoveries on the role of immunity in lung injury and identification of autoimmune phenomena that are integral to fibrosis.[24] Scientific explosion has led to the identification of both novel therapeutic targets and potential biomarkers. Furthermore, autoantibodies that are currently being used in clinical practice are strongly linked with disease presentation and clinical outcomes and thus are valuable in evaluating and treating patients with CTD-ILD. This review article aims to summarize the current state of knowledge on autoimmune biomarkers and highlight future perspectives in the immunologic evaluation of patients with fibrotic lung diseases. The association of autoimmunity with other chronic lung diseases, such as chronic obstructive pulmonary disease and asthma, is outside the scope of this review article.

AUTOIMMUNITY AND LUNG INJURY

Lung injury is thought to be the result of a complex interplay between noxious environmental stimuli, genetic factors, and immune deregulation, repetitive microinjuries of the respiratory epithelium and endothelium, ultimately leading to different phenotypes, such as fibrosis, emphysema, or alveolar hemorrhage, depending on the type of injury and immune response[25] (see **Fig. 1**). Cigarette smoke, in genetically predisposed individuals, has been associated with increased activity

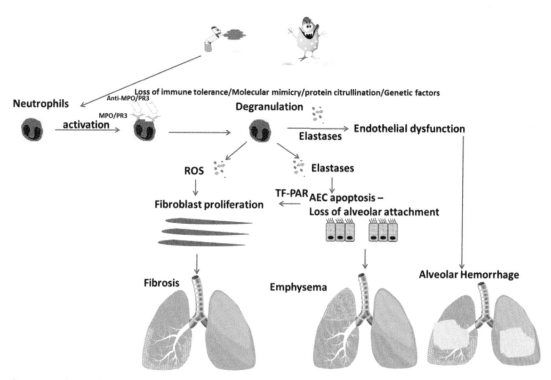

Fig. 1. Simplistic schematic representation of immune-mediated lung injury. Sustained exposure of innate immune cells, that is, neutrophils to repetitive injurious stimuli in genetically predisposed individuals, may lead to neutrophils activation and production of proteolytic enzymes, including proteinase-3 (PR3) and MPO. Prolonged circulation of neutrophilic antigens and loss of immune tolerance may lead to production of ANCA, which target relative antigens on the surface of immune cells, and thus, mediate degranulation of neutrophils and release of (1) reactive oxygen species (ROS) leading to fibroblast activation, myofibroblast proliferation, and ultimately lung fibrosis; (2) elastases causing alveolar epithelial cell apoptosis; and/or (3) endothelial dysfunction, ultimately leading to loss of alveolar attachments and emphysema or alveolar hemorrhage, respectively. AEC, alveolar epithelial cells, TF-PAR, tissue factor and protease-activated receptor.

of peptidyl arginine deiminase enzyme (PAD), the mediator of protein citrullination. Posttranslational modifications of peptidyl arginine lead to loss of immune tolerance, detrimental effects of molecular mimicry, and cross-reactivity with self-antigens.[20,26–28] The generation of anticitrullinated protein antibodies (ACPA), a break in immune tolerance, and upregulation of PADI4 in neutrophils could release neutrophil extracellular traps (NETs) and promote NETosis in response to pathogen recognition patterns, thus leading to tissue damage.[29,30] The role of B cells in lung injury is rather conflicting and controversial. A lymphocytic infiltrate is the hallmark of nonspecific interstitial pneumonia (NSIP) and lymphocytic interstitial pneumonia, 2 pathologic conditions that are prevalent in CTD-ILD, and the presence of germinal centers also suggests the potential of an underlying CTD. Studies have shown that clusters of CD20-positive cells lie immediately adjacent to fibroblastic foci within the fibrotic lung, suggesting a profibrotic role.[31] On the other hand,

experimental studies suggested a protective role for B cells in lung fibrosis as indicated by exacerbated fibrotic responses following depletion of B cells and generation of profibrotic phenotypes of senescent neutrophils in animal models of lung fibrosis.[32] Neutrophils are implicated in autoimmune lung injury: antimyeloperoxidase (MPO) in patients with microscopic polyangitis has been suggested to promote neutrophil activation, migration, and degranulation within vessel walls, release of reactive oxygen species and other toxic metabolites, as well as activation of coagulation cascade, ultimately leading to fibrosis, emphysema, or alveolar hemorrhage.[33–35]

CURRENTLY USED ANTIBODIES AND BIOMARKERS: CLINICAL SETTING
Antinuclear Antibodies

The indirect immunofluorescence test using a human neoplastic cell line has been the most widely used assay for antinuclear antibody (ANA)

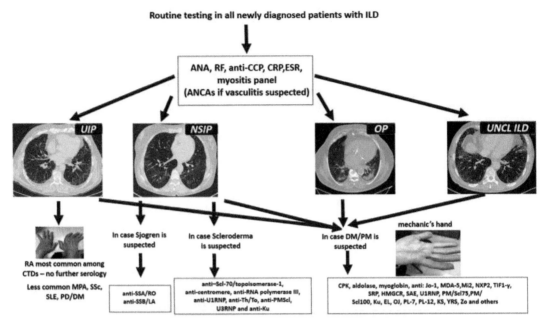

Fig. 2. Immunologic evaluation of the patient with ILD. CRP, C- reactive protein, ESR, erythrocyte sedimentation rate, UNCL, unclassifiable.

detection (**Fig. 2**).[36] The large number of autoantibodies that can be detected represents the most important advantage of this assay. Disadvantages of the indirect immunofluorescence test included the labor intensity of the assay as well as the requirement for experienced technicians to read and interpret the results.[36] ANA staining patterns include homogeneous, heterogeneous, nucleolar, speckled, centromere, rim, and histone and have been loosely associated with underlying autoimmune diseases. However, ANA patterns are not specific for individual autoimmune disorders, and thus, a positive test by indirect immunofluorescence may require additional testing using solid phase assays.[37] Laboratory thresholds for indirect immunofluorescence should be defined by each laboratory and should be chosen so as to detect autoantibodies in approximately 5% of healthy controls; the 1:160 dilution is the most widely used cutoff level for ANA positivity.[38,39] At the 1:160 dilution, the sensitivity of the ANA test for systemic lupus erythematosus (SLE), systemic sclerosis, and Sjögren syndrome (SS) is 95%, 87%, and 74%, respectively. In such patients, ANA titer is recommended only for disease diagnosis and not for monitoring of disease activity.[40,41] ANA positivity is unable to predict risk profiles in patients with IPF, IPAF, and CTD-ILD, although patients with IPAF have an intermediate survival between patients with IPF and different forms of CTD-ILDs.[42] Older cohorts had

suggested that ANA titers ≥1:1280 are associated with improved survival in patients with ILD and autoimmune features.[43]

Systemic Lupus Erythematosus–Specific Autoantibodies

ILDs are relatively uncommon in the context of SLE and usually occur in overlap syndromes. Autoantibodies used for the diagnosis of SLE include the anti-double-stranded (ds) DNA, which are present in 50% to 90% of cases. Anti-dsDNA has a 90% specificity, with a variable sensitivity ranging from 10% to 50%, mainly due to the different detection methods used in clinical practice. Anti-dsDNA are reliably detected by seeing a homogeneous nuclear immunofluorescence pattern, but less specific and more sensitive enzyme-linked immunosorbent assay (ELISA) methods can also be applied.[44] Positive anti-dsDNA represent one of the latest American College of Rheumatology and Systemic Lupus International Collaborating Clinics classification criteria but can be also positive in infections and healthy subjects.[45] Other SLE-specific autoantibodies are those against the Sm protein that is linked to RNA within the nucleus[46] and antiphospholipid syndrome antibodies (lupus anticoagulant, b2-glycoprotein I, and anti-cardiolipin), which are associated with lupus nephritis and thromboembolic disease/pregnancy morbidity, respectively.[47] Anti-dsDNA represent one of the few autoimmune markers with strong association with disease activity. High levels of anti-dsDNA and anti-Sm antibodies are linked to kidney involvement,[48] and they can be used for follow-up and treatment response.

Rheumatoid Arthritis–Specific Autoantibodies

Rheumatoid arthritis (RA) represents the most common cause of CTD-ILD, with usual interstitial pneumonia (UIP) being the most frequently occurring radiological pattern. Mortality of RA-ILD is mainly dependent on the radiological pattern, with UIP presenting with the most dismal prognosis, almost comparable to that of IPF/UIP. Patients with RA-ILD typically present with a positive rheumatoid factor (RF), which is an autoantibody against the Fc fragment of the immunoglobulin G antibodies, and ACPA. Nephelometry and ELISA have gradually replaced other semiquantitative methods for measurement because of their simplicity and greater reproducibility.[49] With regards to ELISA assay for ACPA, arginine residues have been replaced by citrulline in a mixture of cyclic citrullinated peptides, increasing the sensitivity of the assay for ACPA.[50] ACPAs have higher specificity (95%–99% vs 80%–86%, respectively) and similar sensitivity (50%–88%) compared with RF for the diagnosis of RA.[51,52] The positive predictive value of RF is only 24% for RA and 34% for any autoimmune disease, whereas the negative predictive value ranges from 85% to 89%, respectively.[53] RF may also be increased in other autoimmune diseases, including SS and mixed connective tissue diseases, as well as in other conditions such as chronic infections, smoking, and older age.[54] ACPAs have been considered more specific for RA; yet, they may also be positive in SLE, psoriatic arthritis, and tuberculosis.[50] RF and ACPA titers between 1 and 3 times the upper limits are considered to be low. Higher ACPA or RF titers have been associated with ILD development in patients with RA,[55,56] whereas anti-CCP2 antibodies have been suggested as markers of functional severity and radiological extent of RA-ILD.[52,57] Despite diagnostic usefulness, ACPAs present with poor prognostic accuracy in patients with RA-ILD.[58,59] With regards to treatment, RF titers may guide therapeutic decisions, indicating treatment response to rituximab (if high) or antitumor necrosis factor-α regimens (if low).[60,61] Finally, the usefulness of RF and ACPAs for follow-up to predict disease activity is still controversial.[62]

Sjögren Syndrome Associated Autoantibodies

SS is a CTD mainly affecting young women and is characterized by lymphocytic infiltration of exocrine glands causing xerotrachea, xerophthalmia, and xerostomia.[63,64] SS rarely affects the lung and even more rarely causes fibrotic lung disease. The most common ILD patterns are those of lymphocytic interstitial pneumonia (15%–20%) and NSIP (17%). SS is further divided into primary SS and secondary SS, which is associated with other CTDs, mostly RA and SLE. The 2 main antigens recognized by autoantibodies in SS are the SSA/Ro (33%–77%) and SSB/La (23%–48%) ribonucleoproteins (RNP). Their detection is part of the diagnostic criteria for SS, but their presence is not mandatory to confirm the diagnosis.[65] Patients positive for both antibodies are at high risk of developing non-Hodgkin lymphoma, whereas absence of both autoantibodies portends a good prognosis. SS-associated antibodies have been also associated with longer disease duration and more extraglandular manifestations, including life-threatening ventricular arrhythmias, such as QTc prolongation, particularly in the coexistence of Ro52 autoantibodies. RF is also commonly encountered in patients with secondary SS coexisting with RA.[63,64] Their usefulness for disease follow-up is very limited.

Systemic Sclerosis–Associated Autoantibodies

ILD is a frequent manifestation of scleroderma (SSc) occurring in more than 40% of patients, mainly in those with diffuse SSc.[39] Fibrotic nonspecific NSIP is the most common radiographic and histopathologic pattern, although UIP may also be seen.[1] Most of the SSc-associated antibodies are currently detected through ELISA assays.[66] Antitopoisomerase I antibodies (also known as anti-Scl70) are detected in 30% to 40% of SSc sera with a high specificity (90%) and low sensitivity (43%) when using immunodiffusion techniques. Specificity decreases considerably when sensitive ELISA techniques have been applied.[67] Anti-Scl70 antibodies have been associated with diffuse cutaneous form, disease activity, increased risk of pulmonary fibrosis, and worse clinical outcomes. More than 85% of Scl-70 antibody-positive SSc patients will eventually develop pulmonary fibrosis[68] with a sensitivity and specificity for the prediction of ILD of 45% and 81%, respectively.[69] Among anti-Scl70(+) SSc patients, African Americans present with more advanced fibrotic lung disease and worse survival compared with Caucasians.[70] Anticentromere antibodies (ACA) are detected in 30% of SSc patients with low sensitivity (20%–40%) and high specificity (97%). ACA are more frequent in Caucasian women and are associated with limited SSc, higher risk of developing pulmonary arterial hypertension, and lower risk for ILD.[71,72] Similarly, autoantibodies against the 3 mammalian RNA polymerases (RNA pol-I, -II, -III) are highly specific for systemic sclerosis (98%–100%), but not sensitive (~20%).[73] They have been linked with diffuse SSc, higher risk for renal crisis, gastric ectasia, breast cancer, and advanced skin fibrosis. Anti-Th/To antibodies are rarely seen in clinical practice (0.2%–3.4%) and have been associated with development of ILD, pulmonary hypertension, and less joint involvement.[74] Anti-U11/U12 antibodies have also been linked to pulmonary fibrosis development.[75] Anti-PM/Scl antibodies are detected rarely in SSc (3.1%–13% and mainly limited form) and have been associated with lung fibrosis and overlap syndrome with concurrent myositis and digital ulcers.[76] Autoantibodies against small nuclear RNP are detected in patients with mixed CTD (or overlap with SLE) with increased risk for pulmonary arterial hypertension and a controversial link to pulmonary involvement.[77,78]

A small minority of SSc patients (10%) may also present with positive ACPA antibodies, which have been associated with erosive arthritis, diffuse SSc, and fibrotic lung disease. However, their use for assessing disease activity is rather limited.[39] Finally, a recent study showed that a substantial minority of SSc patients (8.9%) presents with ANCA positivity, and these patients (particularly c-ANCA/PR3) have higher risk for development of pulmonary embolism, suggesting the need for perinuclear antineutrophil cytoplasm antibodies (p-ANCA) screening in patients with SSc.[79] Autoantibody positivity is valuable not only for confirmation of SSc diagnosis but also for risk stratification of patients.[74] No usefulness of serum autoantibodies on treatment response has been reported (**Table 2**).

Myositis-Associated Autoantibodies

The idiopathic inflammatory myopathies (IIM) demonstrate heterogeneous phenotypes ranging from polymyositis (PM), dermatomyositis (DM), and antisynthetase syndrome to inclusion body myositis and necrotizing myopathy. ILD represents a relatively common manifestation of the IIMs encountered in almost 25% of patients and is associated with a worse prognosis.[80] The most frequently observed pattern is that of fibrotic NSIP followed by organizing pneumonia.[80] Antibodies detected in myositis can be divided into myositis-specific (mostly non-ANA) and myositis-associated antibodies. The latter can also be observed in other CTDs. Antitransfer RNA (tRNA) synthetase antibodies (Jo-1, PL-7, PL-12, EJ, OJ, KS, Ha, Zo) target enzymes that attach the appropriate amino acid onto its tRNA. They are

Table 2
Circulating autoantibodies in patients with interstitial lung disease

Immune-Autoimmune Markers	Role in Pulmonary Fibrosis	Reference
Cytokeratin 8/18	Autoantibodies in pulmonary fibrosis	Dobashi et al,[121] 2000
Vimentin	Autoantibodies in pulmonary fibrosis	Yang et al,[124] 2002
HSP-70	Autoantibodies in IPF, negative prognosticator	Vuga et al,[129] 2014
KCNRG	Autoantibodies in pulmonary fibrosis	Kahloon et al,[130] 2013
Vomeromodulin	Autoantibodies in pulmonary fibrosis	Shum et al,[131] 2013
Periplakin	Autoantibodies in pulmonary fibrosis, negative prognosticator	Alimohammadi et al,[132] 2009
Annexin	Autoantigen-promoting T-cell response, antibodies in AE-IPF	Shum et al,[133] 2009
Type V collagen	60% of patients with IPF anti-col(V) reactive T cells	Taille et al,[103] 2011
		Kurosu et al,[109] 2008
		Bobadilla et al,[113] 2008
		Hunninghake et al,[19] 2013

Abbreviations: AE, acute exacerbation; BPIFB1, bactericidal/permeability-increasing fold-containing B1; HSP, heat-shock protein; KCNRG, potassium channel regulator.

detected in almost 30% of patients with antisynthetase syndrome and are mainly cytoplasmic. Prognosis of ILD associated with anti-tRNA synthetase antibodies is highly variable and heterogeneous depending on the protein targeted by the autoantibody.[81,82] Anti-Jo1 is the most frequently detected in antisynthetase syndrome (almost 70%), followed by anti-PL12 (15%) and anti-PL7 (10%).[83] Patients with anti-PL7 and PL-12 antibodies have been associated with increased risk for ILD development (mainly OP and NSIP pattern), worse prognosis, and decreased risk for myositis (amyopathic DM with normal levels of aldolase and creatine phosphokinase) as opposed to anti-Jo1(+) patients. Anti-Mi-2 antibody is frequently seen with DM and appears to predict a good response to immunosuppression, whereas anti-SRP, typically seen in PM, often predicts a more treatment-refractory course. Antimelanoma differentiation-associated gene 5/clinically amyopathic DM (CADM140) has been described in CADM and may predict progressive and severe ILD. Transcription intermediary factor 1γ/p155 antibody has been associated with malignancy, and patients carrying this marker should be evaluated thoroughly. Immunoprecipitation analysis of autoantigens using 35S-methionine-labeled cell extract has been considered the most appropriate technique allowing screening for almost all known PM/DM autoantibodies in a single assay.[84]

Antineutrophil Cytoplasmic Antibodies

Indirect immunofluorescence assay with alcohol-fixed buffy coat leukocytes or ELISA using purified specific antigens have been the most widely used antineutrophil cytoplasmic antibody (ANCA) detection assays.[85] The immunofluorescence assay is more sensitive; however, ELISA is more specific.[85] Cytoplasmic-c-ANCA antibodies are highly sensitive (95%) and specific (97%) in active, systemic granulomatosis with polyangiitis (GPA). Positive c-ANCA/anti-PR3, in the appropriate clinical setting, may spare tissue sampling.[86,87] On the contrary, sensitivity and specificity of anti-MPO/perinuclear-p-ANCA for the diagnosis of MPA vasculitis are 31.5% and 99.4%, respectively.[88,89] Recently published data from the multicentric Australian Scleroderma Cohort Study showed that 8.9% of patients with SSc were ANCA positive.[79] ANCA positivity was associated with increased risk for ILD and pulmonary embolism development and thus with worse prognosis.[79] An association between PR3 positivity and treatment response (65% rituximab vs 48% cyclophosphamide) was demonstrated in the RAVE trial; on the contrary, both regimens were similarly effective in patients

with anti-MPO vasculitis.[90,91] Patients with anti-MPO antibodies had less advanced disease, required less frequently immunosuppressive regimens, and presented with reduced relapse risk than patients with anti-PR3.[92–97] Finally, reappearance of anti-MPO or anti-PR3-ANCAs was associated with disease relapse in more than 75% of patients with vasculitis; still this correlation remains controversial.[87,98–102]

AUTOANTIBODIES IN PATIENTS WITH INTERSTITIAL LUNG DISEASE: EXPERIMENTAL SETTING
Innate Immunity

Periplakin
Periplakin represents an intracellular component of adhesion junctions, strongly expressed in the bronchial and alveolar epithelium in both normal and fibrotic lung and is cleaved by caspase 6 during apoptosis (see **Table 2**).[103–107] Circulating antiperiplakin antibodies may be detected in the serum and in bronchoalveolar lavage of patients with IPF. Interestingly, the detection of anti-periplakin antibodies is associated with more severe disease, further supporting the role of autoimmunity in pulmonary fibrosis.[103] Finally, antiperiplakin antibodies have also been detected in nearly 50% of patients with DM and ILD.[106] Thus, further investigation for the role of periplakin in ILD is greatly anticipated.

Annexin
Annexins comprise a group of Ca^{2+}-dependent phospholipid-binding proteins, mainly expressed in alveolar epithelial cells type II and alveolar macrophages.[108,109] Seminal experimental data reported profibrotic properties for both annexin A2 and V.[110,111] Furthermore, annexin 1 has been demonstrated as an autoantigen promoting both T-cell response and antibody production in patients with acute exacerbations of IPF.[109]

Type V collagen
Type V collagen represents a minor collagen normally sequestered within the pulmonary interstitium.[112] Fibrosis-induced remodeling seems to lead to col(V) overexpression and subsequently to the development of anti-col(V) immunity through transforming growth factor-β-related signaling pathways.[112] Up to 60% of patients with IPF present with anti-col(V) reactive T cells, and approximately half of patients will develop specific systemic antibody responses.[113,114] Furthermore, attenuated lung expression of miR-185 and miR-186 has been associated with collagen V overexpression in patients with IPF.[115] Interestingly, experimental data showed that treatment with nebulized col(V) arrested further development of

bleomycin-induced pulmonary fibrosis[112] in a murine model. More importantly, oral immunotherapy with type V collagen in IPF was demonstrated to be safe and well tolerated. Results from larger clinical trials are greatly anticipated.[116]

Interleukin-1α

Interleukin-1α (IL-1α), also known as fibroblast-activating factor, represents one of the major epithelial alarmins, which induces inflammatory mediators release from human lung fibroblasts.[117–119] Increased levels of IL-1α autoantibodies have been obtained from the serum of patients with rapidly progressive IPF.[120]

Cytokeratin 8/18

Cytokeratins are proteins mainly expressed by glandular epithelial cells. Several lines of evidence show that anti-CK8/18 immune complexes might have a role in lung injury and pulmonary fibrosis development.[121,122]

Vimentin

Vimentin is a protein expressed by mesenchymal cells, demonstrating a crucial role for cytoskeletal structure.[123] Serum levels of antivimentin antibody are increased in patients with IPF and NSIP.[124] Most recently, vimentin has been suggested as an independent prognosticator of IPF progression and survival.[125]

Anticitrullinated alpha enolase peptide-1

Anticitrullinated alpha enolase peptide-1 is a specific ACPA. Recent evidence associated their presence with ILD development and bone erosion in patients with RA.[20] Thus, they might be a useful biomarker for stratification of patients with RA and lung involvement.

FUTURE PERSPECTIVES AND CONCLUDING REMARKS

The last few years have demonstrated increased interest in the role of the immune system and chronic lung injury. Despite relative enthusiasm arising from major accomplishments that shifted the understanding on the role of immune-mediated processes in the pathogenesis of lung fibrosis, the specific mechanisms regulating tissue repair by immune cells, including macrophages, neutrophils, and lymphocytes, remain ill defined.[126,127] Although classical autoantibodies may be used as assessment tools for several CTD manifestations, their role in prognosis and as a biomarker to follow treatment response is largely lacking. The mechanisms of inflammation and autoimmunity involved in fibrotic lung disease may be nontraditional. From a prognostic point of view, several autoimmune biomarkers have shown sufficient predictive accuracy in multiple cohorts of patients with IPF; yet, this concept remains experimental. To this end, the ILD patient requires ongoing clinical and immunologic evaluation considering that ILD diagnosis is a process subjected to dynamic alterations. Multidisciplinary approaches involving pulmonologists, rheumatologists, radiologists, and pathologists lie at the core of diagnostic and therapeutic interventions. Biologic enrichment of future large randomized clinical trials is urgently needed to address these uncertainties.[128]

REFERENCES

1. Papiris SA, Manali ED, Kolilekas L, et al. Investigation of lung involvement in connective tissue disorders. Respiration 2015;90(1):2–24.
2. Wells AU, Denton CP. Interstitial lung disease in connective tissue disease—mechanisms and management. Nat Rev Rheumatol 2014;10(12):728–39.
3. Crystal RG, Fulmer JD, Roberts WC, et al. Idiopathic pulmonary fibrosis. Clinical, histologic, radiographic, physiologic, scintigraphic, cytologic, and biochemical aspects. Ann Intern Med 1976; 85(6):769–88.
4. Luzina IG, Todd NW, Iacono AT, et al. Roles of T lymphocytes in pulmonary fibrosis. J Leukoc Biol 2008;83(2):237–44.
5. Idiopathic Pulmonary Fibrosis Clinical Research Network, Raghu G, Anstrom KJ, et al. Prednisone, azathioprine, and N-acetylcysteine for pulmonary fibrosis. N Engl J Med 2012;366(21):1968–77.
6. Antoniou KM, Nicholson AG, Dimadi M, et al. Long-term clinical effects of interferon gamma-1b and colchicine in idiopathic pulmonary fibrosis. Eur Respir J 2006;28(3):496–504.
7. Raghu G, Brown KK, Bradford WZ, et al. A placebo-controlled trial of interferon gamma-1b in patients with idiopathic pulmonary fibrosis. N Engl J Med 2004;350(2):125–33.
8. Bouros D, Antoniou KM, Tzouvelekis A, et al. Interferon-gamma 1b for the treatment of idiopathic pulmonary fibrosis. Expert Opin Biol Ther 2006;6(10): 1051–60.
9. Feghali-Bostwick CA, Tsai CG, Valentine VG, et al. Cellular and humoral autoreactivity in idiopathic pulmonary fibrosis. J Immunol 2007;179(4): 2592–9.
10. Tzouvelekis A, Zacharis G, Oikonomou A, et al. Increased incidence of autoimmune markers in patients with combined pulmonary fibrosis and emphysema. BMC Pulm Med 2013;13:31.
11. Kotsianidis I, Nakou E, Bouchliou I, et al. Global impairment of CD4+CD25+FOXP3+ regulatory T cells in idiopathic pulmonary fibrosis. Am J Respir Crit Care Med 2009;179(12):1121–30.

12. Lee JS, Kim EJ, Lynch KL, et al. Prevalence and clinical significance of circulating autoantibodies in idiopathic pulmonary fibrosis. Respir Med 2013;107(2):249–55.

13. Karampitsakos T, Tzilas V, Tringidou R, et al. Lung cancer in patients with idiopathic pulmonary fibrosis. Pulm Pharmacol Ther 2017;45:1–10.

14. Tzouvelekis A, Herazo-Maya J, Sakamoto K, et al. Biomarkers in the evaluation and management of idiopathic pulmonary fibrosis. Curr Top Med Chem 2016;16(14):1587–98.

15. Oikonomou N, Mouratis MA, Tzouvelekis A, et al. Pulmonary autotaxin expression contributes to the pathogenesis of pulmonary fibrosis. Am J Respir Cell Mol Biol 2012;47(5):566–74.

16. Spagnolo P, Sverzellati N, Rossi G, et al. Idiopathic pulmonary fibrosis: an update. Ann Med 2015; 47(1):15–27.

17. Tzouvelekis A, Aidinis V, Harokopos V, et al. Down-regulation of the inhibitor of growth family member 4 (ING4) in different forms of pulmonary fibrosis. Respir Res 2009;10:14.

18. Desai O, Winkler J, Minasyan M, et al. The role of immune and inflammatory cells in idiopathic pulmonary fibrosis. Front Med (Lausanne) 2018;5:43.

19. Hunninghake GM, Hatabu H, Okajima Y, et al. MUC5B promoter polymorphism and interstitial lung abnormalities. N Engl J Med 2013;368(23): 2192–200.

20. Alunno A, Bistoni O, Pratesi F, et al. Anti-citrullinated alpha enolase antibodies, interstitial lung disease and bone erosion in rheumatoid arthritis. Rheumatology (Oxford) 2018;57(5):850–5.

21. Tzelepis GE, Kokosi M, Tzioufas A, et al. Prevalence and outcome of pulmonary fibrosis in microscopic polyangiitis. Eur Respir J 2010;36(1): 116–21.

22. Tzouvelekis A, Zacharis G, Oikonomou A, et al. Combined pulmonary fibrosis and emphysema associated with microscopic polyangiitis. Eur Respir J 2012;40(2):505–7.

23. Fischer A, Antoniou KM, Brown KK, et al. An official European Respiratory Society/American Thoracic Society research statement: interstitial pneumonia with autoimmune features. Eur Respir J 2015; 46(4):976–87.

24. Gieseck RL 3rd, Wilson MS, Wynn TA. Type 2 immunity in tissue repair and fibrosis. Nat Rev Immunol 2018;18(1):62–76.

25. Fernandez IE, Eickelberg O. New cellular and molecular mechanisms of lung injury and fibrosis in idiopathic pulmonary fibrosis. Lancet 2012; 380(9842):680–8.

26. Lugli EB, Correia RE, Fischer R, et al. Expression of citrulline and homocitrulline residues in the lungs of non-smokers and smokers: implications for autoimmunity in rheumatoid arthritis. Arthritis Res Ther 2015;17:9.

27. Klareskog L, Catrina AI. Autoimmunity: lungs and citrullination. Nat Rev Rheumatol 2015;11(5):261–2.

28. Mahdi H, Fisher BA, Källberg H, et al. Specific interaction between genotype, smoking and auto-immunity to citrullinated α-enolase in the etiology of rheumatoid arthritis. Nat Genet 2009;41:1319. Available at: https://www.nature.com/articles/ng.480#supplementary-information.

29. Samara KD, Trachalaki A, Tsitoura E, et al. Upregulation of citrullination pathway: from autoimmune to idiopathic lung fibrosis. Respir Res 2017;18(1):218.

30. Narasaraju T, Yang E, Samy RP, et al. Excessive neutrophils and neutrophil extracellular traps contribute to acute lung injury of influenza pneumonitis. Am J Pathol 2011;179(1):199–210.

31. Xue J, Kass DJ, Bon J, et al. Plasma B lymphocyte stimulator and B cell differentiation in idiopathic pulmonary fibrosis patients. J Immunol 2013; 191(5):2089–95.

32. Kim JH, Podstawka J, Lou Y, et al. Aged polymorphonuclear leukocytes cause fibrotic interstitial lung disease in the absence of regulation by B cells. Nat Immunol 2018;19(2):192–201.

33. Schwarz M, Brown K. Small vessel vasculitis of the lung. Thorax 2000;55(6):502–10.

34. Frankel SK, Schwarz MI. The pulmonary vasculitides. Am J Respir Crit Care Med 2012;186(3): 216–24.

35. Miao D, Li DY, Chen M, et al. Platelets are activated in ANCA-associated vasculitis via thrombin-PARs pathway and can activate the alternative complement pathway. Arthritis Res Ther 2017;19(1):252.

36. Agmon-Levin N, Damoiseaux J, Kallenberg C, et al. International recommendations for the assessment of autoantibodies to cellular antigens referred to as anti-nuclear antibodies. Ann Rheum Dis 2014;73(1):17–23.

37. Meroni PL, Schur PH. ANA screening: an old test with new recommendations. Ann Rheum Dis 2010;69(8):1420–2.

38. Solomon DH, Kavanaugh AJ, Schur PH. Evidence-based guidelines for the use of immunologic tests: antinuclear antibody testing. Arthritis Rheum 2002; 47(4):434–44.

39. Didier K, Bolko L, Giusti D, et al. Autoantibodies associated with connective tissue diseases: what meaning for clinicians? Front Immunol 2018;9:541.

40. Mittoo S, Gelber AC, Christopher-Stine L, et al. Ascertainment of collagen vascular disease in patients presenting with interstitial lung disease. Respir Med 2009;103(8):1152–8.

41. Jee AS, Adelstein S, Bleasel J, et al. Role of autoantibodies in the diagnosis of connective-tissue disease ILD (CTD-ILD) and interstitial pneumonia

with autoimmune features (IPAF). J Clin Med 2017; 6(5). https://doi.org/10.3390/jcm6050051.

42. Oldham JM, Adegunsoye A, Valenzi E, et al. Characterisation of patients with interstitial pneumonia with autoimmune features. Eur Respir J 2016; 47(6):1767–75.

43. Vij R, Noth I, Strek ME. Autoimmune-featured interstitial lung disease: a distinct entity. Chest 2011; 140(5):1292–9.

44. Enocsson H, Sjowall C, Wirestam L, et al. Four anti-dsDNA antibody assays in relation to systemic lupus erythematosus disease specificity and activity. J Rheumatol 2015;42(5):817–25.

45. Ines L, Silva C, Galindo M, et al. Classification of systemic lupus erythematosus: Systemic Lupus International Collaborating Clinics versus American College of Rheumatology criteria. A comparative study of 2,055 patients from a real-life, international systemic lupus erythematosus cohort. Arthritis Care Res (Hoboken) 2015;67(8):1180–5.

46. Janwityanuchit S, Verasertniyom O, Vanichapuntu M, et al. Anti-Sm: its predictive value in systemic lupus erythematosus. Clin Rheumatol 1993;12(3):350–3.

47. Ruiz-Irastorza G, Egurbide MV, Ugalde J, et al. High impact of antiphospholipid syndrome on irreversible organ damage and survival of patients with systemic lupus erythematosus. Arch Intern Med 2004;164(1):77–82.

48. Vitali C, Bencivelli W, Isenberg DA, et al. Disease activity in systemic lupus erythematosus: report of the consensus study group of the European Workshop for Rheumatology Research. I. A descriptive analysis of 704 European lupus patients. European Consensus Study Group for disease activity in SLE. Clin Exp Rheumatol 1992;10(5):527–39.

49. Ulvestad E, Wilfred LL, Kristoffersen EK. Measurement of IgM rheumatoid factor by ELISA. Scand J Rheumatol 2001;30(6):366.

50. Whiting PF, Smidt N, Sterne JA, et al. Systematic review: accuracy of anti-citrullinated peptide antibodies for diagnosing rheumatoid arthritis. Ann Intern Med 2010;152(7):456–64. w155-66.

51. Bridges SL. Update on autoantibodies in rheumatoid arthritis. Curr Rheumatol Rep 2004;6(5): 343–50.

52. Rodriguez-Mahou M, Lopez-Longo FJ, Sanchez-Ramon S, et al. Association of anti-cyclic citrullinated peptide and anti-Sa/citrullinated vimentin autoantibodies in rheumatoid arthritis. Arthritis Rheum 2006;55(4):657–61.

53. Shmerling RH, Delbanco TL. How useful is the rheumatoid factor? An analysis of sensitivity, specificity, and predictive value. Arch Intern Med 1992; 152(12):2417–20.

54. Nell VP, Machold KP, Stamm TA, et al. Autoantibody profiling as early diagnostic and prognostic tool for rheumatoid arthritis. Ann Rheum Dis 2005;64(12): 1731–6.

55. Reynisdottir G, Karimi R, Joshua V, et al. Structural changes and antibody enrichment in the lungs are early features of anti-citrullinated protein antibody-positive rheumatoid arthritis. Arthritis Rheumatol 2014;66(1):31–9.

56. Yin Y, Liang D, Zhao L, et al. Anti-cyclic citrullinated peptide antibody is associated with interstitial lung disease in patients with rheumatoid arthritis. PLoS One 2014;9(4):e92449.

57. Giles JT, Danoff SK, Sokolove J, et al. Association of fine specificity and repertoire expansion of anticitrullinated peptide antibodies with rheumatoid arthritis associated interstitial lung disease. Ann Rheum Dis 2014;73(8):1487–94.

58. Minnis P, Henry K, Clark B, et al. Predicting progression of RA-ILD using anti-CCP. Eur Respir J 2015;46(suppl 59):PA3801.

59. Assayag D, Lubin M, Lee JS, et al. Predictors of mortality in rheumatoid arthritis-related interstitial lung disease. Respirology 2014;19(4):493–500.

60. Edwards JC, Cambridge G. Prospects for B-cell-targeted therapy in autoimmune disease. Rheumatology (Oxford) 2005;44(2):151–6.

61. Takeuchi T, Miyasaka N, Inui T, et al. High titers of both rheumatoid factor and anti-CCP antibodies at baseline in patients with rheumatoid arthritis are associated with increased circulating baseline TNF level, low drug levels, and reduced clinical responses: a post hoc analysis of the RISING study. Arthritis Res Ther 2017;19(1):194.

62. Chou C, Liao H, Chen C, et al. The clinical application of anti-CCP in rheumatoid arthritis and other rheumatic diseases. Biomark Insights 2007;2: 165–71.

63. Papiris SA, Tsonis IA, Moutsopoulos HM. Sjogren's syndrome. Semin Respir Crit Care Med 2007;28(4): 459–71.

64. Papiris SA, Maniati M, Constantopoulos SH, et al. Lung involvement in primary Sjogren's syndrome is mainly related to the small airway disease. Ann Rheum Dis 1999;58(1):61–4.

65. Shiboski CH, Shiboski SC, Seror R, et al. 2016 American College of Rheumatology/European League against Rheumatism classification criteria for primary Sjogren's syndrome: a consensus and data-driven methodology involving three international patient cohorts. Ann Rheum Dis 2017;76(1):9–16.

66. Homer KL, Warren J, Karayev D, et al. Performance of anti-topoisomerase I antibody testing by multiple-bead, enzyme-linked immunosorbent assay and immunodiffusion in a university setting. J Clin Rheumatol 2018. https://doi.org/10.1097/rhu.0000000000000971.

67. Basu D, Reveille JD. Anti-scl-70. Autoimmunity 2005;38(1):65–72.

68. Briggs DC, Vaughan RW, Welsh KI, et al. Immuno-genetic prediction of pulmonary fibrosis in systemic sclerosis. Lancet 1991;338(8768):661–2.

69. Reveille JD, Solomon DH. Evidence-based guidelines for the use of immunologic tests: anticentromere, Scl-70, and nucleolar antibodies. Arthritis Rheum 2003;49(3):399–412.

70. Steen V, Domsic RT, Lucas M, et al. A clinical and serologic comparison of African American and Caucasian patients with systemic sclerosis. Arthritis Rheum 2012;64(9):2986–94.

71. Karampitsakos T, Tzouvelekis A, Chrysikos S, et al. Pulmonary hypertension in patients with interstitial lung disease. Pulm Pharmacol Ther 2018;50:38–46.

72. Mehra S, Walker J, Patterson K, et al. Autoantibodies in systemic sclerosis. Autoimmun Rev 2013;12(3):340–54.

73. Koenig M, Dieude M, Senecal JL. Predictive value of antinuclear autoantibodies: the lessons of the systemic sclerosis autoantibodies. Autoimmun Rev 2008;7(8):588–93.

74. Nihtyanova SI, Denton CP. Autoantibodies as predictive tools in systemic sclerosis. Nature reviews. Rheumatology 2010;6(2):112–6.

75. Fertig N, Domsic RT, Rodriguez-Reyna T, et al. Anti-U11/U12 RNP antibodies in systemic sclerosis: a new serologic marker associated with pulmonary fibrosis. Arthritis Rheum 2009;61(7):958–65.

76. Hanke K, Bruckner CS, Dahnrich C, et al. Antibodies against PM/Scl-75 and PM/Scl-100 are independent markers for different subsets of systemic sclerosis patients. Arthritis Res Ther 2009;11(1):R22.

77. Tall F, Dechomet M, Riviere S, et al. The clinical relevance of antifibrillarin (anti-U3-RNP) autoantibodies in systemic sclerosis. Scand J Immunol 2017;85(1):73–9.

78. Aggarwal R, Lucas M, Fertig N, et al. Anti-U3 RNP autoantibodies in systemic sclerosis. Arthritis Rheum 2009;60(4):1112–8.

79. Moxey J, Huq M, Proudman S, et al. Significance of anti-neutrophil cytoplasmic antibodies in systemic sclerosis. Arthritis Res Ther 2019;21(1):57.

80. Marie I, Hachulla E, Cherin P, et al. Interstitial lung disease in polymyositis and dermatomyositis. Arthritis Rheum 2002;47(6):614–22.

81. Yamakawa H, Hagiwara E, Kitamura H, et al. Predictive factors for the long-term deterioration of pulmonary function in interstitial lung disease associated with anti-aminoacyl-tRNA synthetase antibodies. Respiration 2018;96(3):210–21.

82. Tzilas V, Tzouvelekis A, Bouros E, et al. Prognosis of interstitial lung disease associated with anti-aminoacyl-tRNA synthetase antibodies: look in the middle. Respiration 2018;96(3):207–9.

83. Cruellas MG, Viana Vdos S, Levy-Neto M, et al. Myositis-specific and myositis-associated autoantibody profiles and their clinical associations in a large series of patients with polymyositis and dermatomyositis. Clinics (Sao Paulo) 2013;68(7):909–14.

84. Satoh M, Tanaka S, Ceribelli A, et al. A comprehensive overview on myositis-specific antibodies: new and old biomarkers in idiopathic inflammatory myopathy. Clin Rev Allergy Immunol 2017;52(1):1–19.

85. Merkel PA, Polisson RP, Chang Y, et al. Prevalence of antineutrophil cytoplasmic antibodies in a large inception cohort of patients with connective tissue disease. Ann Intern Med 1997;126(11):866–73.

86. Brown KK. Pulmonary vasculitis. Proc Am Thorac Soc 2006;3(1):48–57.

87. Cornec D, Cornec-Le Gall E, Fervenza FC, et al. ANCA-associated vasculitis—clinical utility of using ANCA specificity to classify patients. Nat Rev Rheumatol 2016;12(10):570–9.

88. Choi HK, Liu S, Merkel PA, et al. Diagnostic performance of antineutrophil cytoplasmic antibody tests for idiopathic vasculitides: metaanalysis with a focus on antimyeloperoxidase antibodies. J Rheumatol 2001;28(7):1584–90.

89. Mandl LA, Solomon DH, Smith EL, et al. Using antineutrophil cytoplasmic antibody testing to diagnose vasculitis: can test-ordering guidelines improve diagnostic accuracy? Arch Intern Med 2002;162(13):1509–14.

90. Stone JH, Merkel PA, Spiera R, et al. Rituximab versus cyclophosphamide for ANCA-associated vasculitis. N Engl J Med 2010;363(3):221–32.

91. Unizony S, Villarreal M, Miloslavsky EM, et al. Clinical outcomes of treatment of anti-neutrophil cytoplasmic antibody (ANCA)-associated vasculitis based on ANCA type. Ann Rheum Dis 2016;75(6):1166–9.

92. Slot MC, Tervaert JW, Boomsma MM, et al. Positive classic antineutrophil cytoplasmic antibody (C-ANCA) titer at switch to azathioprine therapy associated with relapse in proteinase 3-related vasculitis. Arthritis Rheum 2004;51(2):269–73.

93. Sanders JS, de Joode AA, DeSevaux RG, et al. Extended versus standard azathioprine maintenance therapy in newly diagnosed proteinase-3 anti-neutrophil cytoplasmic antibody-associated vasculitis patients who remain cytoplasmic antineutrophil cytoplasmic antibody-positive after induction of remission: a randomized clinical trial. Nephrol Dial Transplant 2016;31(9):1453–9.

94. Jayne D, Rasmussen N, Andrassy K, et al. A randomized trial of maintenance therapy for vasculitis associated with antineutrophil cytoplasmic autoantibodies. N Engl J Med 2003;349(1):36–44.

95. Puechal X, Pagnoux C, Perrodeau E, et al. Long-term outcomes among participants in the WEGENT trial of remission-maintenance therapy for

granulomatosis with polyangiitis (Wegener's) or microscopic polyangiitis. Arthritis Rheumatol 2016;68(3):690–701.

96. Chang DY, Li ZY, Chen M, et al. Myeloperoxidase-ANCA-positive granulomatosis with polyangiitis is a distinct subset of ANCA-associated vasculitis: a retrospective analysis of 455 patients from a single center in China. Semin Arthritis Rheum 2018. https://doi.org/10.1016/j.semarthrit.2018.05.003.

97. Schirmer JH, Wright MN, Herrmann K, et al. Myeloperoxidase-antineutrophil cytoplasmic antibody (ANCA)-positive granulomatosis with polyangiitis (Wegener's) is a clinically distinct subset of ANCA-associated vasculitis: a retrospective analysis of 315 patients from a German Vasculitis Referral Center. Arthritis Rheumatol 2016;68(12): 2953–63.

98. Fussner LA, Specks U. Can antineutrophil cytoplasmic antibody levels be used to inform treatment of pauci-immune vasculitis? Curr Opin Rheumatol 2015;27(3):231–40.

99. Specks U. Accurate relapse prediction in ANCA-associated vasculitis—the search for the Holy Grail. J Am Soc Nephrol 2015;26(3):505–7.

100. Tomasson G, Grayson PC, Mahr AD, et al. Value of ANCA measurements during remission to predict a relapse of ANCA-associated vasculitis–a meta-analysis. Rheumatology 2012;51(1):100–9.

101. Kemna MJ, Damoiseaux J, Austen J, et al. ANCA as a predictor of relapse: useful in patients with renal involvement but not in patients with nonrenal disease. J Am Soc Nephrol 2015;26(3):537–42.

102. Fussner LA, Hummel AM, Schroeder DR, et al. Factors determining the clinical utility of serial measurements of antineutrophil cytoplasmic antibodies targeting proteinase 3. Arthritis Rheumatol 2016;68(7):1700–10.

103. Taille C, Grootenboer-Mignot S, Boursier C, et al. Identification of periplakin as a new target for autoreactivity in idiopathic pulmonary fibrosis. Am J Respir Crit Care Med 2011;183(6):759–66.

104. Mignot S, Taille C, Besnard V, et al. Detection of anti-periplakin auto-antibodies during idiopathic pulmonary fibrosis. Clin Chim Acta 2014;433:242.

105. Aho S. Plakin proteins are coordinately cleaved during apoptosis but preferentially through the action of different caspases. Exp Dermatol 2004; 13(11):700–7.

106. Feghali-Bostwick CA, Wilkes DS. Autoimmunity in idiopathic pulmonary fibrosis: are circulating autoantibodies pathogenic or epiphenomena? Am J Respir Crit Care Med 2011;183(6):692–3.

107. Besnard V, Dagher R, Madjer T, et al. Identification of periplakin as a major regulator of lung injury and repair in mice. JCI Insight 2018;3(5). https://doi.org/10.1172/jci.insight.90163.

108. Nagase T, Uozumi N, Aoki-Nagase T, et al. A potent inhibitor of cytosolic phospholipase A2, arachidonyl trifluoromethyl ketone, attenuates LPS-induced lung injury in mice. Am J Physiol Lung Cell Mol Physiol 2003;284(5):L720–6.

109. Kurosu K, Takiguchi Y, Okada O, et al. Identification of annexin 1 as a novel autoantigen in acute exacerbation of idiopathic pulmonary fibrosis. J Immunol 2008;181(1):756–67.

110. Schuliga M, Jaffar J, Berhan A, et al. Annexin A2 contributes to lung injury and fibrosis by augmenting factor Xa fibrogenic activity. Am J Physiol Lung Cell Mol Physiol 2017;312(5):L772–82.

111. Buckley S, Shi W, Xu W, et al. Increased alveolar soluble annexin V promotes lung inflammation and fibrosis. Eur Respir J 2015;46(5):1417–29.

112. Vittal R, Mickler EA, Fisher AJ, et al. Type V collagen induced tolerance suppresses collagen deposition, TGF-beta and associated transcripts in pulmonary fibrosis. PLoS One 2013;8(10): e76451.

113. Bobadilla JL, Love RB, Jankowska-Gan E, et al. Th-17, monokines, collagen type V, and primary graft dysfunction in lung transplantation. Am J Respir Crit Care Med 2008;177(6):660–8.

114. Burlingham WJ, Love RB, Jankowska-Gan E, et al. IL-17-dependent cellular immunity to collagen type V predisposes to obliterative bronchiolitis in human lung transplants. J Clin Invest 2007;117(11): 3498–506.

115. Lei GS, Kline HL, Lee CH, et al. Regulation of collagen V expression and epithelial-mesenchymal transition by miR-185 and miR-186 during idiopathic pulmonary fibrosis. Am J Pathol 2016;186(9):2310–6.

116. Wilkes DS, Chew T, Flaherty KR, et al. Oral immunotherapy with type V collagen in idiopathic pulmonary fibrosis. Eur Respir J 2015;45(5):1393–402.

117. Dong J, Porter DW, Batteli LA, et al. Pathologic and molecular profiling of rapid-onset fibrosis and inflammation induced by multi-walled carbon nanotubes. Arch Toxicol 2015;89(4):621–33.

118. Suwara MI, Green NJ, Borthwick LA, et al. IL-1alpha released from damaged epithelial cells is sufficient and essential to trigger inflammatory responses in human lung fibroblasts. Mucosal Immunol 2014;7(3):684–93.

119. Tracy EC, Bowman MJ, Henderson BW, et al. Interleukin-1alpha is the major alarmin of lung epithelial cells released during photodynamic therapy to induce inflammatory mediators in fibroblasts. Br J Cancer 2012;107(9):1534–46.

120. Ogushi F, Tani K, Endo T, et al. Autoantibodies to IL-1 alpha in sera from rapidly progressive idiopathic pulmonary fibrosis. J Med Invest 2001; 48(3–4):181–9.

121. Dobashi N, Fujita J, Murota M, et al. Elevation of anti-cytokeratin 18 antibody and circulating cytokeratin 18: anti-cytokeratin 18 antibody immune complexes in sera of patients with idiopathic pulmonary fibrosis. Lung 2000;178(3):171–9.

122. Dobashi N, Fujita J, Ohtsuki Y, et al. Circulating cytokeratin 8:anti-cytokeratin 8 antibody immune complexes in sera of patients with pulmonary fibrosis. Respiration 2000;67(4):397–401.

123. Tzouvelekis A, Toonkel R, Karampitsakos T, et al. Mesenchymal stem cells for the treatment of idiopathic pulmonary fibrosis. Front Med (Lausanne) 2018;5:142.

124. Yang Y, Fujita J, Bandoh S, et al. Detection of anti-vimentin antibody in sera of patients with idiopathic pulmonary fibrosis and non-specific interstitial pneumonia. Clin Exp Immunol 2002;128(1): 169–74.

125. Surolia R, Li H, Kulkarni T, et al. Identification of Pathogenic and Prognostic Anti-Vimentin Antibodies in Idiopathic Pulmonary Fibrosis. D21. Immune pathways in acute lung injury and fibrosis: A7069-A69.

126. Bouros D, Tzouvelekis A. Idiopathic pulmonary fibrosis: on the move. Lancet Respir Med 2014; 2(1):17–9.

127. Hoyne GF, Elliott H, Mutsaers SE, et al. Idiopathic pulmonary fibrosis and a role for autoimmunity. Immunol Cell Biol 2017. https://doi.org/10.1038/icb.2017.22.

128. Karampitsakos T, Vraka A, Bouros D, et al. Biologic treatments in interstitial lung diseases. Front Med (Lausanne) 2019;6:41.

129. Vuga LJ, Tedrow JR, Pandit KV, et al. C-X-C motif chemokine 13 (CXCL13) is a prognostic biomarker of idiopathic pulmonary fibrosis. Am J Respir Crit Care Med 2014;189. https://doi.org/10.1164/rccm.201309-1592OC.

130. Kahloon RA, Xue J, Bhargava A, et al. Patients with idiopathic pulmonary fibrosis with antibodies to heat shock protein 70 have poor prognoses. Am J Respir Crit Care Med 2013;187(7):768–75.

131. Shum AK, Alimohammadi M, Tan CL, et al. BPIFB1 is a lung-specific autoantigen associated with interstitial lung disease. Sci Transl Med 2013;5(206): 206ra139.

132. Alimohammadi M, Dubois N, Skoldberg F, et al. Pulmonary autoimmunity as a feature of autoimmune polyendocrine syndrome type 1 and identification of KCNRG as a bronchial autoantigen. Proc Natl Acad Sci U S A 2009;106(11):4396–401.

133. Shum AK, DeVoss J, Tan CL, et al. Identification of an autoantigen demonstrates a link between interstitial lung disease and a defect in central tolerance. Sci Transl Med 2009;1(9):9ra20.

Moving?

Make sure your subscription moves with you!

To notify us of your new address, find your **Clinics Account Number** (located on your mailing label above your name), and contact customer service at:

Email: journalscustomerservice-usa@elsevier.com

800-654-2452 (subscribers in the U.S. & Canada)
314-447-8871 (subscribers outside of the U.S. & Canada)

Fax number: 314-447-8029

Elsevier Health Sciences Division
Subscription Customer Service
3251 Riverport Lane
Maryland Heights, MO 63043

*To ensure uninterrupted delivery of your subscription, please notify us at least 4 weeks in advance of move.

Printed and bound by CPI Group (UK) Ltd, Croydon, CR0 4YY

08/05/2025

01864747-0019